Toward Universal Health Coverage and
Equity in Latin America and the Caribbean

DIRECTIONS IN DEVELOPMENT
Human Development

Toward Universal Health Coverage and Equity in Latin America and the Caribbean

Evidence from Selected Countries

Tania Dmytraczenko and Gisele Almeida, Editors

WORLD BANK GROUP

Pan American
Health
Organization

World Health
Organization

REGIONAL OFFICE FOR THE **Americas**

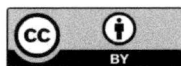

Contents

Boxes

Figures

Tables

Foreword

Over the past quarter century, the countries of Latin America and the Caribbean (LAC) have experienced rising incomes, with corresponding reductions in levels of poverty. At the same time, countries have achieved improvements in health and well-being for all segments of the population: average life expectancy has risen significantly, more children live to see their first and fifth birthdays, and fewer mothers are dying from complications of childbirth. Nonetheless, health inequities persist between and within countries, and some health outcomes are still unacceptable, challenging health systems to develop innovative approaches that will improve responsiveness and address people's changing needs.

Universal health coverage (UHC) has been at the center of the global public health agenda in recent years. As one of the overarching goals of health systems, UHC provides countries a way forward to address unmet needs and health inequities. The World Bank has embraced UHC as part of its mission to eliminate absolute poverty by 2030 and to boost shared prosperity. The Pan American Health Organization (PAHO) in October 2014 adopted a regional Strategy for Universal Access to Health and Universal Health Coverage, which expresses the commitment of PAHO Member States to strengthen health systems, expand access to comprehensive quality health services, provide financial protection, and adopt integrated, comprehensive policies to address the social determinants of health and health inequities.

For the past two years, the World Bank and PAHO have engaged in a collaborative effort to examine policies and initiatives in LAC aimed at achieving UHC. This report is one product of that collaboration. It includes contributions from professionals from both institutions and it has received the support of researchers from several countries in the region. The report provides insight on different approaches and progress being made by selected countries over the past quarter century to increase population coverage, services covered, and financial protection, with a special focus on reductions in health inequities.

The report shows that countries have made meaningful progress toward UHC, with increases in population coverage and access to health services, a rise in public spending on health, and a decline in out-of-pocket payments, which can result in catastrophic spending and impoverishment for many households. Expanded health services, including preventive, curative, and specialized services, have also been observed in most countries, and service utilization has become less inequitable over the years. The gap between rich and poor has also narrowed on a number of key health outcomes. Despite the advances, much remains to be done to close the equity gap and address new health challenges in the region.

As many countries in LAC adopt policies, plans, and strategies to move rapidly toward universal access to health and universal health coverage, continuous assessment of progress will be required to build the evidence base to inform policies and decision-making processes at the national level. Priority should be placed on the analysis of critical factors such as governance and stewardship in health, social participation and accountability, equity in access to quality services, health financing, and the intersectoral approach to address the social determinants of health, among others.

National policies and strategies promoting universal access to health and universal health coverage should be firmly anchored in the premise that the enjoyment of the highest attainable standard of health is one of the fundamental rights of every human being. This report reaffirms that policies oriented toward the achievement of UHC can improve equity, promote development, and increase social cohesion, ultimately leading to improved health and well-being for all.

Carissa Etienne
Director
Pan American Health Organization

Jorge Familiar
Vice President of the Latin America and
Caribbean Region
The World Bank

James Fitzgerald
Director of the Department of Health
Systems and Services
Pan American Health Organization

Tim Evans
Senior Director of the Health, Nutrition,
and Population Global Practice
The World Bank

Acknowledgments

This report is the culmination of more than two years of collaborative effort between the World Bank and the Pan American Health Organization (PAHO). Both organizations have embraced universal health coverage as an integral part of their work to strengthen health systems and improve the health of the world's people. The studies conducted for this report extend and complement those developed under PAHO's EquiLAC project.

The technical team was led by Tania Dmytraczenko of the World Bank's Health, Nutrition, and Population Global Practice and Gisele Almeida of PAHO's Department of Health Systems and Services. The team included Heitor Werneck, research analyst; Eleonora Cavagnero, economist; Magnus Lindelow, program leader; Fernando Montenegro Torres, senior economist; Evan Sloane Seely, junior professional associate; and Steven Kennedy, editor; with logistic and administrative support from Marise de Fátima Santos, Claudia Patricia Pacheco Florez and Isabel Nouel, administrative assistants. The work was conducted under the helpful guidance of Joana Godinho, practice manager, Health, Population, and Nutrition Global Practice, World Bank; and James Fitzgerald, director, Department of Health Systems and Services at PAHO.

This study stems from a concept originally developed by Joana Godinho and Christoph Kurowski. It was presented to the Chief Economist's Office of the Latin America and the Caribbean Region of the World Bank in July 2011. The authors thank the chief economist, Augusto de la Torre, and Tito Cordella for endorsing the concept and funding it. We are grateful as well to Daniel Lederman for guiding it to completion and to Adam Wagstaff for initiating the interinstitutional collaboration.

This report draws on commissioned background papers prepared by Flávia Mori Sarti, Terry Macedo Ivanauskas, Maria Dolores Montoya Diaz, Antonio Carlos Coelho Campino (Brazil), Guillermo Paraje, Felipe Vásquez (Chile); Fernando Ruiz, Teana Zapata Jaramillo (Colombia); James Cercone, Silvia Molina (Costa Rica and Guatemala); Ewan Scott (Jamaica); John Scott, Yadira Díaz (Mexico); Martín Valdivia, and Juan Pablo Ocampo (Peru). It also draws on papers prepared under the leadership of Daniel Cotlear for the Universal Health Coverage Studies Series (UNICO) by Rafael Cortez, Daniela Romero (Argentina); Bernard Couttolenc, Tania Dmytraczenko (Brazil); Ricardo Bitran (Chile); Fernando Montenegro Torres (Costa Rica and Colombia);

Oscar Bernal-Acevedo (Colombia); Christine Lao Pena (Guatemala); Shiyan Chao (Jamaica); María Eugenia Bonilla-Chacín, Nelly Aguilera (Mexico); and Pedro Francke (Peru).

The study benefited from the notable contributions of Joana Godinho, Margaret Grosh, Adam Wagstaff, Caryn Bredenkamp, Leander Buisman, Michele Gragnolati, Alexo Esperato, Oce Ozcelik, Molly Bode, Victor Valdívia, Javier Vasquez, Maria Eugenia Bonilla-Chacín, Shiyan Chao, Katharina Ferl, André Medici, Christine Lao Pena, Fernando Lavadenz, Sunil Rajkumar, Vanina Camporeale, Luis Orlando Perez and Dov Chernichovsky, as well as from the peer reviewers Tim Evans, James Fitzgerald, Christian Baeza, Daniel Cotlear, Amalia Del Riego, Pablo Gottret, Jack Langenbrunner, Akiko Maeda, Jed Friedman, Carlos Ocke-Reis, and Cristian Morales. We are also thankful to Zurab Sajaia for providing technical support related to the ADePT software.

About the Contributors

About the Editors

Tania Dmytraczenko, a senior economist with the World Bank's Health, Nutrition, and Population Global Practice, has extensive experience as a researcher and technical advisor working on health policy, health financing, and health systems strengthening in Latin America, Africa, and Asia. Before joining the World Bank, she was a principal at Abt Associates, where she provided technical assistance on United States Agency for International Development (USAID), the World Health Organization, the United Nations Population Fund, and the Joint UN Programme on HIV/AIDS projects. Before that, she had a joint appointment with the Department of Economics and the Center for Latin American Studies at Tulane University in New Orleans, Louisiana. She holds a PhD in economics from the University of North Carolina at Chapel Hill.

Gisele Almeida is an advisor in Health Systems and Services Analysis and coordinator of the EquiLAC Project at the Pan American Health Organization/ World Health Organization in Washington, DC, where she provides technical cooperation to member countries on monitoring and evaluation processes, use of evidence in public policies, and assessment of health systems performance. She has extensive expertise in health systems research, health services management tools, evaluation methods, and project management. She received a doctor of public health with specialization in health policy and a master of science in information management from the George Washington University. She has published in books and peer-reviewed journals.

About the Authors

Airlane Alencar earned her master's degree and PhD in statistics from the Institute of Mathematics and Statistics of the University of São Paulo in Brazil. She is a professor of statistics at the University of São Paulo, where she specializes in time series analysis. Airlane Alencar has been working as an advisor to the Ministry of Health of Brazil in the areas of data analysis and time trends analysis. She has worked as a consultant at the Pan American Health Organization on statistical analysis of pneumonia and influenza trends in several countries of the Americas.

Adam M. Aten is a researcher at the Brookings Institution's Engelberg Center for Health Care Reform, where he focuses on evidence development and biomedical innovation. Before joining Brookings, he was a civil servant at the U.S. Department of Health and Human Services working in the areas of health insurance for low-income populations, digital information systems and information governance, and cost-effectiveness of public health programs. He received an MPH from Des Moines University, Des Moines, Iowa, and an MSc in health economics from the Barcelona Graduate School of Economics in Barcelona, Spain. He also did graduate work in public health informatics at the Johns Hopkins University.

Eleonora Cavagnero, an economist, joined the World Bank in 2010. She has worked in the South Asia and Latin America and the Caribbean regions. Before joining the Bank, she worked for six years in the Department of Health Systems Financing at the World Health Organization in Geneva. She has published extensively, including books and articles in peer-reviewed journals about health financing, health system strengthening, and the socioeconomic and poverty impact of health payments, among other topics. She is an Argentinian national and holds a PhD from the University of Antwerp.

James A. Cercone, president and founder of Sanigest Internacional, is a mathematical economist from the University of Michigan. Over 20 years, he has worked extensively with the World Bank, Inter-American Development Bank (IDB), and other organizations on a wide range of social and public sector projects. His experience covers more than 60 countries through the development of health systems, establishing health insurance and financing reforms, monitoring and evaluation frameworks, economic analysis, and impact evaluations. He lectures frequently and publishes extensively on public sector reform, the design and implementation of insurance systems, resource allocation mechanisms, hospital management, contracting, and monitoring and evaluation.

Yadira Díaz is a PhD candidate in economics at the Institute for Social and Economic Research at the University of Essex. Her research interests are poverty, inequality, and health economics, with a focus on quantitative research methods. She has experience working on Colombia and other Latin American and Caribbean countries during the past 14 years. Her expertise includes the design of poverty and inequality measurement tools, the study of the Colombian health reform impact on health services use and health status, and the design of public policy impact evaluations. She has been a consultant for several developing countries' governments and international organizations.

Magnus Lindelow coordinates the World Bank's program on health, education, social protection, and poverty in Brazil. He holds a doctorate in economics from Oxford University. At the World Bank, he has been involved in projects and research in various regions, including Africa, East Asia and, most recently, Latin America. He has published books and research articles on health system reform, distributional issues in the health sector, public finance, service delivery, poverty, and other topics. Before joining the World Bank, he worked as an economist in the Ministry of Planning and Finance in Mozambique.

Daniel Maceira has a PhD in economics from Boston University and is a senior researcher at the Center for the Study of State and Society, independent researcher of the National Council of Scientific and Technological Research, and professor in the Department of Economics at the University of Buenos Aires, as well as in several postgraduate programs in Latin America. He collaborates with the World Bank, the Pan American Health Organization, the World Health Organization, the United Nations Development Programme, the United Nations Children's Fund, Economic Commission for Latin America and the Caribbean, the Inter-American Development Bank, the International Development Research Centre, the United States Agency for International Development, the Inter-American Foundation, the Gates Foundation, the Global Development Network, and the Global Fund. He has numerous peer-reviewed publications and coordinates research projects in Latin America and other developing countries.

Fatima Marinho obtained an MD from the Federal University of Rio de Janeiro, and an MPH and PhD in preventive medicine and epidemiology from the University of São Paulo, where she worked as a medical researcher until she became coordinator for epidemiological analyses at the Brazilian Ministry of Health. From 2008 to 2012, she worked at the Pan American Health Organization in Washington, DC, where she continues to serve as an advisor to the Pan American Health Organization's Regional Health Observatory. In 2014, she returned to the Brazilian Ministry of Health and currently provides technical assistance on the Burden of Disease Project and on strengthening Brazil's vital statistics system.

Silvia Molina is an economist from the National University of Costa Rica with extensive experience in the areas of planning, accounting, internal control, risk management research, and statistics. As part of the Sanigest International consulting team, she collaborates in research, benchmarking analyses, preparation of technical documents, survey planning and fieldwork, monitoring, and assessment. She has supported projects in health, education, health financing, monitoring and evaluation, impact evaluation, equity, AIDS, health reforms, and insurance coverage in Latin America and the Caribbean, Asia, and Eastern Europe. She also works on the firm's Quality Management System.

Fernando Montenegro Torres, a senior economist and medical doctor, has worked for various international organizations on universal health coverage policies and projects, including leading the health sector portfolio of the World Bank in Colombia, Costa Rica, and the Dominican Republic. He obtained an MD at Ecuador's Central University, an MSc in health systems at Heidelberg Universtaet, and an MA and PhD in health economics at the Johns Hopkins University. Fernando Montenegro Torres leads a results-based program for noncommunicable diseases and a Nordic Trust Fund grant on the right to health. He is a member of the World Bank multisectoral team on new digital tools for social sector information systems.

Flávia Mori Sarti has been a professor of economics applied to public policy management at the University of São Paulo since 2006. Her research areas are health economics (focusing on public health and nutrition policies) and complex systems modeling (focusing on health systems evaluation). Her main research projects include health technology assessment, food security, public policies of health and nutrition, and economic evaluation. Flávia Mori Sarti has a bachelor's in economics, a bachelor's in nutrition, and a PhD in Applied Human Nutrition from the University of São Paulo.

Saskia Nahrgang is a public health advisor at the World Health Organization's Regional Office for Europe. She trained as medical doctor at Ruperto Carola University in Heidelberg and holds a master of public health degree from Johns Hopkins University. At the World Bank, she has worked as health specialist on health system reform, service delivery, and chronic noncommunicable diseases and was involved in projects in Brazil, Nicaragua, and Panama. Over the past few years, she has been involved in design and evaluation of health sector programs, health policy planning, and research in Albania, Burkina Faso, Georgia, Nepal, Tanzania, Turkmenistan, and Uzbekistan.

Guillermo Paraje is an economist with expertise in the areas of development and health economics. Before joining Universidad Adolfo Ibáñez, he spent three years as an economist at the World Health Organization. He has been a consultant for several international organizations and national health ministries. Also, he has published several research articles on health economics topics and presented in international conferences. In addition, he has led international research teams, funded by the International Development Research Centre. Recently, he was part of the Presidential Advisory Committee for the Private Health System Reform in Chile. He has a DPhil in economics from the University of Cambridge.

Fernando Ruiz is the Colombian Deputy Minister of Public Health and Health Services. He was director for Cendex, a health services research center at Javeriana University in Bogotá, Colombia, and a cofounder of the Colombian Health Economics Association. He has been working on design, management, and evaluation of health projects in Colombia and other Latin American countries. He received an MPH from the Harvard School of Public Health. He holds an MA in health economics and a PhD in public health from the Instituto Nacional de Salud Pública of Mexico.

Ewan Scott holds a PhD in food and resource economics from the University of Florida and has been a lecturer in the Department of Economics at the University of the West Indies in St. Augustine since 2001. Ewan Scott's research interests have spanned a wide range of topics related to the economics of poverty, labor, public finance, and health; he has collaborated actively with researchers in other disciplines such as medicine and agriculture.

John Scott is a professor-researcher in the Economics Department at the Centro de Investigación y Docencia Económicas in Mexico City, Mexico, and an academic researcher of the Consejo Nacional de Evaluación de la Política de Desarrollo Social, a public institution responsible for poverty measurement and the evaluation of social programs in Mexico. He holds a BA in philosophy from New York University and an MPhil in economics and doctoral studies from the University of Oxford. His principal research areas include the distributive incidence of social spending, poverty and inequality analysis, evaluation of social policy, rural development policies, and health.

Evan Sloane Seely has an MPH from Dartmouth College in Hanover, New Hampshire, and is a junior health professional at the World Bank with experience working in the areas of child and adolescent obesity and fragile states. He has been a member of the Latin America and the Caribbean Health team at the World Bank since 2013.

Martín Valdivia has a PhD in applied economics from the University of Minnesota. He is currently a senior researcher at the Grupo de Análisis para el Desarrollo in Lima, Peru, and the current director of the Latin American office of the Poverty and Economic Policy Research Network. He works on economic development and has done several studies on the social determinants of health, the most recent focusing on issues such as the long-term effects of economic recessions on child health, and the role of culture in explaining patterns of teen pregnancy. He is also an active member of professional associations such as the Latin American and Caribbean Economic Association and the Global Development Network.

Heitor Werneck is a dentist by training with seven years of clinical experience with undeserved communities in Brazil. He has an MPH from Brazil's National School of Public Health and is now pursuing his PhD in public health at the George Washington University. As part of his doctoral training, he worked as a research assistant with the EquiLAC Project at the Pan American Health Organization. He currently works for ANS, a Brazilian federal regulatory agency that oversees private health insurance in the country.

Abbreviations

ANC	Antenatal care
CI	Concentration index
CONAPO	Consejo Nacional de Población
CSO	Civil society organization
CVD	Cardiovascular disease
DHS	Demographic and Health Survey
GDP	Gross domestic product
GHE	Government health expenditure
HI	Horizontal inequity index
ICESCR	International Covenant of Economic, Social and Cultural Rights
IDB	Inter-American Development Bank
IHME	Institute of Health Metrics and Evaluation
LAC	Latin America and the Caribbean
MDG	Millennium Development Goal
MoH	Ministry of health
NCD	Noncommunicable disease
NHF	National Health Fund
OECD	Organisation for Economic Co-operation and Development
ORS	Oral rehydration salts
PAHO	Pan American Health Organization
PEC	Program of Expansion of Coverage
PHE	Public health expenditure
PPP	Purchasing power parity
SAH	Self-assessed health
STEMI	ST Elevation Myocardial Infarction
THE	Total health expenditure
UDHR	Universal Declaration of Human Rights
UHC	Universal health coverage
USAID	United States Agency for International Development
WHO	World Health Organization

Overview

Recognizing and Fulfilling the Right to Health

Over the past three decades, many countries of Latin America and the Caribbean (LAC) have recognized health as a human right and acted on that recognition. Several have amended their constitutions to guarantee their citizens the right to health.[1] Most have ratified international conventions that define the progressive and equitable implementation of the right to health as an obligation of the state.[2] Grounded in the expanded legal framework regulating these new rights, demands have grown steadily for health systems to become more responsive in delivering affordable care that meets the needs of the population. Accordingly, countries have implemented policies and programs aimed at achieving universal health coverage (UHC)—that is, ensuring that all people can obtain the services they need without suffering financial hardship.

Key to those policies has been a concern for greater equity. While LAC has seen tremendous gains in health outcomes in the past century, inequities in health among and within the countries persist. In most countries of the region, the poor are more likely than the rich to experience worse health and less likely to make use of basic health services, such as preventive care, needed to avoid health problems and detect diseases early. At the same time, the region's changing demographic and epidemiological profiles—notably its aging population and the shift of the burden of disease toward chronic illness, which has been increasing in all income groups—create greater demand for health services.

The focus on equity is not unique to the health sector. Over the past decade, LAC, a region long plagued by persistent inequalities in the distribution of wealth, has seen a dramatic social transformation. Social policies encompassing reforms in the health sector have been implemented in a context of redemocratization and stable economic growth that have brought rising household incomes, drastic drops in poverty, and declining income inequality in most countries. A rising middle class and empowered electorate have demanded greater and more effective investments in health and other social sectors that, once fulfilled, have the potential to increase human capital and spur further growth and poverty reduction, creating a virtuous cycle. (Ferreira and others 2013)

What is clear from previous research (Savedoff and others 2012) and confirmed by the findings in this report is that larger quantities of pooled financing and a focus on equity are necessary conditions to progress toward UHC. All study countries saw an increase in public financing for health as a share of gross domestic product (GDP), and most scaled up coverage of pooling mechanisms, financed largely if not entirely from general revenues that prioritized or explicitly targeted populations lacking the capacity to pay. In most countries, political commitment translated not only into larger budget allocations but also into the passage of legislation that ring-fenced funding for health by establishing minimum levels of health spending, labeling or earmarking taxes for health. Even countries that did not take such permanent measures moved partially away from input-based, line-item budgets toward per capita transfers, sometimes derived from actuarial cost calculations. Such mechanisms are known to reduce uncertainty in financing.

From Segmentation to UHC

Historically, most countries of the LAC region maintained a two-tiered system of health care: one for those employed in the formal sector and another, delivered through ministries of health, for the poor and uninsured (Baeza and Packard 2006). During the 1980s and 1990s, several countries (beginning with Chile, Costa Rica, Brazil, and Colombia) embarked on reforms to minimize fragmentation of health services created by the two-tiered systems. Since then, Argentina, Guatemala, Jamaica, Mexico, Peru, and Uruguay have implemented a much broader array of policies to improve the incentives and governance framework with the objective of increasing efficiency and expanding access to health care, particularly among the poor and those at risk of falling into poverty because of health care costs. New policy iterations are emerging in the early reform countries of Brazil, Chile, Colombia, and Costa Rica as well.

After nearly a quarter-century of experience with reforms to advance UHC in LAC,[3] it is a good time to take stock of progress made in improving population health and access to health services. This is particularly timely in light of global momentum toward UHC—recently accelerated by the publication of the World Health Report *Health Systems Financing: The Path to Universal Coverage* (WHO 2010). The adoption in 2011 of the World Health Assembly resolution WHA 64.9 urging countries to aim for affordable universal coverage is further evidence of progress. In 2012, the United Nations General Assembly encouraged member states to pursue the transition to universal coverage, recommending that UHC be considered for inclusion in the post-2015 development agenda. In 2014, the members of the Pan American Health Organization (PAHO) unanimously approved a resolution to implement the Strategy for Universal Access to Health and UHC, A/67/L.36 (PAHO 2014). The World Bank has also embraced UHC as integral to its mission to eliminate absolute poverty by 2030 and to boost shared prosperity.

It is within this context that this study addresses the following questions:

- Have the above referenced reforms reduced inequality in health outcomes, service utilization, and financial protection?
- What measures can be reliably used across countries over time to monitor progress toward UHC?
- What regional trends, if any, emerge from implementation of policies to advance UHC?

To analyze the range of reforms in LAC and measure progress toward UHC, we use as the organizing framework the "WHO cube" proposed by Busse, Schreyögg, and Gericke (2007). We apply an equity lens to assess the extent to which countries are moving along three dimensions: population coverage, service coverage, and financial protection. For purposes of monitoring progress toward UHC, we conclude that utilization rates are not a sufficient measure. Making health services available and more affordable does not automatically translate into improved health outcomes. We propose that better methods for collecting and reporting measures of timeliness and quality of care need to be developed. Our conclusions and recommendations are substantiated by an extensive literature review and primary analyses of nationally representative household surveys.

While the WHO cube is a useful construct for reviewing progress toward UHC, it is not a framework for analyzing health system performance. A limitation of this report is that it does not provide a comprehensive assessment of policies and programs to strengthen health systems. Nonetheless, we do review key policies and programs aimed at advancing UHC, drawing on papers produced for nine LAC countries (Argentina, Brazil, Chile, Colombia, Costa Rica, Guatemala, Jamaica, Mexico, and Peru) under the Universal Health Coverage Studies Series (UNICO). The UNICO Series applies a structured protocol for reviewing policies implemented to: (1) manage the benefits package; (2) manage inclusion of the poor and vulnerable groups; (3) improve efficiency in the provision of care; (4) address challenges in primary care; and (5) adjust financing mechanisms to better align incentives.

Looking Back: Common Approaches

The countries of the LAC region have taken various paths toward UHC, and achieved varying levels of success. Some have attained outcomes comparable with Organisation for Economic Co-operation and Development (OECD) countries despite getting a much later start establishing programs and policies to improve population coverage, access to health services and financial protection. While the countries studied represent a diverse set of experiences, a review of the evidence and policies implemented to advance toward UHC reveals some common features in the approaches taken.

Steady Gains in the Scope and Equity of Health Programs with Increases in Public Spending

The share of the region's population covered by health programs with explicit guarantees of affordable care has increased considerably. Since the early 2000s, 46 million additional people in the countries analyzed are nominally covered by health programs and policies aimed at advancing UHC. At the same time, equity has improved. Several countries have implemented subsidized programs (mostly insurance schemes with proactive enrollment of beneficiaries) that target specific populations, such as those not covered by contributory social health insurance schemes, whereas others have extended coverage to vulnerable groups within universal programs. Even in countries that have maintained health systems where subsidized and contributory schemes coexist, overall coverage rates have become more equal across income groups. Though employment-based social health insurance remains heavily skewed toward the rich, subsidized schemes that are, at least initially, targeted to the poor have provided a counterbalance.

From a financing perspective, reforms have been accompanied by a rise in public spending on health and, in most cases, a decline in the share of out-of-pocket payments in total health expenditures. Though not all reforms had an explicit stated objective to extend financial protection, most countries saw a reduction in catastrophic health expenditures and in impoverishment owing to outlays for health.

No consistent picture emerges regarding catastrophic payments and equity. This may reflect limitations in the measure of out-of-pocket expenditures, which cannot capture individuals who did not seek care because of financial barriers; nor is there enough granularity regarding the nature of the expenditure, in particular, whether the care paid for was necessary or elective. It should be noted that while the rate of impoverishment owing to health care (including catastrophic) expenditures is low in relative terms and generally declining, there are 2–4 million people in the countries analyzed who have been driven into poverty due to out-of-pocket health spending. Despite the improvements, the share of out-of-pocket payments in total spending is still relatively high in the study countries compared with OECD averages. Expenditures on medicines absorb by far the largest share of direct payments across income groups, but they pose a particularly heavy burden for the poor.

Variability in Benefits Packages and a Coming Crisis as Health Needs Change

Nominal service coverage has also expanded during the period analyzed. Subsidized schemes cover maternal and child interventions at the very least, while most go beyond that to include comprehensive primary care. Half the countries covered in this study offer extensive benefits ranging from low- to high-complexity care.

The evidence corroborates that investments in extending health care, with particular attention to reaching vulnerable populations, are yielding positive results. The expansion of programs to advance UHC has coincided with a reduction of the gap between the rich and the poor in health outcomes and service utilization, particularly for targets specified in the Millennium Development Goals.

Prioritization of cost-effective primary care is the common denominator across all countries, whether they start small and gradually expand the benefits package, as in Argentina and Peru, or offer comprehensive coverage from the onset, as was the case in Brazil, Costa Rica, and Uruguay. The approach of prioritizing primary care has improved the comparative position of the poor, who were more likely than wealthier people to lack access to the first level of care. Benefits coverage is more comprehensive in countries with integrated health systems and in those that are further along the path to integration. Although most countries have a positive list of services covered, Brazil, Colombia, and Costa Rica have open-ended benefits.

Countries with greater population coverage and more extensive benefits packages have achieved near universal utilization of maternal health services, with high levels of utilization and virtually no difference across income quintiles. Where a pro-rich gradient in service utilization remains, it is narrowest for services delivered through traditionally vertical programs such as immunization and family planning. The pro-rich gradient has also been successfully minimized for services provided mostly at lower levels of the health services network (for example, antenatal care, medical treatment of acute respiratory infections). Rich–poor gaps are wider for deliveries, which are done in hospitals.

The picture is more nuanced, and not nearly as positive, for chronic conditions and illnesses that are the most important causes of mortality and morbidity in the middle to late stages of life. The share of the population reporting less-than-good health status has not declined markedly or consistently in most countries; and the indicator is highly skewed, with the poor uniformly reporting the worst outcomes.[4] Further, diagnosed chronic conditions such as diabetes, ischemic heart disease, and asthma have been increasing for all income groups in several countries, as are associated risk factors such as obesity and hypertension.

No clear gradient emerges in diagnosed chronic conditions and associated risk factors among income groups, despite the available evidence showing higher mortality rates for these conditions among the poor (Di Cesare and others 2013). A likely explanation is that the poor have less access to health care, particularly diagnostic services, and therefore are less likely to be diagnosed when compared to the rich. Evidence from cancer screening suggests that this may indeed be the case. Utilization of such diagnostics is generally pro-rich, with the gradient being particularly pronounced for breast cancer screening, which requires access to specialist care. The trend in level and equity is positive, however: Countries with high levels of population coverage, with the exception of Brazil, have greatly reduced the rich-poor gap, especially for cervical cancer screening, but also for mammography in the cases of Colombia and Mexico.

Toward Universal Health Coverage and Equity in Latin America and the Caribbean
http://dx.doi.org/10.1596/978-1-4648-0454-0

Reducing Fragmentation of Health Systems

Few countries have followed the path of full integration by creating a system in which all mandatory contributions—whether financed from payroll levies and general revenues, as in Costa Rica, or only the latter, as in Brazil—are pooled so as to offer access to the entire population through a common network of providers. Most countries have opted to maintain, to a greater or lesser extent, a segmented system in which a subsidized subsystem exists in parallel with a subsystem financed entirely or mostly through payroll contributions, with beneficiaries generally having access to different networks of providers.

Historically, large discrepancies in the benefits package, and in the quality of care, have been present across schemes. But more recently, pooling arrangements that broadened the risk pool and facilitated cross-subsidization between contributing and subsidized beneficiaries, accompanied by regulations that equalized benefits packages and provided explicit guarantees to timely access to services meeting specified standards of care (thus closing off avenues used to ration care in the resource-poor public sector), have been effective in reducing disparities in financing and service provision across subsystems—for example, in Chile, Colombia, and Uruguay.

Data from selected countries, though limited, bolstered by available research, demonstrate that many health systems face serious challenges in these areas that are likely to grow in importance as health care needs become more complex and population expectations of the health system grow. To date, because of data limitations, efforts to monitor progress toward UHC do not capture dimensions of need, quality, and timeliness well enough to determine whether access to *effective* coverage is improving.

Separating Financing and Provision in the Public Sector

Despite wide variability in the extent to which countries have moved away from highly integrated service delivery and finance toward separation of these functions, there is a common trend of adopting purchasing methods that incentivize efficiency and accountability for results, and that give stewards of the health sector greater leverage to steer providers to deliver on public health priorities. One way in which countries have created a separation of functions is by establishing contractual relationships between finance and provision, either through legally binding contracts or through explicit agreements that specify the roles and responsibilities of each party as well as expected results. Payment mechanisms vary considerably, from capitation to fee-for-services to case-based payments, but as a rule the mechanisms incentivize providers to satisfy demand by tying the flow of funds to enrollment of beneficiaries or to services actually rendered. Increasingly, countries are instituting pay-for-performance mechanisms that reward achievement of specific targets linked to population health needs.

By eliminating the rigidities of line-item budgets, the new financing modalities offer providers greater autonomy in managing inputs to achieve efficiency gains.

In decentralized (federal) systems, similar arrangements that promote the achievement of national policy priorities are being applied to fund transfers to subnational governments. Even in countries where the volume of resources that flow through the new payment mechanisms is relatively small, the reforms introduce a platform on which to build systems that rely more heavily on strategic purchasing.

Looking Ahead: The Unfinished Agenda

Raising Revenue in a Narrowing Fiscal Space

Protecting achievements to date and tackling the challenges that remain will require sustained investments in health. Delivering on the commitment to UHC will require concerted efforts to improve revenue generation in a fiscally sustainable manner and to increase the efficiency of expenditures. Both will be particularly important as countries move further along the demographic transition and begin to face the challenges of gradually rising population dependency ratios and, eventually, shrinking tax bases.

Throughout the region, countries have ramped up public financing for health, though these expenditures still represent less than 5 percent of GDP in half the study countries.[5] Nonetheless, in eight of the 10 countries the health sector already absorbs more than 15 percent of the public budget (the OECD average) and in three of the eight the share exceeds 20 percent. This is of concern because the middle-income countries of the region may not have the fiscal space to allow health expenditures to rise faster than economic growth.

As countries look for ways to finance public health expenditures, it will be important to assess the effectiveness and fairness of financing measures. Many countries in the region rely on levies on wage income to finance health, but it would be worth exploring options that have been implemented elsewhere. Including rental or interest income in the calculation simultaneously generates revenue while improving progressivity in financing, as nonwage earnings represent a larger share of wealthier households' total revenue.

While earmarking taxes for health has been widely used in the region to finance expansion of coverage, this type of measure may reduce flexibility to reallocate resources for meeting changing population needs across all sectors. Regardless of source, levying new taxes for health will be difficult for some countries, such as Argentina and Brazil, where the tax burden is already at OECD levels.[6]

Improving the Efficiency of Health Spending

While prioritizing cost-effective primary care and reforming arrangements for pooling and purchasing undoubtedly contribute to improving the effectiveness of investments in health, much more needs to be done to contain cost escalation and increase efficiency in spending.

- First, *strategic purchasing reforms* must be deepened and their scope extended beyond primary care to yield greater gains in technical and allocative efficiency.

Toward Universal Health Coverage and Equity in Latin America and the Caribbean
http://dx.doi.org/10.1596/978-1-4648-0454-0

- Second, countries must establish *formal and transparent priority-setting systems for selecting service coverage* based on well-defined criteria grounded in scientific evidence of effectiveness and cost, as well as in social preferences. In the absence of such systems, several countries in the region have seen a "judicialization" of the right to health, whereby disputes over what the state must legally provide are often resolved though litigation, which can lead to public subsidization of ineffective or inefficient care and have the added adverse effect of increasing inequality, since the wealthy can better afford legal counsel.
- Third, in a region where the share of out-of-pocket payments in total health expenditures still exceeds 30 percent in many countries, efforts to *contain rising input costs* in the public sector cannot work in isolation. This is particularly, though not exclusively, relevant to the adoption of new medical technologies in the private sector, an area where supplier-induced demand was shown to be an important driver of cost escalation in developed countries.

Managing Quality Differences across Subsystems

Substantial differences persist in the quality of providers across subsystems. Initiatives emphasizing quality of care, supply-side readiness, integration of service delivery, and eHealth can play important roles in narrowing these gaps.

The existing gap in per capita financing and quality of services delivered across the subsystems, while suboptimal from an equity perspective, provides a powerful incentive for individuals to buy into the contributory regime, which offers a more generous benefit package and better care. As the differential between subsystems narrows, there is a risk that this incentive will be eroded. In Chile, where workers have an option to apply their mandatory contribution toward a private health plan or enroll in the public plan, our data show a migration of people away from the first and into the second alternative. The evidence thus far suggests that extension of insurance coverage to those outside the formal sector, such as Mexico's Seguro Popular, has had only a marginal impact on informality (Reyes, Hallward-Driemeier, and Pages 2011).

To sustain the effort to provide affordable health care to the entire population in the face of these uncertainties, countries will need to remain vigilant about capturing the contributions of those who can afford to pay but are unwilling to do so voluntarily, while also targeting public subsidies to those who cannot afford to pay. Compulsion and subsidization are both necessary (and sufficient) conditions for universal coverage (Fuchs 1996).

Gathering Better Data and Devising Better Processes for Monitoring Quality

As the international community prepares for the 2015 World Summit, which will define the goals and targets for the post–Millennium Development Goals era, we will need better tracking indicators. These challenges go beyond national aggregates. Fortunately, our study demonstrates that, despite shortcomings, one can measure progress in service utilization and financial protection.

With few exceptions (for example, for cancer diagnoses), available surveys generally do not provide the level of granularity needed to determine whether individuals are receiving the care they need. Administrative records provide better medical detail but are weak in capturing socioeconomic information, are not publicly available, and raise privacy concerns. The complexity of managing large data systems from multiple institutions containing highly sensitive medical information makes this a difficult area to tackle within the resource-constrained public sector. Partnerships with research institutions domestically and abroad could be a way for the ministries of health to mine the vast amount of information being generated on health financing, service provision, and outcomes to inform policy decision making and strengthen governance over the sector.

A Preview, by Chapter

Chapter 2: The Emergence of Reforms to Advance UHC

In recent decades, UHC has emerged in the context of health as a fundamental human right and been closely linked to broader social reforms to improve living conditions and access to health services for vulnerable groups. These social reforms happened in parallel with a democratization process during a period of sustained economic growth and improved equity in the region. Social policies, including those that expand coverage and access to health services and ensure financial protection for the population, have emerged as an important topic on the political agenda. Demographic changes have also fueled societal demands for more comprehensive health coverage and services to cope with the rise in chronic conditions, which poses special challenges in the health system and its financial sustainability.

The results show that the 10 countries under study generally fall behind the high-performing OECD countries but ahead of most less-developed countries. The LAC countries have also shown a tendency to perform better than expected, which can be partly attributed to better public policies and increased public health expenditure. The region continues to show improved health outcomes, positive trends, and stronger economies. Despite the progress, however, inequality remains high. To counter inequality, countries must maintain their macroeconomic stability and monitor changing demographics, which fuel demands for more comprehensive health coverage. The region must find a way to continue to grow. A slowing of the population growth of recent decades is almost certain, but countries will continue to age, challenging the region to become more creative in sustaining the expansion of policies to advance UHC in order to deal with both NCDs and infectious diseases. NCDs pose challenges for both the delivery and the financing of health care due to the epidemiological transitions underway and the increasingly aging populations. LAC countries face the challenge need to sustain the progress already achieved, improve equitable access to health services, and improve the quality of services. By working in tandem, public agencies, academia, and the private sector can tackle the main constraints in moving toward UHC.

Toward Universal Health Coverage and Equity in Latin America and the Caribbean
http://dx.doi.org/10.1596/978-1-4648-0454-0

Chapter 3: A Comparative Analysis of Policies to Advance UHC in the Region

Over the past few decades various governments across LAC have acted to strengthen the performance of their health systems by developing new policies and interventions aimed at realizing the vision of UHC. Governments' focus has been on reducing fragmentation in the financing and organization of health systems, harmonizing the scope and quality of services across subsystems, leveraging public sector financing in a more comprehensive and integrated manner, and creating incentives that promote achievement of improved health outcomes and financial protection. Health policies have emphasized making entitlements explicit; establishing enforceable guarantees; and instituting supply side incentives aimed at improving quality of care and reducing geographical barriers to access. To a lesser extent, governments have also made efforts to enhance governance and accountability. This chapter takes stock of these changes and identifies key trends in policies to advance UHC across the region in countries with diverse health systems facing distinct challenges.

Some key themes emerge from our review of the implementation experiences of policies to advance UHC in the LAC countries analyzed for this study:

- Leveraging public financing to reach the poor
- A pragmatic and contextual approach to defining (or not) the benefits package
- An increase in public financing for health
- Reforms in the way providers are paid and managed
- Emphasis on primary care
- Tackling equalization across subsystems

The review and analysis of policies of the cases used in this study suggest that tackling regulation to reduce inequalities in differences in the quality, timeliness, and scope of services can be carried out once the traditional public sector has improved its performance and responsiveness through not only increased financing but other policy aspects. Positive results have been achieved by introducing new mechanisms to align incentives and monitoring timeliness, accessibility, and quality of services so that patients can navigate the systems without breaking the continuity of health care and improving patient satisfaction.

Chapter 4: The Results of Measurements of Progress toward UHC in the Countries Studied

Analysis of population coverage, health outcomes, service coverage, and financial protection measures over time and across socioeconomic groups show that the region has made considerable progress in extending population coverage to schemes aimed at advancing UHC and improvements in equity have been identified during the same period. Socioeconomic gradients are clearly observed in health status, with the poor having worse health outcomes than the rich, though disparities have narrowed considerably particularly in the early stage of the life course. Countries have reached high levels of coverage of maternal and child health services but, despite narrowing inequality, services remain pro-rich. Coverage of noncommunicable disease interventions is not as high and service utilization is skewed toward the better off, though disparities are lessening over time. Primary care services are in general more equally distributed across income groups than specialized care. Disease prevalence has not behaved as expected given the drop in mortality. Better access to services, and hence diagnosis, among wealthier individuals may be masking changes in actual prevalence. Catastrophic health expenditures have declined in most countries. The picture regarding equity, however, is mixed, pointing to limitations in the measure.

Chapter 5: Beyond Utilization and Health Outcomes: looking at quality of health services

Assessments of UHC tend to focus on the utilization of health services, formal entitlement, or eligibility to access services and measures of financial protection. But if our concern is to assess to what extent all persons can get the health care they need without financial hardship, indicators in these areas have important limitations. Indeed, expansion of health care coverage, in the sense of making health services available and more affordable, does not automatically translate into improved health outcomes. With this issue in mind, chapter 5 complements analyses of patterns of utilization, coverage, and financial protection in LAC with a review of what is known about the links between utilization and health outcomes. In doing so, it looks at questions of unmet need for health care, timeliness of care, and quality of health services. These are areas in which measurement tends to be more difficult than it is with utilization and financial protection. Nonetheless, although there are limited routine data that are comparable across countries, studies and monitoring data from selected countries provide enough of a picture to highlight the importance of these issues and hopefully to stimulate efforts to develop more systematic approaches for collecting and reporting on timeliness and quality of care in the region.

Chapter 6: Conclusions

The concluding chapter summarizes the main findings, discusses policy implications, and points to areas where further research is needed.

Notes

1. The establishment of a constitutional or legal right to health reflects political commitment. But rights do not automatically translate into higher coverage and may not be a sufficient condition for achieving it. In fact, several countries in and outside the region that are considered to be farther along the path to UHC do not have the right to health enshrined in their constitutions (for example, Canada and Costa Rica).

2. We refer here to the American Convention on Human Rights, "Pact of San Jose, Costa Rica," and the Protocol of San Salvador.

3. We use "advance UHC" as shorthand for "advance the goal of UHC."

4. There are severe limitations to analyzing differences in adult health outcomes by socioeconomic strata. Data for analysis of mortality trends generally come from civil vital registration statistics that typically do not contain information on socioeconomic status. Educational attainment can be used as a proxy, but among the countries studied only Chile and Mexico had reliable data for this type of analysis to be carried out. Self-assessed health status is an indicator that has its shortcomings but is measured in the surveys reviewed (Lora 2012).

5. Below the 5–6 percent threshold of public expenditures as a share of GDP countries struggle to ensure health service coverage for the poor (WHO 2010).

6. Tax revenue as a share of GDP is 36 and 37 percent, respectively, in Brazil and Argentina, compared with the OECD average of 34 percent.

References

Baeza, C., and T. Packard. 2006. *Beyond Survival: Protecting Households from Health Shocks in Latin America*. Washington, DC: World Bank.

Busse, R., J. Schreyögg, and C. Gericke. 2007. "Analyzing Changes in Health Financing Arrangements in High-Income Countries: A Comprehensive Framework Approach." HNP Discussion Paper, World Bank, Washington, DC.

Di Cesare, Mariachiara, Young-Ho Khang, Perviz Asaria, Tony Blakely, Melanie J. Cowan, Farshad Farzadfar, Ramiro Guerrero, Nayu Ikeda, Catherine Kyobutungi, Kelias P. Msyamboza, Sophal Oum, John W. Lynch, Michael G. Marmot, and Majid Ezzati, on behalf of The Lancet NCD Action Group. 2013. "Inequalities in Non-Communicable Diseases and Effective Responses." *The Lancet* 381 (9866): 585–97.

Ferreira, F. H. G., J. Messina, J. Rigolini, L. F. López-Calva, M. A. Lugo, and R. Vakis. 2013. *Economic Mobility and the Rise of the Latin American Middle Class*. Washington, DC: World Bank.

Fuchs, Victor. 1996. "What Every Philosopher Should Know about Health Economics." *Proceedings of the American Philosophical Society* 140 (2): 186–96.

Lora, Eduardo. 2012. "Health Perceptions in Latin America." *Health Policy and Planning* 27 (7): 555–69.

PAHO (Pan American Health Organization). 2014. "Strategy for Universal Access to Health and Universal Health Coverage." Document CD53/5, Rev 2, 53rd Directing Council, PAHO, Washington, DC.

Reyes, A., M. Hallward-Driemeier, and C. Pages. 2011. "Does Expanding Health Insurance beyond Formal-Sector Workers Encourage Informality? Measuring the Impact of Mexico's Seguro Popular." Policy Research Working Paper 5785, World Bank, Washington, DC.

Savedoff, William, David de Ferranti, Amy L. Smith, and Victoria Fan. 2012. "Political and Economic Aspects of the Transition to Universal Health Coverage." *The Lancet* 380: 924–32.

WHO (World Health Organization). 2010. *The World Health Report 2010: Health Systems Financing—The Path to Universal Coverage*. Geneva: WHO.

CHAPTER 1

Introduction

Gisele Almeida and Tania Dmytraczenko

Summary

Countries in Latin America and the Caribbean (LAC) are increasingly embracing the notion of health as a human right. Several have even amended their constitutions to guarantee their citizens the right to health. Most have also ratified international conventions that define the progressive and equitable implementation of the right to health as an obligation of the state.[1] In an effort to realize this right, countries have been implementing policies and programs aimed at achieving universal health coverage (UHC)—that is, ensuring that all people can obtain the services they need without financial hardship. The ultimate goal of UHC is to improve the health of the entire population, leaving no one behind, by ensuring access to quality health services without financial hardship.

LAC has a long history of implementing health policies to deliver on this promise of UHC. In the 1980s and 1990s, a number of countries embarked on reforms that sought to minimize fragmentation of health financing and care introduced through the two-tiered systems then in place. Earlier policies have created health systems with one tier for those employed in the formal sector and another tier, managed through ministries of health, primarily for the poor and uninsured (Baeza and Packard 2006). Most such policies did not succeed in reducing fragmentation. This early wave of reforms began with Chile, Costa Rica, Brazil, and Colombia. Since then countries in the region have implemented a much broader array of policies. The goal has been to improve the incentives and governance framework in order to increase efficiency and to expand equitable access to health care, particularly among the poor or those at risk of falling into poverty due to spending on health care. These reforms are being implemented in Argentina, Guatemala, Jamaica, Mexico, Peru, and Uruguay; new policy iterations are also emerging in the early reform countries of Brazil, Chile, Colombia, and Costa Rica.

The focus on equity is not unique to the health sector. Over the past decade, LAC, a region long plagued by persistent inequalities in the distribution of wealth, has seen a dramatic social transformation. Millions have moved out of the ranks of the poor and are joining the middle class (Ferreira and others 2013). This has been spurred by a shift in government policies that now favor the delivery of social programs, which along with economic stability have worked to produce higher incomes and less income inequality. Health reforms that promote universality through inclusion of the poor must be seen in this context.

After nearly a quarter-century of experience implementing reforms aimed at achieving UHC in LAC, it is a good time to take stock of how well countries have fared in improving the health of their populations. This is particularly relevant in light of global momentum toward UHC—momentum that has taken on greater force since publication of the World Health Report *Health Systems Financing: The Path to Universal Coverage* (WHO 2010). The adoption in 2011 of the World Health Assembly resolution, WHA64.9, urging countries to aim for affordable universal coverage is further evidence of progress. In 2012, the United Nations General Assembly encouraged member states to pursue the transition to universal coverage, recommending that UHC be considered for inclusion in the post-2015 development agenda (A/67/L.36). In 2014, the members of the Pan American Health Organization (PAHO) unanimously approved a resolution to implement the Strategy for Universal Access to Health and UHC (PAHO 2014). The World Bank has also embraced UHC as integral to its mission to eliminate absolute poverty by 2030 and to boost shared prosperity.

In reviewing the experiences of LAC, this study hopes to contribute to the global knowledge base about the pathways to UHC. The main objectives of this report are to (1) describe the reforms intended to advance UHC that have taken place in the region, and (2) measure progress toward this goal. We seek to answer these questions in particular: Have the reforms reduced inequality in health outcomes, service utilization, and financial protection? What measures can be reliably used across countries over time to monitor progress toward universal coverage? What regional trends, if any, emerge from implementation of policies to advance UHC?

To analyze the range of reforms in LAC and measure progress toward UHC, this report uses, as its organizing framework, the "WHO cube" proposed by Busse, Schreyögg, and Gericke (2007), which appears in the 2008 World Health Report and, in a slightly modified version, in the 2010 report. We apply an equity lens to assess how countries are managing progress toward UHC along three dimensions: population coverage, service coverage, and financial protection. We also postulate that implicit in the definition of UHC is the notion that the population must have access to *quality* services that address health needs. And, in monitoring progress toward UHC, we conclude that it is not sufficient to track utilization and financial protection. Making health services available and more affordable does not automatically translate into improved health outcomes. We propose that the region needs to develop more systematic approaches for collecting and reporting on measures of timeliness and quality of care.

While the WHO cube is a useful construct for reviewing progress toward UHC, it is not a framework for analyzing health system performance. A limitation of this report is that it does not provide a comprehensive assessment of policies and programs to strengthen health systems; it does not review aspects of governance, health workforce, or medical products and technologies. Further, the report does not delve deeply into issues of efficiency and sustainability, although these areas merit critical attention if countries in the region hope to maintain gains already achieved and make further progress toward the realization of the right to health.

As the international community prepares for the 2015 World Summit, which will define the goals and targets for the post–Millennium Development Goals era, we hope to illustrate the feasibility and highlight the challenges of tracking indicators that go beyond national aggregates. We build on previous studies by demonstrating that, despite the shortcomings, countries can measure progress in financial protection and service utilization—at various stages of the life course—by using existing, routine national household surveys (Almeida and others 2013; Barraza-Lloréns, Panopoulou, and Díaz 2013; Bredenkamp and others 2013; Gómez, Jaramillo, and Beltrán 2013; Knaul, Wong, and Arreola-Ornelas 2012; Petrera, Martín, and Almeida 2013; Scott and Theodore 2013; Vásquez, Paraje, and Estay 2013).

In addition to the literature review and data analyses, the authors draw on background papers produced for nine LAC countries (Argentina, Brazil, Chile, Colombia, Costa Rica, Guatemala, Jamaica, Mexico, and Peru) under the Universal Health Coverage Studies Series (UNICO). The UNICO Series applies a structure protocol for reviewing policies implemented to (1) manage the benefits package, (2) manage inclusion of the poor and vulnerable groups, (3) improve efficiency in provision of care, (4) address challenges in primary care, and (5) adjust financing mechanisms to better align incentives.

Health policies do not happen in a vacuum. They are shaped by their political, economic, demographic, and epidemiological environments. Chapter 2 describes the emergence of UHC in the context of health as a fundamental human right. In addition, it describes how democratization, a commitment to implement social policies, and the sustained and more equitable economic growth of the past decade all fed into the progressive realization of the right to health. Chapter 3 offers a comparative analysis of policies to advance UHC in the region, identifying common traits across countries. In chapter 4, we present the results of our measurement of progress toward UHC in the nine countries studied. It begins by describing population coverage by different schemes, followed by an analysis of how health outcomes, service coverage, and financial protection measures have changed over time and across socioeconomic groups. Chapter 5 complements these analyses with a review of what is known about the links between utilization and health outcomes. In doing so, it looks at questions of unmet need for health care, timeliness of care, and quality of health services. The concluding chapter summarizes the main findings, discusses policy implications, and points to areas where further research is needed.

Note

1. We refer here to the American Convention on Human Rights, "Pact of San Jose, Costa Rica," and the Protocol of San Salvador.

References

Almeida, G., F. Mori Sari, F. F. Ferreira, M. D. Montoya Diaz, and A. C. Campino. 2013. "Analysis of the Evolution and Determinants of Income-Related Inequalities in the Brazilian Health System, 1998–2008." *Pan American Journal of Public Health* 33 (2): 90–7.

Baeza, C., and T. Packard. 2006. *Beyond Survival: Protecting Households from Health Shocks in Latin America*. Washington, DC: World Bank.

Barraza-Lloréns, M., G. Panopoulou, and B. Y. Díaz. 2013. "Income-Related Inequalities and Inequities in Health and Health Care Utilization in Mexico, 2000–2006." *Pan American Journal of Public Health* 33 (2): 122–30.

Bonilla-Chacín, M. E., and N. Aguilera. 2013. *The Mexican Social Protection System in Health*. UNICO Study Series 1, World Bank, Washington, DC.

Bredenkamp, C., A. Wagstaff, L. Buisman, and L. Prencipe. 2013. *Health Equity and Financial Protection Datasheets—Latin America*. Washington, DC: World Bank.

Busse R., J. Schreyögg, and C. Gericke. 2007. "Analyzing Changes in Health Financing Arrangements in High-Income Countries: A Comprehensive Framework Approach." HNP Discussion Paper, World Bank, Washington, DC.

Chao, S. 2013. *Jamaica's Effort in Improving Universal Access within Fiscal Constraints*. UNICO Study Series 6, World Bank, Washington, DC.

Commission on Social Determinants of Health. 2008. *Closing the Gap in a Generation: Health Equity through Action on the Social Determinants of Health*. Geneva: WHO.

Ferreira, F. H. G., J. Messina, J. Rigolini, L. F. López-Calva, M. A. Lugo, and R. Vakis. 2013. *Economic Mobility and the Rise of the Latin American Middle Class*. Washington, DC: World Bank.

Gómez, F. Ruiz, T. Zapata Jaramillo, and L. Garavito Beltrán. 2013. "Colombian Health Care System: Results on Equity for Five Health Dimensions, 2003–2008." *Pan American Journal of Public Health* 33 (2): 107–15.

Knaul, F. M., R. Wong, and H. Arreola-Ornelas, eds. 2012. *Household Spending and Impoverishment*. Vol. 1 of *Financing Health in Latin America Series*. Cambridge, MA: Harvard Global Equity Initiative, in collaboration with Mexican Health Foundation and International Development Research Centre; distributed by Harvard University Press.

PAHO (Pan American Health Organization). 2014. "Strategy for Universal Access to Health and Universal Health Coverage." Document CD53/5, Rev 2, 53rd Directing Council, PAHO, Washington, DC.

Petrera, M., V. Martín, and G. Almeida. 2013. "Equity in Health and Health Care in Peru, 2004–2008." *Pan American Journal of Public Health* 33 (2): 131–6.

Scott, Ewan, and Karl Theodore. 2013. "Measuring and Explaining Health and Health Care Inequalities in Jamaica, 2004 and 2007." *Pan American Journal of Public Health* 33 (2): 116–21.

Vásquez, F., G. Paraje, and M. Estay. 2013. "Income-Related Inequality in Health and Health Care Utilization in Chile, 2000–2009." *Pan American Journal of Public Health* 33 (2): 98–106.

WHO (World Health Organization). 2010. *The World Health Report 2010: Health System Financing—The Path to Universal Coverage.* Geneva: WHO.

Setting the Context for Universal Health Coverage Reforms in Latin America and the Caribbean

Eleonora Cavangero, Gisele Almeida, Evan Sloane Seely, and Fatima Marinho

Abstract

Over the past decades, universal health coverage has emerged in the context of health as a fundamental human right and been closely linked to broader social reforms to improve living conditions and access to health services for vulnerable groups. These social reforms happened in parallel with a democratization process during a period of sustained economic growth and improved equity in the region. Social policies, including those that expand coverage and access to health services and ensure financial protection for the population, have emerged as an important topic on the political agenda. Demographic changes have also fueled societal demands for more comprehensive health coverage and services to cope with the rise in chronic conditions, which poses special challenges for the health system and its financial sustainability.

Introduction

The path to universal health coverage (UHC) in Latin America and the Caribbean (LAC) has a long and diverse history, marked with important milestones. Although not common to all countries, four factors assured the advent of UHC. They are (1) the enactment of international and national legal instruments to the right to health, (2) the achievement of democracy, (3) sound economic growth, and (4) the political commitment to improve the health of the population by increasing its access to health care.

The Right to Health in Latin America and the Caribbean

From 1946 to 1966, the right to health was inscribed in important international instruments, from the Constitution of the World Health Organization to the Universal Declaration of Human Rights and the International Covenant of Economic, Social and Cultural Rights. These instruments became the backbone of important international strategies that sought to improve the health of the population and inspired the inclusion of the right to health in many national constitutions, establishing a commitment between governments and their citizens and promoting enforcement of these rights.

The commitment to the right to health began more than 68 years ago when it was asserted as a social right in the 1946 World Health Organization (WHO) Constitution, which states that "[t]he enjoyment of the highest attainable standard of health is one of the fundamental rights of every human being without distinction of race, religion, political belief, economic or social condition" (WHO 1946). WHO's Constitution came into force in 1948, the same year the right to health was proclaimed in the Universal Declaration of Human Rights (UDHR). This historic United Nations Declaration was passed with the vote of 48 countries of the world (19 of them from Latin America and the Caribbean—see table 2.1), bringing together countries from the Eastern and Western blocs, divided by World War II but committed to secure inalienable human rights for their people. Article 25 of the Declaration, which states that "[e]veryone has the right to a standard of living adequate for the health and well-being of himself and of his family, including food, clothing, housing and medical care and necessary social services, and the right to security in the event of unemployment, sickness, disability, widowhood, old age or other lack of livelihood in circumstances beyond his control," supplied important normative guidelines to public policy and health systems, paving the way to the goal of UHC (United Nations 1949).

The right to health was codified in 1966 with the International Covenant of Economic, Social and Cultural Rights (ICESCR), which claimed "the right of everyone to the enjoyment of the highest attainable standard of physical and mental health." Now signed, ratified, or accessed by all but three LAC countries (table 2.1), the ICESCR sets out four specific steps that signatories must take to realize this right, including (1) reduction of stillbirth and infant mortality and provision for the healthy development of the child; (2) improvement of environmental and industrial hygiene; (3) prevention, treatment, and control of epidemic, endemic, occupational, and other diseases; and (4) access to medical care to all in the event of sickness (United Nations 1976).

Since the 1970s, backed by the adoption of the international instruments mentioned above, the right to health became the legal foundation for important strategies of WHO and its regional offices—from the "Health for All by the Year 2000," established under the 1978 Alma-Ata Declaration, to the 2014 Pan American Health Organization (PAHO) "Strategy for Universal Access to Health and UHC." Passed unanimously by all the member countries, the PAHO strategy specifies four ways to advance the goal of universal access to health and UHC

Table 2.1 Constitutional Provisions and International Instruments Concerning the Right to Health in Latin America and the Caribbean

Country	Constitutional right to health provision	Universal Declaration of Human Rights[a]	International Covenant on Economic, Social and Cultural Rights[b]
Antigua and Barbuda			
Argentina		✓	✓
Bahamas			✓
Barbados			✓
Belize			✓
Bolivia	✓	✓	✓
Brazil	✓	✓	✓
Chile	✓	✓	✓
Colombia		✓	✓
Costa Rica		✓	✓
Cuba	✓	✓	✓
Dominica			✓
Dominican Republic	✓	✓	✓
Ecuador	✓	✓	✓
El Salvador	✓	✓	✓
Grenada			✓
Guatemala	✓	✓	✓
Guyana	✓		✓
Haiti	✓	✓	✓
Honduras	✓		✓
Jamaica			✓
Mexico	✓	✓	✓
Nicaragua	✓	✓	✓
Panama	✓	✓	✓
Paraguay	✓	✓	✓
Peru	✓	✓	✓
Saint Kitts and Nevis			
Saint Lucia			
Saint Vincent and the Grenadines			✓
Suriname	✓		✓
Trinidad and Tobago			✓
Uruguay	✓	✓	✓
Venezuela, RB	✓	✓	✓

Sources: PAHO 2010; United Nations 1949, n.d.

Note: This table includes only independent countries and island nations of Latin America and the Caribbean region.

a. When the Universal Declaration of Human Rights was drafted in 1948, most of the English Caribbean islands, Guyana, and Suriname were not independent countries and therefore could not vote.

b. Belize and Cuba have signed the International Covenant on Economic, Social, and Cultural Rights but have not ratified or accessed the Covenant. Signature expresses intention to become a party to the Covenant, while ratification and accession involve the legal obligation to apply it.

while promoting the right to health, including (1) expanding equitable access to comprehensive, quality, people- and community-centered health services; (2) strengthening stewardship and governance; (3) increasing and improving financing, with equity and efficiency, and advancing toward the elimination of direct payment at the point of service; and (4) strengthening intersectoral coordination to address social determinants of health (PAHO 2014).

Notwithstanding its strong international support, the UDHR (and the ICESCR, for that matter) does not afford constitutional rights to the citizens of signatory countries in Latin America. Argentina is the sole exception, granting these and other related international treaties the same legal status as its national constitution (Zuniga, Marks, and Gostin 2013). Seventeen of the 20 countries of the region have enshrined the right to health in their national constitutions (see table 2.1)—those that have not extended the right to health to their citizens have extended related rights, such as the right to life (HIV and cancer care) in Colombia and Costa Rica, which are enforced through judicial processes. The landmark ruling, T-760/2008, in Colombia consolidated claims for the right to health, signaling the need for reforms to address health system shortcomings that were leading to excessive legal disputes. Colombia's constitutional court was fielding about 90,000 right-to-health legislation cases per year. Approximately 80 percent of the cases were decided in favor of those who could not afford care, including those petitioning for: (1) the right to life (such as HIV/AIDS and cancer treatments); (2) assistance with health conditions afflicting pregnant women, children, and the elderly; and (3) health benefits ascribed to individuals under the contributory or subsidized system (Yamin and Parra-Vera 2009). The Costa Rican constitutional court has consistently upheld the right to life in court cases, protected under Article 21, which recognizes that human life is inviolable and one that guarantees the right to the protection of health (Sáenz, Bermúdez, and Acosta 2010).

Although essential, constitutional and other rights do not automatically translate into actions that protect the health of individuals. Information gathered from a number of countries suggests that even those with constitutionally enshrined rights to health and signed international treaties on human rights struggle to bring about the health system transformations needed to improve health care for all their citizens (World Policy Forum 2014; Zuniga, Marks, and Gostin 2013). When individuals have been denied their right to health, legal frameworks allow them to find judicial protection. In these situations, the courts have become the guarantors not only of the right to health but also of government accountability—witness the increasing judicial health processes filed in Argentina, Brazil, Colombia, Costa Rica, and Uruguay. Although litigation plays a legitimate role in enforcing the right to health, there are some unintended distributional consequences. Evidence suggests that legal processes originate mostly with individuals and regions that are better off. This makes sense. Those who already have better access to health services will also have better access to the judicial system, mirroring inequities found throughout society (Iunes, Cubillos-Turriago, and Escobar 2012).

By way of contrast, the absence of constitutional or legal rights to health in other countries—Canada, the Netherlands, and the United Kingdom, to name three notable examples—has not precluded them from implementing programs and initiatives to strengthen their health systems, target social determinants of health, and produce excellent health outcomes for their populations. Securing constitutional or legal rights to health, while important, may be insufficient on its own. In Latin America, democratization and increased social participation have also been essential factors in propelling governments to implement national programs to deliver better health care with improved financial protection. The adoption of these policies was facilitated by a period of economic stability.

The Redemocratization Process in the Region

After two decades of dictatorship in the region, democracy started to be reestablished in the 1980s. A period of approximately 25 years of uninterrupted democracy ensued, allowing for important institutional reforms to take place in government and for social participation in policy making to reshape the political agenda. Democratization has also allowed for the creation of civil society organization, which has been playing a prominent role in assuring government's response to population needs and demands.

During the 1960s, when right-to-health instruments were being drafted and presented to the international community, dictatorship was spreading throughout Latin America. As per figure 2.1, between 1960 and 1985, 13 countries transitioned from democracy to dictatorship, most of them military regimes.

Figure 2.1 Dictatorships in Latin America and the Caribbean, 1934–92

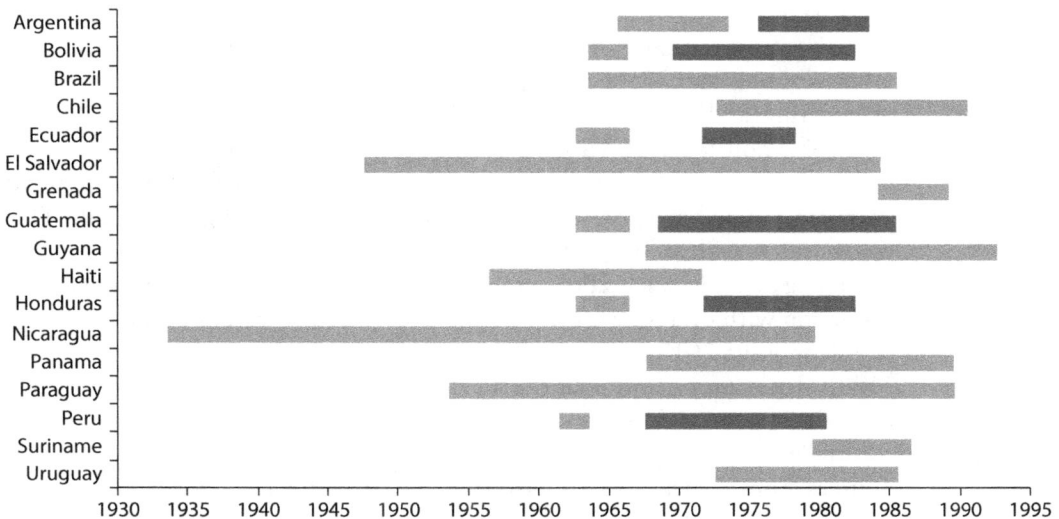

Sources: World Bank calculations, with information from Anderson 1988; Catoggio 2010; Conaghan and Espinal 1990; Dangl 2007; Doumerc 2003; Harding 2006; Kolb 1974; Lambert 2000; Rutgers and Rollins 1998; Schiller 2005; Singh 2008; Skidmore 2009; Sondrol 1992; Valenzuela, and Valenzuela 1986; Youngers 2000.
Note: In Argentina, Bolivia, Ecuador, Guatemala, Honduras, and Peru, there were two segments of dictatorship.

The English Caribbean Islands, which transitioned from colonial status to become democracies during the same period, have remained democracies, with the exception of Grenada and Suriname, which experienced periods of dictatorship from 1979 to 1983 and 1980 to 1986, respectively.

Transitions from democracy to dictatorship were not unique to Latin America. Many countries in Europe and Asia also moved from democracy to dictatorship, including those with histories of sustained democratic government such as India and the Philippines. Likewise, Chile and Uruguay had long-term democratic regimes before devolving into military dictatorship (Huntington 1991).

In the 1970s, only Colombia, Costa Rica, and República Bolivariana de Venezuela had democratic governments. By way of contrast, in 1992, all the LAC countries were democracies. Only Cuba and Haiti had one-party rule (Mainwaring and Pérez-Liñan 2005). Restoration of democracy in the region started in 1979 in Ecuador, followed by Peru, Honduras, Argentina, El Salvador, Brazil, Uruguay, and Guatemala in the early 1980s and Panama, Paraguay, Chile, and Guyana in the late 1980s and the early 1990s. This movement toward democracy brought important social reforms and a period of sustained progress that have reshaped the political, economic, and social development in the region. The democratization of Latin America and the Caribbean has taken place as part of a third wave of democratization worldwide since the nineteenth century—the first taking place from approximately 1828 to 1926 and the second, roughly, from 1943 to 1962 (Huntington 1991).

The region has now enjoyed nearly 25 years of uninterrupted democracy, the lengthiest span of democracy so far. Nondemocratic countries are now a rarity in the region. Some authors argue that democracy's long-term regional success stems from (1) the decreasing polarization of political views, (2) international community support for democratization and less tolerance for authoritarian regimes, and (3) a more favorable popular perception of democracy (Mainwaring and Pérez-Liñan 2005). The latter trend is confirmed by the results of a poll taken in 18 LAC countries since 1996 and published in *The Economist*. Close to 80 percent of respondents agreed with the statement: "Democracy may have problems but it is the best system of government." This demonstrates a clear support for democracy. Pro-democracy sentiment has been rising steadily since 2003 and is consistent with the rise in respondents' satisfaction with everyday life, registered at around 77 percent in the same poll (The Economist 2013).

With democracy came political freedoms and popular demands for government reform. One such reform implemented in many countries of the region was decentralization, where countries ascribing to it transferred responsibilities and resources from central to local governments to better respond to the specific needs of the population. There were exceptions. In Chile, for example, decentralization was part of a pro-privatization policy that began in the early 1980s during the dictatorship. This new environment has also promoted social participation and allowed for the establishment of civil society organizations (CSOs) that have led to the creation of social networks, self-help initiatives, and mutual support groups (Carrión 2001).

Civil society has increasingly become more involved in politics and taken new responsibilities in government processes, and governments are supporting and promoting their participation in the policy-making process. Bolivia, Ecuador, and República Bolivariana de Venezuela, for example, have inscribed social participation in their new constitutions as a means of reducing social and economic inequality. In Brazil, social participation was considered a democratic method of governing and an important governmental tool for the design, implementation, and evaluation of public policies (Pogrebinschi 2013).

The uninterrupted cycle of democracy in Latin America and the Caribbean, coupled with the implementation of important institutional reforms and social participation in government, has coincided with a period of economic growth and development in the region, which will be discussed in the next section.

Economic Growth, Income Distribution, and Social Policies

Countries in LAC have experienced a period of sustained economic improvement during the past two decades, marked by higher gross domestic products (GDPs) and less poverty, unemployment, and inequalities. Governments have invested more to improve the health of their population, changing the composition of health financing. Government health expenditures have increased as a percentage of GDP and total health expenditure in most countries, while the out-of-pocket share has decreased.

Figure 2.2 GDP Growth in Latin America and in the High-Income Countries (Cyclically Adjusted Growth Computed Using Band-Pass Filter)

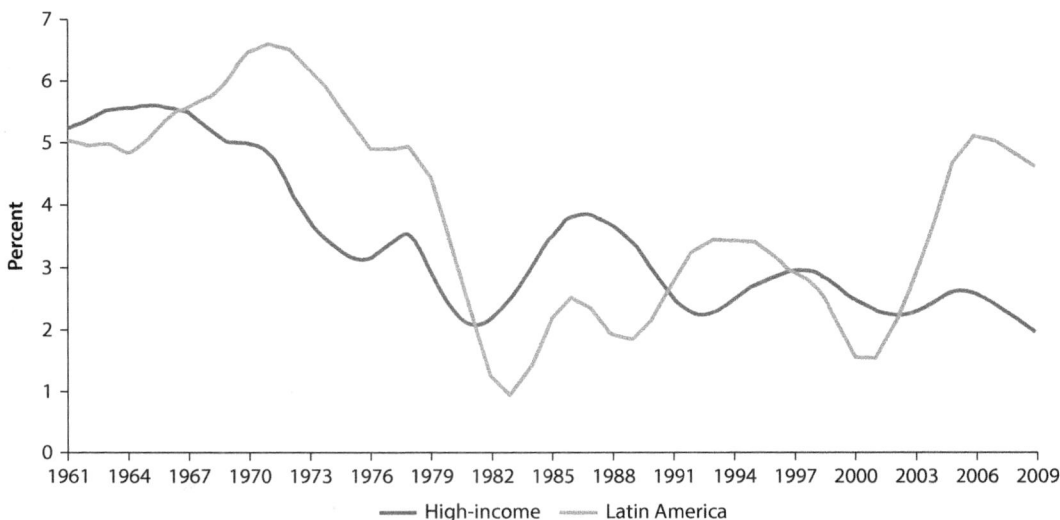

Source: World Bank 2011.

In addition to the political changes and the democratic governments established in the region over the past few decades, the economies of Latin America and the Caribbean have also experienced healthy growth, coupled with reductions in poverty and inequality (World Bank 2011). The region's economic performance has mirrored and sometimes outperformed that of high-income countries (figure 2.2) and created jobs at a faster pace than the growth in the labor force, resulting in historically low unemployment rates. Some countries are reported to be operating "at or near potential." Although these are considerable achievements, the region is still marked by great socioeconomic inequalities between and within countries (IMF 2013).

In the beginning of the twenty-first century, stable growth in Latin America reached its highest peak since the early 1970s owing to solid external demand, ample global liquidity, and positive terms-of-trade shocks (De la Torre and Yeyati 2013). These factors led to declines in poverty and income inequality (Ferreira and others 2013), which ultimately reduced the impact of the financial crisis of 2008. Except for the countries with the worst macro outcomes, poverty continued to decline during the global financial crisis (Grosh, Fruttero, and Oliveri 2013).

Per capita GDP growth shows a direct correlation to poverty reduction in the region for a 15-year period from 1995 to 2010 (figure 2.3). Economic growth allowed for better incomes, which in turn increased the size of the middle class, identified as those living on at least US$10 a day (figure 2.4). Per capita GDP rose from less than US$4,000 in 1995 to almost US$9,000 in 2010, and the middle class became larger than the population living in poverty—that is, those who live on less than US$4 a day.

Figure 2.3 Per Capita GDP Growth and Poverty in Latin America and the Caribbean, 1995–2010

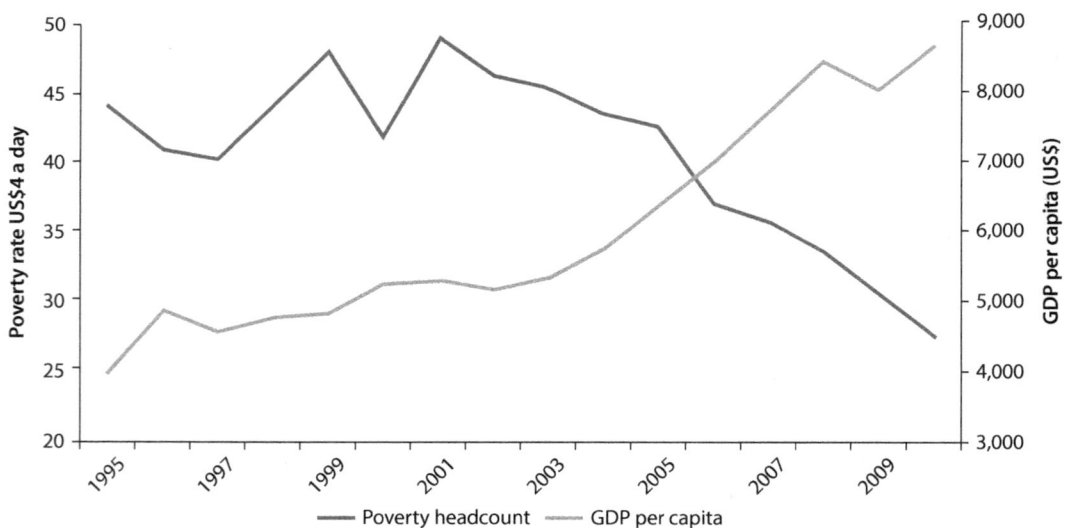

Source: World Bank 2012.

Figure 2.4 Reduction of Poverty and Expansion of the Middle Class in Latin America and the Caribbean, 1992–2010

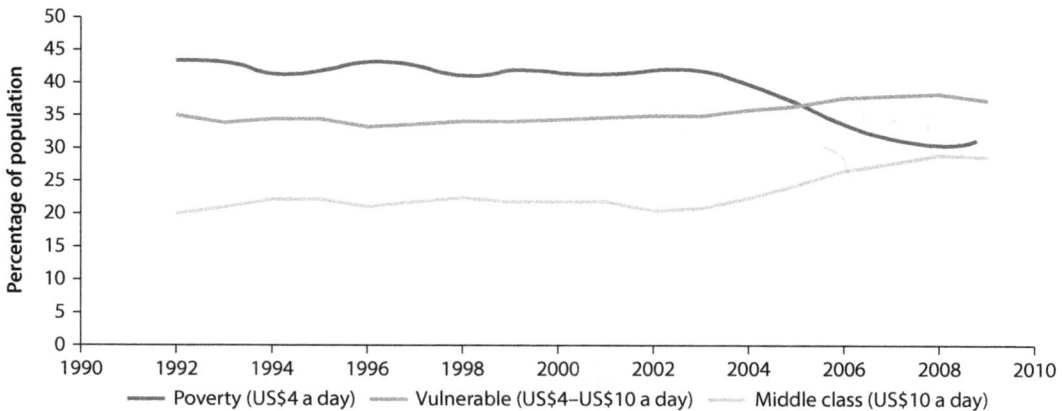

Poverty (US$4 a day)   Vulnerable (US$4–US$10 a day)   Middle class (US$10 a day)

Source: World Bank 2012.

Although increased compensation for labor was the main driver of declines in extreme and moderate poverty, income transfers and pensions also played important roles (Cord, Lucchetti, and Rodriquez-Castelan 2013). With consistent, sustained growth, the countries of the region have been able to expand their fiscal space and increase investments in their social sectors, targeting the poorest population groups and reducing inequalities (figure 2.5). Although most countries have cut income disparities, inequality in the region is still high, ranging from Honduras with a Gini coefficient of 57.40 to Uruguay at 41.32 (World Bank 2012).

External factors that aided growth in the region before the crisis (notably demand from China and the advanced economies, as well as low financial risk) have been muted—neither aiding nor restricting growth—which may affect future growth in LAC. Global forces cannot be relied on for the region to return to precrisis growth rates of 5–6 percent. The region needs to locate internal growth engines (Cord, Lucchetti, and Rodriquez-Castelan 2013). This may pose a challenge for the expansion of health coverage, although in the past economic growth has not necessarily been a precondition for the adoption of policies to advance UHC—for instance, Brazil's commitment to UHC occurred during slow economic growth (Maeda 2014).

In the 10 countries under study, the emergence of policies to advance UHC occurred with a rise of public social spending (health, education, and social protection) from 2000 to the present (figure 2.6). Further, many countries in the LAC region were quite active in their social protection policies during the last economic crisis, which entailed taking advantage of programs built in precrisis years, and launching new programs that will serve in future crises (Grosh, Fruttero, and Oliveri 2013). This can be observed by the dip around the time of the crisis and the quick recovery by every country.

Toward Universal Health Coverage and Equity in Latin America and the Caribbean
http://dx.doi.org/10.1596/978-1-4648-0454-0

Figure 2.5 Cumulative Changes in Gini Coefficient of Inequality, 2011 over 1995

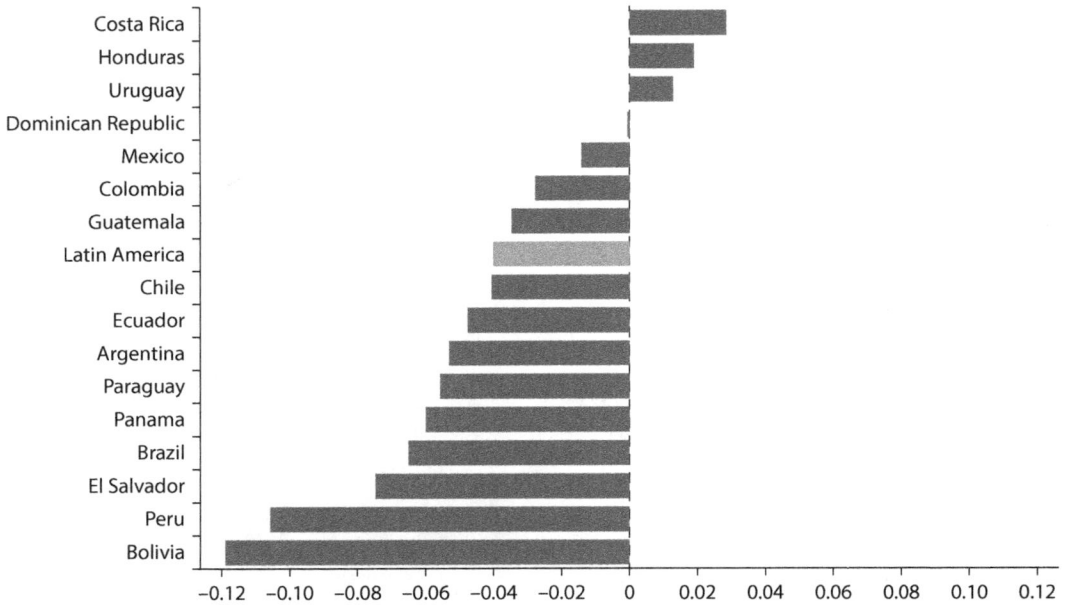

Source: World Bank World Development Indicators Data Bank 2012.
Note: Bolivia—1997; Chile, Colombia, Dominican Republic—1996; Guatemala and Peru—1998; Mexico—1996 and 2010.

Progressive fiscal policy has also improved the lives of the poor. Over the past few years, governments have extended social assistance to those outside of the formal labor market; this includes transfer programs designed to reduce poverty and inequality, such as conditional cash transfers or school nutrition programs (Draaisma and Zamecnik 2014). Under the social assistance umbrella, some programs also focus on health services. For example, most conditional cash transfers include stipulations linked to use of health services; the literature shows that conditional cash transfer programs can yield health benefits (Fiszbein, Schady, and Ferreira 2009). Public expenditure on health as a percentage of GDP increased in the 10 LAC countries over the previous decade. In some cases the expansion of coverage was responsible, and in others the rise of expenditure on chronic diseases was the cause. In any case, increases in social spending reflect the growing importance of social policy in political agendas.

Many of the countries that implemented broader UHC health reforms saw their government health expenditure[1] (GHE) as percentage of GDP increase throughout the 2000s (figure 2.7). Argentina, Brazil, Uruguay, and Costa Rica saw their GHEs increase the most, with Costa Rica seeing more than a 2 percentage-point increase between 2005 and 2012. Other countries, such as Jamaica Chile and Jamaica, saw increases of 1 percentage point, while a final group had a rise of around half a percentage point of the GDP (figure 2.7).

Figure 2.6 Public Health, Education, and Social Protection Spending as a Share of GDP, 2000–09

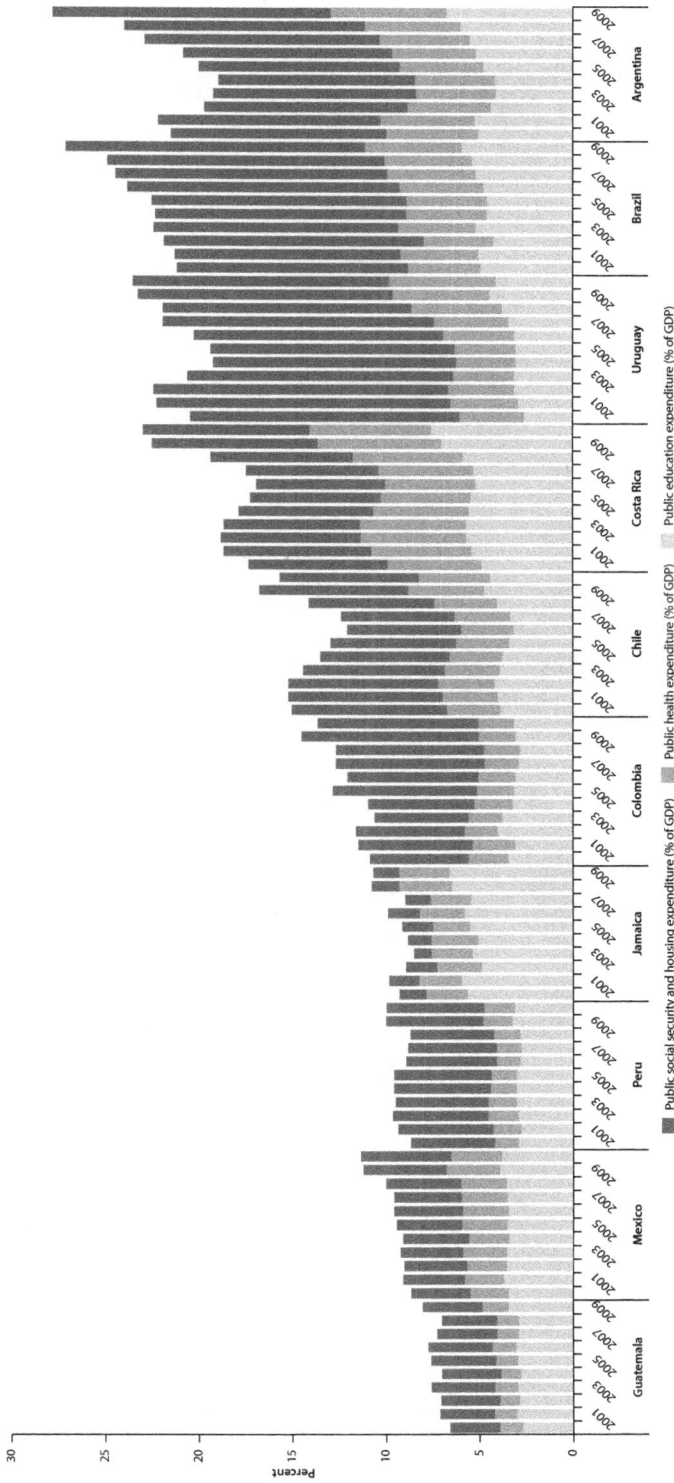

Source: Economic Commission for Latin America and the Caribbean (ECLAC)—Social Development Division. Social Expenditure Database.
Note: Data for 2010–12 was not readily available for all countries. Peru did not have data for public health expenditure.

Figure 2.7 Government Health Expenditure as a Share of GDP, 2005–12

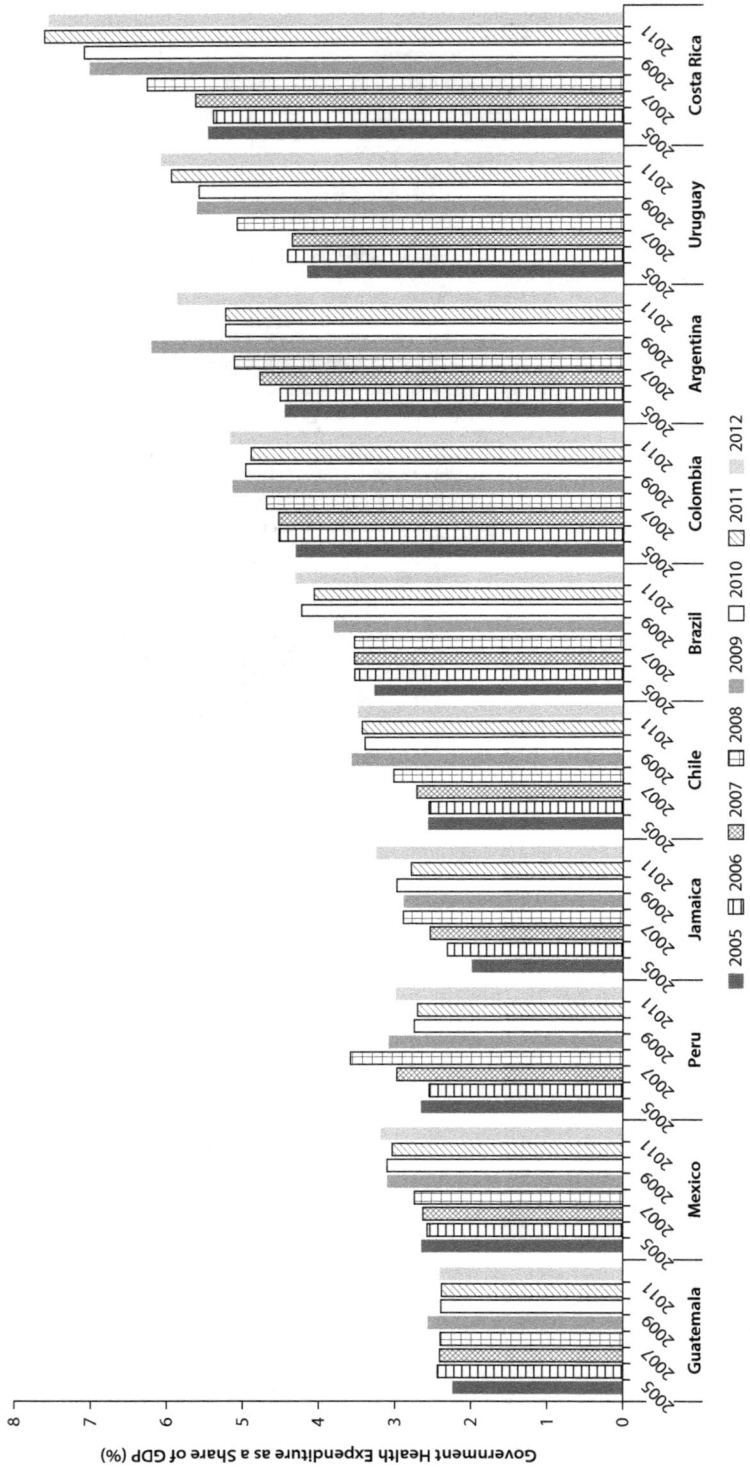

Source: World Bank World Development Indicators Data Bank 2012.

Figure 2.8 Government Health Expenditure as a Share of General Government Expenditure, 2005–12

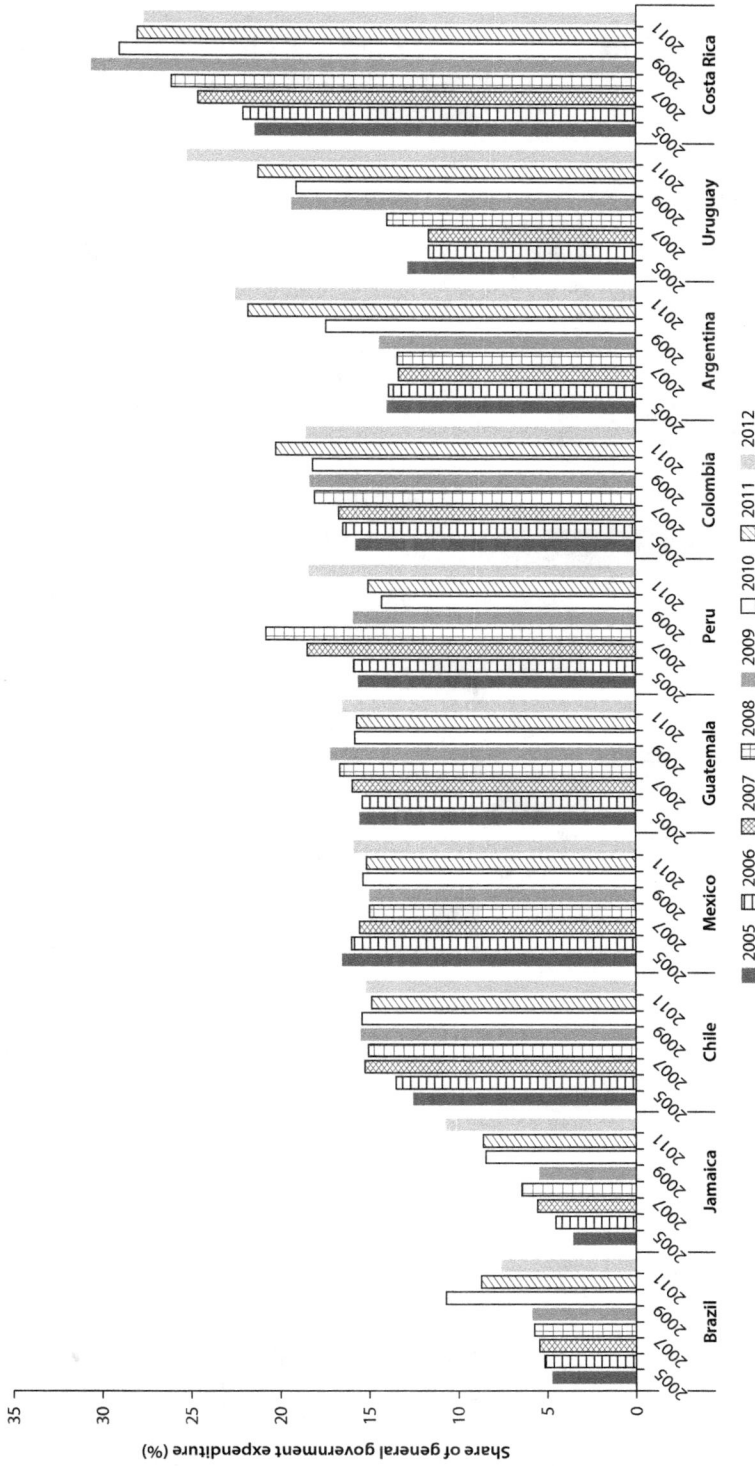

Legend: ■ 2005 ▦ 2006 ▦ 2007 ▦ 2008 ▦ 2009 ☐ 2010 ▨ 2011 ▨ 2012

Source: World Bank World Development Indicators Data Bank 2012.

Figure 2.9 Total Health Expenditure per Capita by Source (PPP in Constant International $), 2001–12

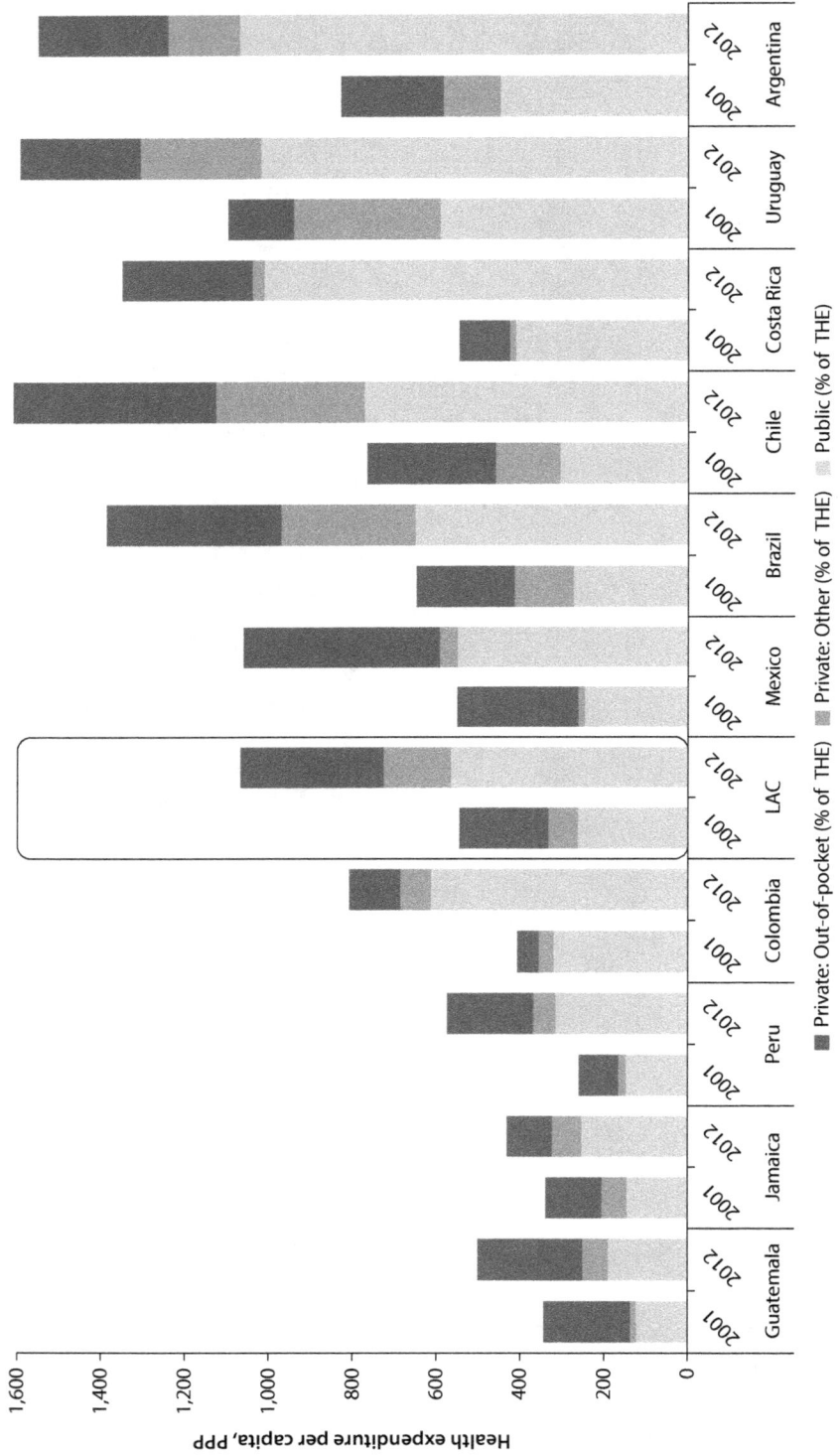

Source: World Bank World Development Indicators Data Bank 2012.
Note: THE = Total health expenditure; PPP = Purchasing power parity.

GHE as a proportion of general government expenditure is often used in international comparisons as a measure of government commitment to health investment (Cavagnero and others 2008). Although a higher proportion does not necessarily imply better health outcomes, research has shown an association between general government expenditure on health and infant mortality rate (Bhutta 2004). Over the period 2005 to 2012, the ratio of GHE to general government expenditure increased in Argentina, Brazil, Chile (to a lesser extent), Colombia, Costa Rica, Jamaica, and Uruguay; it remained stable in Guatemala and Mexico. In general, GHE is higher in LAC than in other regions. Indeed, most LAC countries are already above the 15 percent threshold required by the Abuja Declaration.[2] Although Brazil and Jamaica have not met the 15 percent goal, both have shown strong improvement over the past five years (figure 2.8).

As shown in figure 2.9, total health expenditure (THE)[3] across countries differs substantially—Argentina has the highest per capita spending on health (US$1,434), while Guatemala has the lowest (US$334). Government health expenditure has increased in all countries and, in most, it has outstripped the growth in out-of-pocket spending. Across the region, roughly 32 percent of THEs were out-of-pocket payments in 2011, down about 7 percentage points from 2001 but still above the 20 percent recommended by the *World Health Report* (WHO 2010).

Some countries that undertook reforms have been able to reduce their out-of-pocket expenditure—especially Argentina, Chile, Colombia, Guatemala, and Mexico (figure 2.10). Guatemala and Mexico had the highest out-of-pocket shares, at 60 and 52 percent of total health spending in the beginning of the period. Of the 10 countries, only Argentina, Colombia, Costa Rica, Jamaica and Uruguay have out-of-pocket spending below 30 percent.

Demographic and Epidemiological Transition and Implications for UHC

Population aging and lower fertility rates have drastically changed the population pyramid in all countries of LAC. Population aging has also contributed to the epidemiological change observed in the region, which transitioned from high prevalence and mortality due to infectious disease at the beginning of the last century to high prevalence and mortality due to noncommunicable diseases (NCDs) from the end of last century to the present day.

Over the past 50 years, populations have grown and aged in LAC. The region's population is now almost twice what it was in the 1970s, and the aging populations are posing new challenges such as the increase in chronic diseases (Marinho and others 2013). During this period, the share of the population older than 60 increased more than five times and is expected to quadruple by 2040. The fertility rate has fallen nearly everywhere, reducing the share of children in the population and raising that of the elderly. Life expectancy in the region has increased 15 years in the period between 1960 and 2012, with wide variations across countries: Guatemala's life expectancy is just over 70 and Costa Rica's is just under 80 years of age (figure 2.11).

Figure 2.10 Out-of-Pocket Health Expenditures as a Share of Total Health Expenditure, 1995–2012

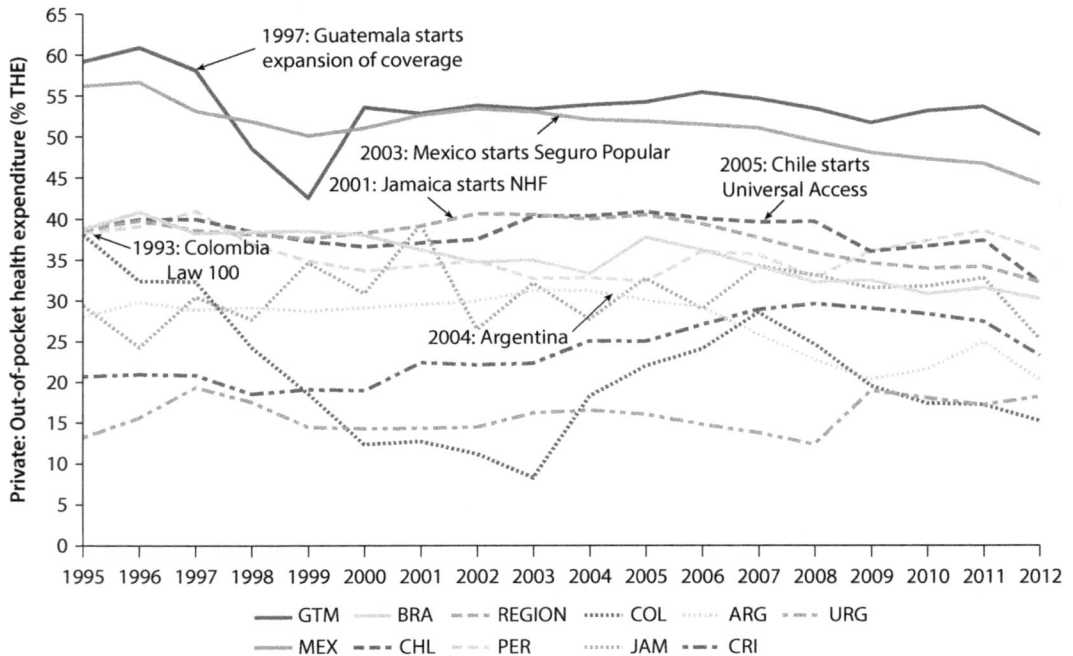

Source: World Bank World Development Indicators Data Bank 2012.

Countries are in different phases of the demographic transition. Some have relatively older populations (Argentina and Uruguay), while others have younger profiles (Guatemala and Peru), but with falling fertility rates. All countries are trending toward a larger elderly population, as seen in figure 2.12. Overall improvements in income, environment, lifestyles, and medical advances have increased life expectancy in the region, creating a greater demand for long-term medical care (Marinho and others 2013).

Although improvements in life expectancy have occurred with relative uniformity, the countries have experienced the epidemiological transition at different times. Aging populations, changing lifestyles, and modifiable risk factors are increasing the role of noncommunicable diseases (NCDs) in mortality, which accounted for 78 percent, or 4.5 million deaths, in 2007. However, in 2010 some countries are still registering high mortality in the younger populations (Marinho and others 2013).

The burden of mortality has also shifted, a trend that is producing at least three distinct stages along the epidemiological transition. The advanced stage carries a high burden of NCDs and low burden of infectious diseases, seen in Uruguay, where NCDs accounted for 79 percent of deaths. The middle stage reveals a dual burden of NCDs and infectious diseases in countries where NCD mortality increased substantially in the 1980s and 1990s. An example is Mexico, where in the mid-1950s the proportion of infectious diseases was around 61

Figure 2.11 Life Expectancy in Study Countries and Regional Average, 1960–2012

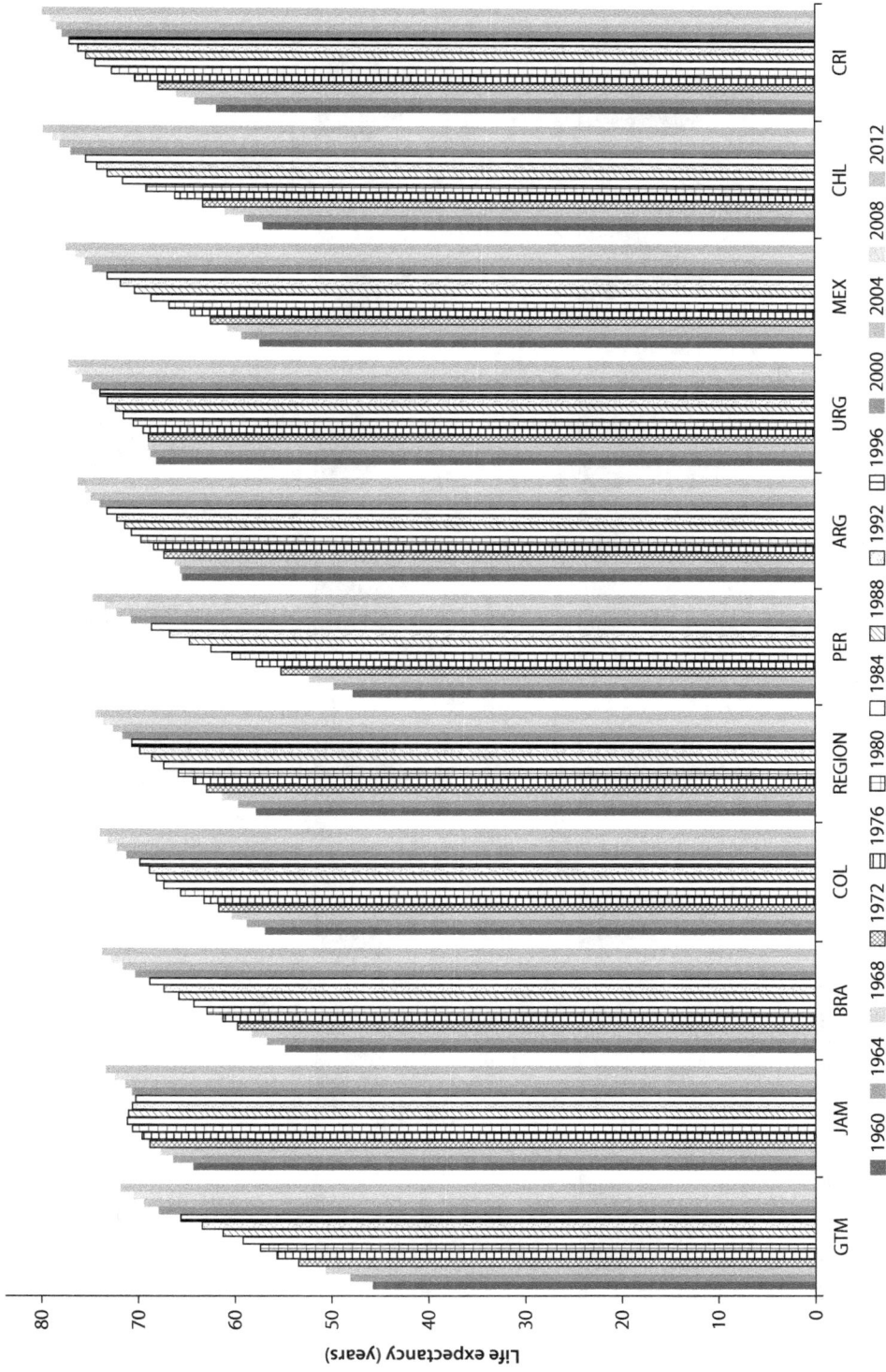

Life expectancy (years)

GTM JAM BRA COL REGION PER ARG URG MEX CHL CRI

■ 1960 ■ 1964 ■ 1968 ▨ 1972 ▨ 1976 ▦ 1980 □ 1984 ▨ 1988 □ 1992 ▥ 1996 ▨ 2000 ▨ 2004 ▨ 2008 ▨ 2012

Source: World Bank World Development Indicators Data Bank 2012.

Figure 2.12 Demographic Age Change, 1950–2040

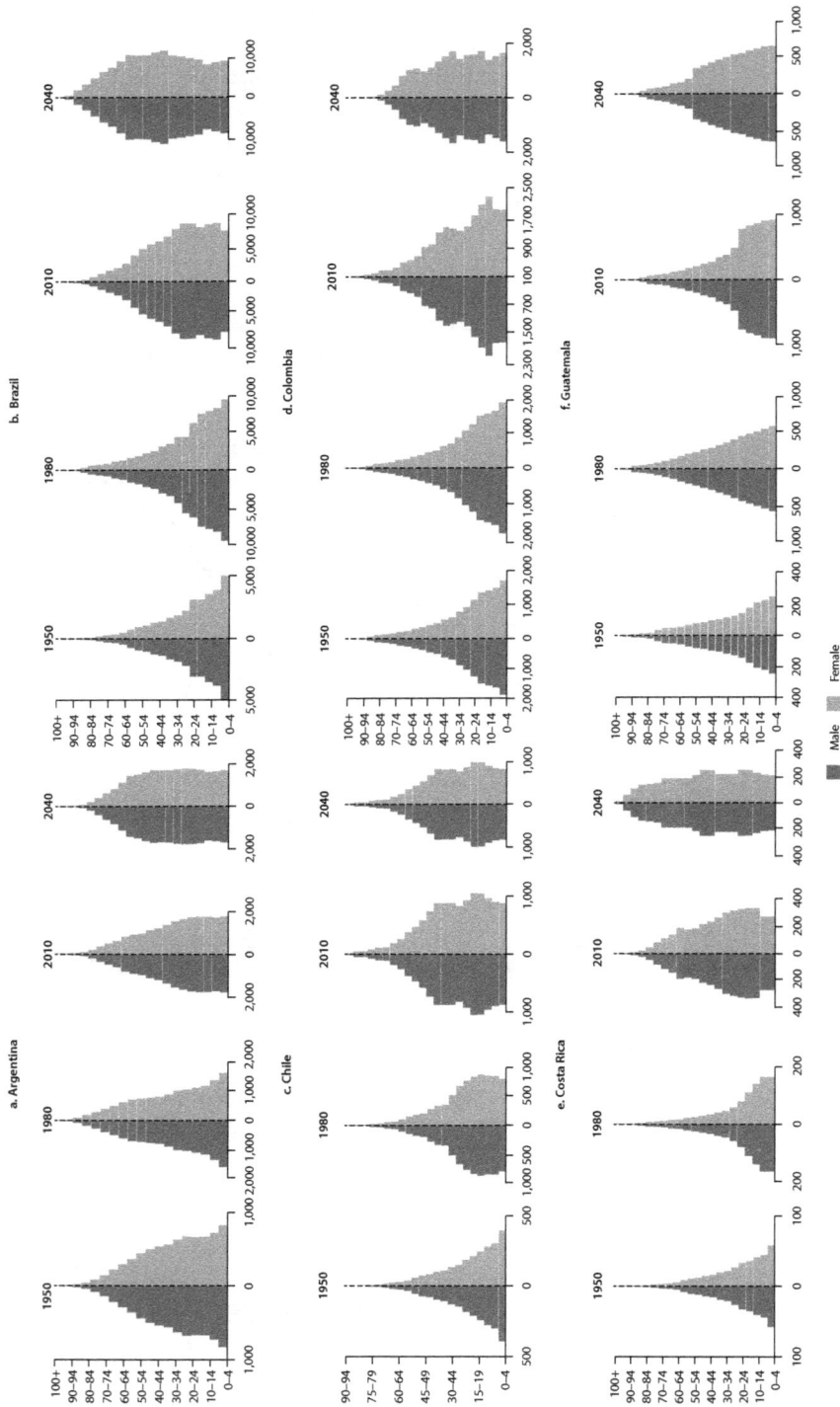

a. Argentina

b. Brazil

c. Chile

d. Colombia

e. Costa Rica

f. Guatemala

Male   Female

figure continues next page

Figure 2.12 Demographic Age Change, 1950–2040 (*continued*)

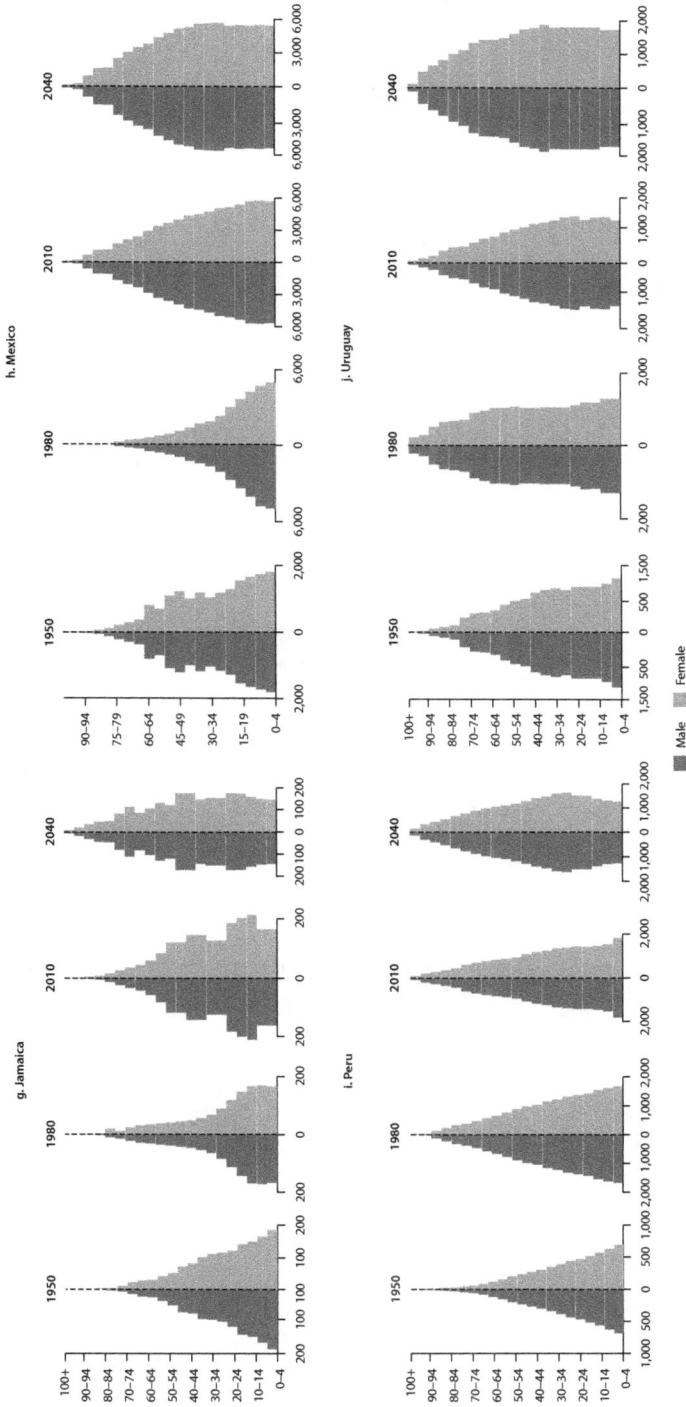

g. Jamaica

h. Mexico

i. Peru

j. Uruguay

Male   Female

Source: World Bank World Development Indicators Data Bank 2012.

percent while the share of NCDs was much lower (22 percent); now, the proportion of infectious diseases decreased by four-fifths, and NCDs shot up to 75 percent. The early stage shows a low burden of NCDs and high proportion of infectious diseases. In Guatemala, in 1980, the proportion of infectious diseases was high (55 percent) relative to that of NCDs (31 percent). Undoubtedly, infectious diseases have been falling in Guatemala, but not as rapidly as in LAC countries that are farther along their epidemiological transitions (Marinho and others 2013). Examples of each of these stages can be seen in figure 2.13.

Figure 2.13 Epidemiological Transitions in Latin America and Causes of Death, 1955–2009 (or Nearest Year)

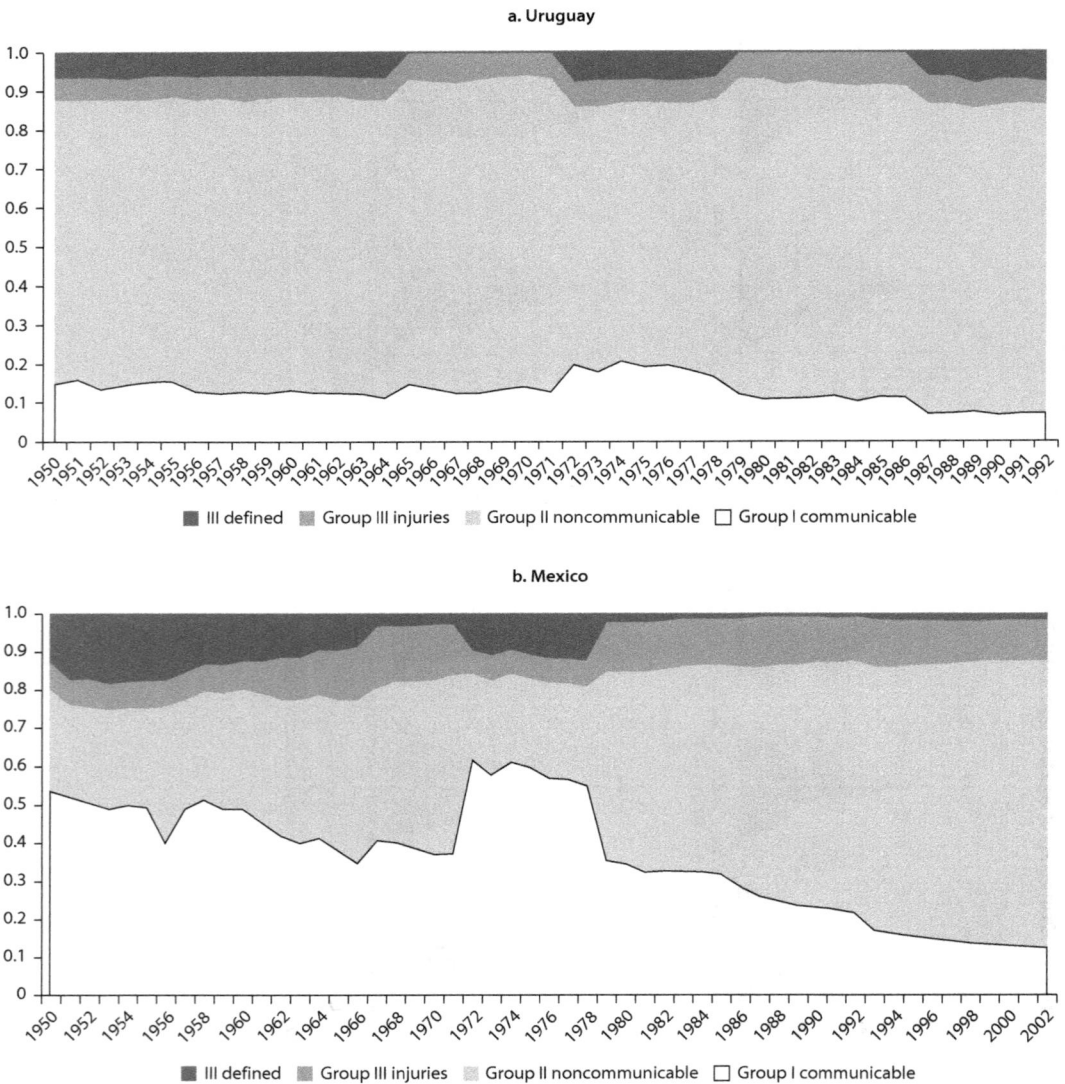

a. Uruguay

III defined   Group III injuries   Group II noncommunicable   Group I communicable

b. Mexico

III defined   Group III injuries   Group II noncommunicable   Group I communicable

figure continues next page

Figure 2.13 Epidemiological Transitions in Latin America and Causes of Death, 1955–2009 (or Nearest Year)
(continued)

c. Guatemala

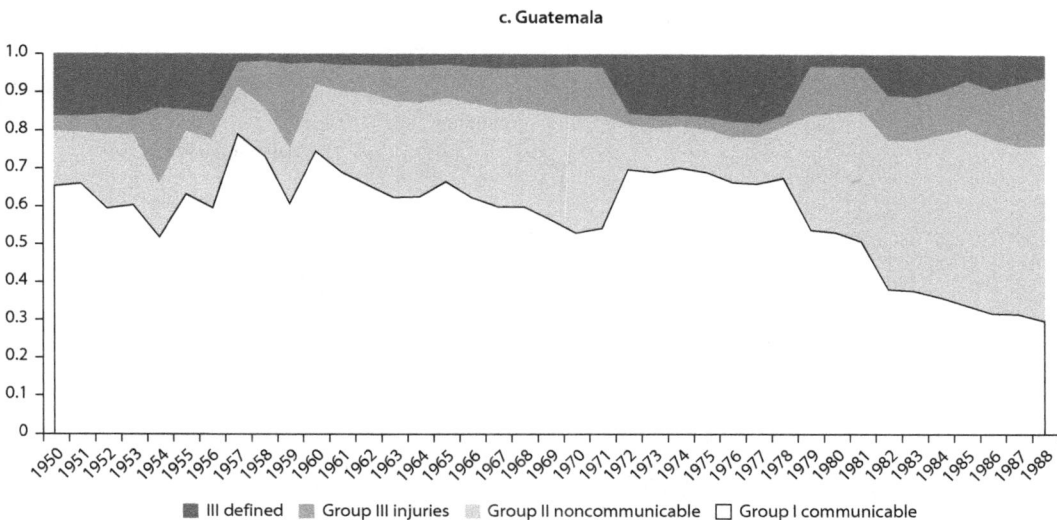

III defined   Group III injuries   Group II noncommunicable   Group I communicable

Some countries in LAC are still in the early and middle stages of epidemio-logical transition, such as Guatemala and Mexico (WHO 2014). Guatemala is drastically different from the other nine countries under study, mainly in the percentage of cardiovascular deaths (16 percent below the regional average) and communicable disease deaths (19 percent above the regional average), and has the highest percentage of deaths owing to injuries, at 18 percent. This is what we would expect of an early-stage country (see figure 2.13). The 10 countries differ greatly in terms of the share of communicable disease and injury-related deaths: more than 50 percent of Guatemalan deaths fall under these two categories, while less than 20 percent of deaths in Argentina and Costa Rica are due to com-municable diseases and injuries.

With an aging population comes a greater need to treat NCDs. The need to care for the elderly is not new, but the sheer numbers of elderly people requiring care will stress existing health systems. The economic and health burdens imposed by NCDs are costly to individuals and to the system. Cardiovascular diseases and cancer are the two main causes of deaths in LAC (figure 2.14). The region can also claim some of the highest diabetes death rates in the world. The rising incidence of diabetes stems in part from urban-ization and lifestyle changes. Urbanization and changes in forms of land trans-portation have led to greater numbers of injuries over the past 40 years; injuries as a cause of death in the region stabilized in the 2000s (Bonilla-Chacín 2014).

A quarter of deaths owing to NCDs occur in people under 60 years of age (Le Gales-Camus and Epping-Jorda 2005), making disease prevention para-mount, along with monitoring risk factors and early diagnosis and treatment for

Figure 2.14 Main Causes of Death in Latin America and the Caribbean (Age-Standardized), 2008

Percent

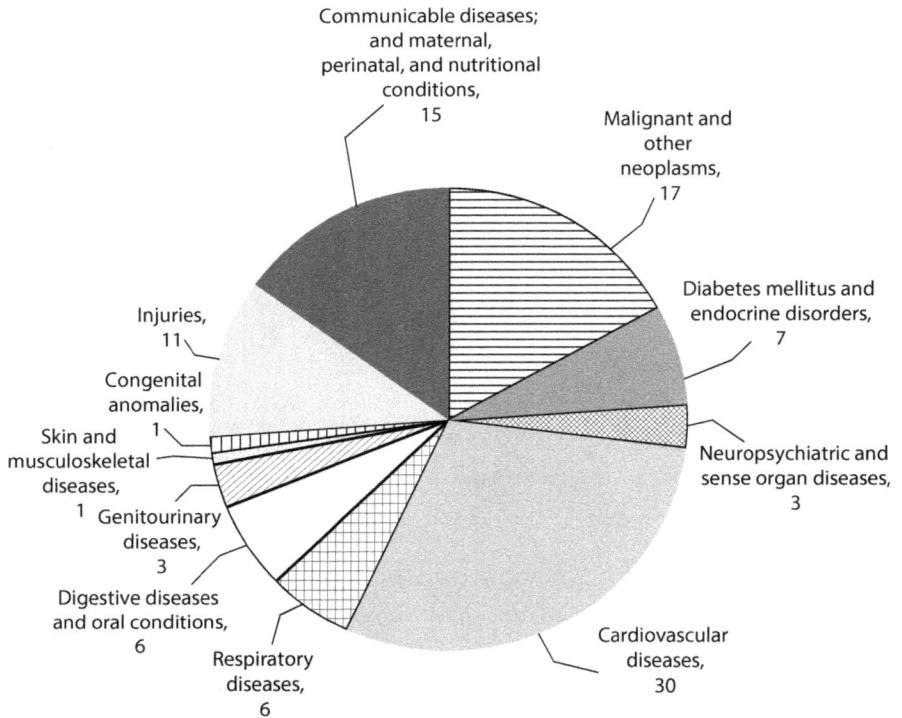

Source: Bonilla-Chacín 2014.

all segments of the population. One way to reduce intermediate risk factors and death rates from NCDs is through strong policies, such as antismoking initiatives that countries like Uruguay have used to reduce the number of smokers and related health problems (Godinho 2013).

Countries will face challenges sustaining UHC-advancement programs over the long term, particularly given the epidemiological transition and aging populations. The need to capitalize on the demographic dividend while their populations are still young will become even more critical in countries like Brazil where the proportion of the over-65 population is expected to double in the next 20 years. This transition took place in high-income countries over the course of a century. Unhealthy aging will bring out significant economic and social pressure and will compress the timeline available for effective action.

Some countries face the paradoxical double burden of malnourishment and obesity, which are related to a series of changes, namely, the nutrition transition, the demographic transition, and the epidemiological transition countries undergo (Shrimpton and Rokx 2012). Three of the four countries in the world with the highest percentage of overweight mothers and malnourished children are found in the LAC region: Guatemala (13 percent of households), Bolivia (11 percent), and Nicaragua (10 percent) (Garret and Ruel 2003). These conditions are often linked, as malnourished children are at an increased risk of hypertension, cardiovascular diseases, and diabetes (Bonilla-Chacín 2014) as well as a decreased likelihood of finishing school and reduced economic success later in life (Shrimpton and Rokx 2012).

Indeed, LAC faces challenges of both low- and high-income countries. While improvements have been made in maternal and childcare, the region as a whole will not achieve the Millennium Development Goals related to the reduction of the maternal mortality rate (MDG5). The region also must address both infectious and NCDs, which require health systems capable of providing both preventive and curative care. Many challenges come with this epidemiological change, one of which is the sustainability of health systems and social programs and their ability to respond to an ever-increasing and more demanding population.

Health Service Delivery and Its Evolution Toward Universality

Provision of health services in LAC has been changing over time to accommodate population demands and needs. Health services have been expanding and reaching more of those in need. While charitable organizations were responsible for the provision of services in the 19th century, especially for the poor, increased public investment and political commitment have allowed for the expansion and delivery of health services through other arrangements, including public systems/programs and social security.

To appreciate the influence that the political landscape has on health service delivery in LAC, it is important to understand how it has changed over time. During the nineteenth century, charitable organizations provided health services to the majority of the population in LAC (Canal 1984; Flisser 2009; Landivar 2004; Tobar 2001). Funding for these services, delivered mostly through hospitals, was organized by religious entities at the national level; at the municipal level services were provided by civil society and charitable organizations. In the first half of the last century most countries in the region established ministries of health (MoHs), with a mandate to take over the provision of health care from traditional providers—private charitable organizations—and to improve access to basic services. They were also generally in charge of certifying medical professions, licensing medicines for the national market, and establishing public hygiene guidelines, including standards for safe water and sanitation (which in many countries was functionally a department of the MoH). In some cases, the health facilities of charitable organizations were incorporated into the public sector (at the national, state, or municipal levels) or regulated by the MoHs and subsidized with public funds. These providers had the mandate to deliver health services to the entire population.

Toward Universal Health Coverage and Equity in Latin America and the Caribbean
http://dx.doi.org/10.1596/978-1-4648-0454-0

The most notable progress in health outcomes took place in the mid-20th century after public sector investments in safe water and sanitation infrastructure, vector control, vaccinations, health promotion, and the expansion of education centers for physicians, nurses, and other medical professionals. During the first half of the 20th century, PAHO and its predecessor, the Health Secretariat of the Americas, played a key role in vector and communicable-disease control. In the second half of the century, public health interventions expanded to include vaccinations, safe drinking water, and sanitation. After the Alma Ata Declaration of 1978, many governments focused on programs to expand primary health care services in sparsely populated rural and remote areas. Training of health workers to serve in rural areas was a frequent approach to expand access to basic services. As the scope and sophistication of health technologies and services grew, existing inequalities were exacerbated, due in part to the poor distribution of human resources, which remained highly concentrated in larger urban centers (Cetrangolo and others 2006).

Social security institutions were founded in the first half of the previous century and were based on the German model of employment-based mandatory health insurance. These institutions, generically known as social security systems, also provided pensions and typically covered public sector employees. They rapidly expanded to workers in other formal sectors, including large state-owned enterprises and publicly funded but privately owned companies (typically extractive industries, railroads, and electricity). Social security institutions provided costly services, which included specialized diagnostic and therapeutic care. These institutions typically owned a national network of health facilities, with a concentration of specialized services in large urban areas, whereas the MoH's network typically encompassed a broader range of facilities, including both hospitals and basic health centers in rural areas. This meant that in urban centers one would see an inefficient duplication of high-complexity inpatient services (Cetrangolo and others 2006).

The expansion of social security enrollment varies greatly across the region. Several countries with large public sectors or those that experienced early industrialization—namely, Argentina, Brazil, Chile, Mexico, and Uruguay—saw steady expansions in the enrollment of blue- and white-collar workers and their dependents. In other countries, coverage expanded not by virtue of extending coverage to the formal sector but through inclusion of family members of the employee or progressive agreements with workers from the agricultural or service sectors. This was the case in Costa Rica and Panama. In other countries, expansion of social security coverage was minimal (for example, Colombia, Guatemala, Ecuador, and Peru) (Rofman 2005).

In more recent times, Latin Americans have demanded more responsive health systems, compelling their countries' governments to explore reforms to advance UHC. Efforts to improve system responsiveness include developing clear medical guidelines and standards, linking resources to incentives for providers, and implementing information systems that improve strategic decision-making. The experiences of 10 countries—Argentina, Brazil, Chile, Colombia, Costa Rica,

Table 2.2 Policies and Programs to Advance UHC in Latin America and the Caribbean

Country	Reforms	Year
Argentina	Plan Nacer	2004
	Plan Sumar	2012
Brazil	Unified Health System (SUS)	1988
	Scale-up of Family Health Program (FHP)	1998
Chile	FONASA	1981
	Universal Access with Explicit Guarantees (AUGE)	2005
Colombia	National Health Insurance System	1993
Costa Rica	Special regime for the indigent	1984
	Transfer of health services from MoH to CCSS	1993
	Mandatory enrollment of the self-employed	2006
Guatemala	Program of Expansion of Coverage (PEC)	1997
Jamaica	National Health Fund (NHF)	2003
	User fees abolished	2008
Mexico	Social Protection System in Health (SPSS)/Seguro Popular	2003
Peru	Maternal and Child Health Insurance	1999
	Comprehensive Health Insurance (SIS)	2002
	Universal Health Insurance (AUS)	2009
Uruguay	FONASA	2007
	Integrated National Health System (SNIS)	2007

Guatemala, Jamaica, Mexico, Peru, and Uruguay—in implementing such policies are reviewed in this study. Table 2.2 presents these experiences, which are discussed in the next chapter.

How Does the Region Compare in the Global Context?

Many low- and middle-income countries in LAC have embraced policies to advance UHC in the past few decades. As we have seen in previous sections, these movements were closely linked to broader social reforms and also accompanied by a process of democratization and a period of sustained and more equitable economic growth. The reforms to advance UHC also translated into changes in health financing, in most cases increasing government expenditures on health. To better understand this progress within a global perspective, we will benchmark the LAC countries against other countries. These results show where the LAC countries are lagging, or excelling, given their demographic profile and level of development.

This exercise compares projected outcomes for all 187 countries for which data are available for 2012. The outcomes used for the analysis—which assess health and financial protection—were regressed on a set of demographic and economic variables.[4] Through this approach countries can be compared in terms of their actual and expected levels of performance.[5]

Although all countries with available data have been used to produce the expected levels, only some will be used for comparison in the following tables.

Toward Universal Health Coverage and Equity in Latin America and the Caribbean
http://dx.doi.org/10.1596/978-1-4648-0454-0

The results compare the 10 selected LAC countries with a random selection of OECD countries, the 4C countries (Chile, China, Costa Rica, and Cuba), and other similar countries (table 2.3).[6]

In the models, most of the 10 countries under study have THE per capita below their expected levels. Argentina is the exception, since its THE per capita is higher than expected; it should be noted that of all countries used in the exercise, Argentina has one of the lowest expected values. Furthermore, THEs per capita in the countries under study are significantly lower than OECD countries. As an example, the United States has THE per capita three times its expected value. Although actual expenditure for the LAC countries ranges from US$350 to US$1,750, which is higher than other regions, expenditures in the OECD countries range between US$1,750 and US$9,000 (figure 2.15).

Government health expenditure as a percentage of general government expenditure is the variable with the most variance among the 10 LAC countries. With the exception of Brazil and Jamaica, all the LAC countries have higher than expected values. In these relative terms, Costa Rica, Argentina, and Uruguay invest the most in health as a proportion of their government expenditure. The other countries fall in the middle and are in line with many of the OECD countries. The expected government health expenditure as a percentage of government expenditure falls between 10 and 13 percent for nearly all the countries (figure 2.16).

The 10 LAC countries have generally high levels of out-of-pocket spending compared with most selected OECD countries, with the exception of the Republic of Korea. However, as figure 2.17 shows, out-of-pocket spending as a percentage of THE in Argentina, Brazil, Colombia, Costa Rica, Jamaica, and Uruguay is lower than expected for their economic and demographic status. Chile, Guatemala, Mexico, and Peru spend more out of pocket than expected. If a large portion of THE in a country is financed out of pocket, more people face the risk of financial catastrophe and may forgo health care. Lower out-of-pocket expenditures reduce this problem and may lead to a healthier population.

As indicated above, the majority of countries under study have higher government health expenditures as a percentage of general government expenditures than expected. When comparing with GDP, half of the 10 countries have greater government health expenditure as a percentage of GDP than expected (figure 2.18). Argentina, Brazil, Colombia, Costa Rica, and Uruguay each spend more on government health expenditure than expected; Costa Rica comes closest to

Table 2.3 Countries Used in the Analysis

Ten selected countries in LAC	OECD countries (randomly selected)	Other countries (randomly selected)
Argentina, Brazil, Chile, Colombia, Costa Rica, Guatemala, Jamaica, Mexico, Peru, Uruguay	Australia, Austria, Belgium, Canada, Denmark, Estonia, France, Germany, Hungary, Israel, Japan, Korea, Rep., New Zealand, Sweden, Turkey, United States	Bolivia, China, Cuba, Dominican Republic, Haiti, India, Russian Federation, South Africa, Thailand

Figure 2.15   Actual and Expected Total Health Expenditure Per Capita in PPP

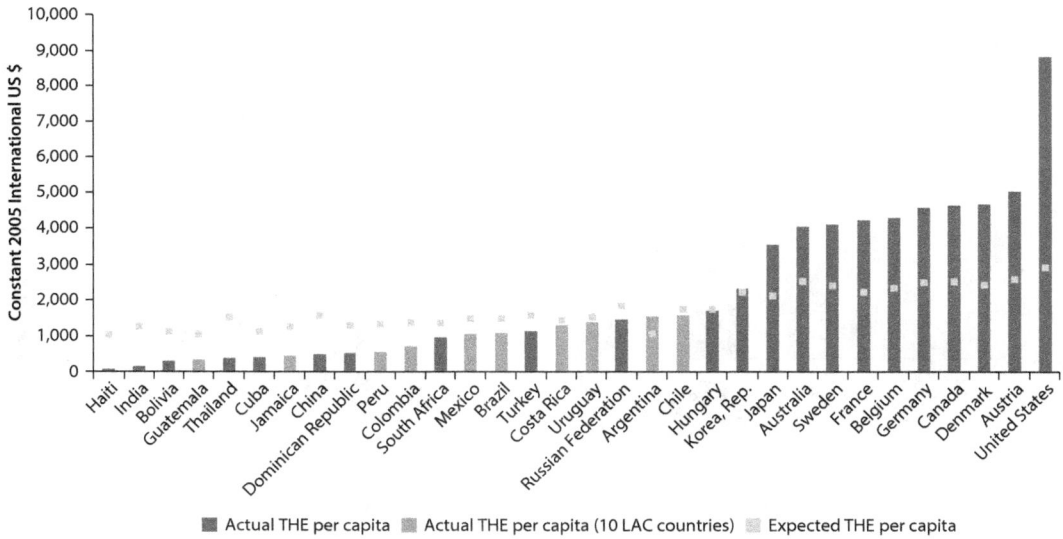

Source: World Bank calculations with data from World Bank World Development Indicators Data Bank 2012.
Note: LAC = Latin America and the Caribbean; PPP = purchasing power parity; THE = total health expenditure.

Figure 2.16   Actual and Expected Government Health Expenditure as a Share of General Government Expenditure

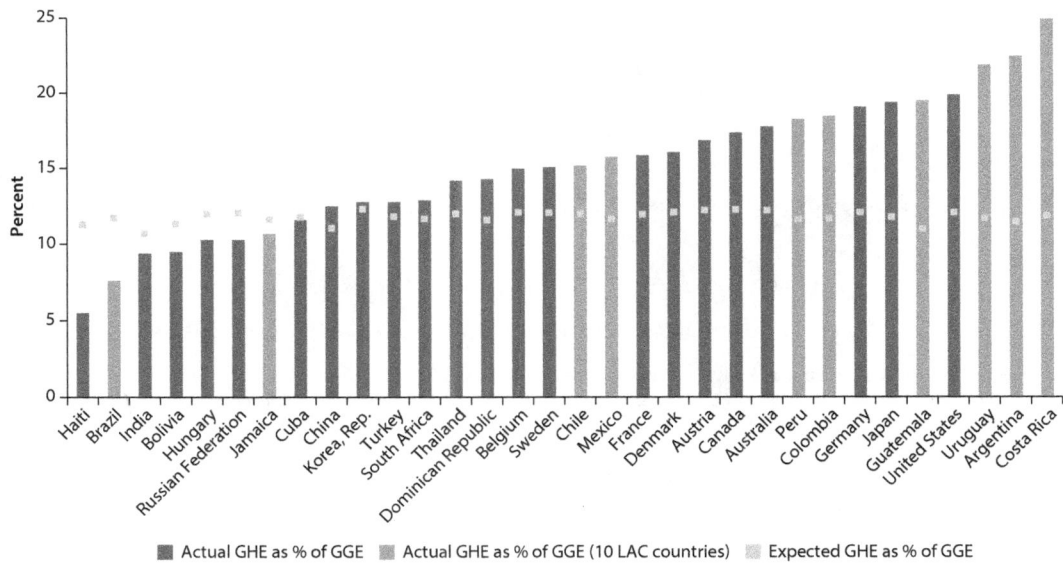

Source: World Bank calculations with data from World Bank World Development Indicators Data Bank 2012.
Note: GHE = government health expenditure; GGE = general government expenditure; LAC = Latin America and the Caribbean.

Toward Universal Health Coverage and Equity in Latin America and the Caribbean
http://dx.doi.org/10.1596/978-1-4648-0454-0

Figure 2.17 Actual and Expected Out-of-Pocket Health Expenditure as a Share of Total Health Expenditure

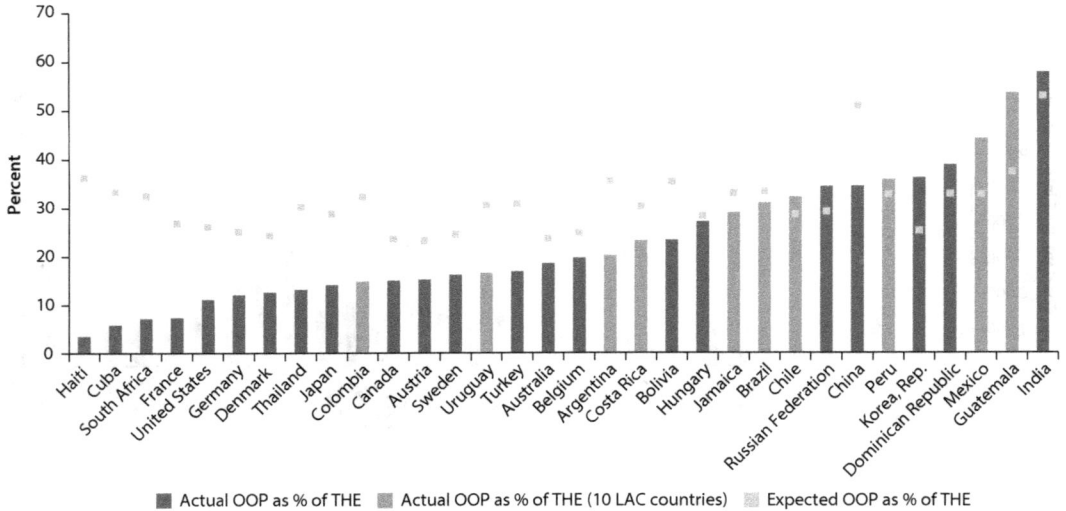

Source: World Bank calculations with data from World Bank World Development Indicators Data Bank 2012.
Note: LAC = Latin America and the Caribbean; OOP = out-of-pocket health expenditures; THE = total health expenditure.

Figure 2.18 Actual and Expected Government Health Expenditure as a Share of Gross Domestic Product

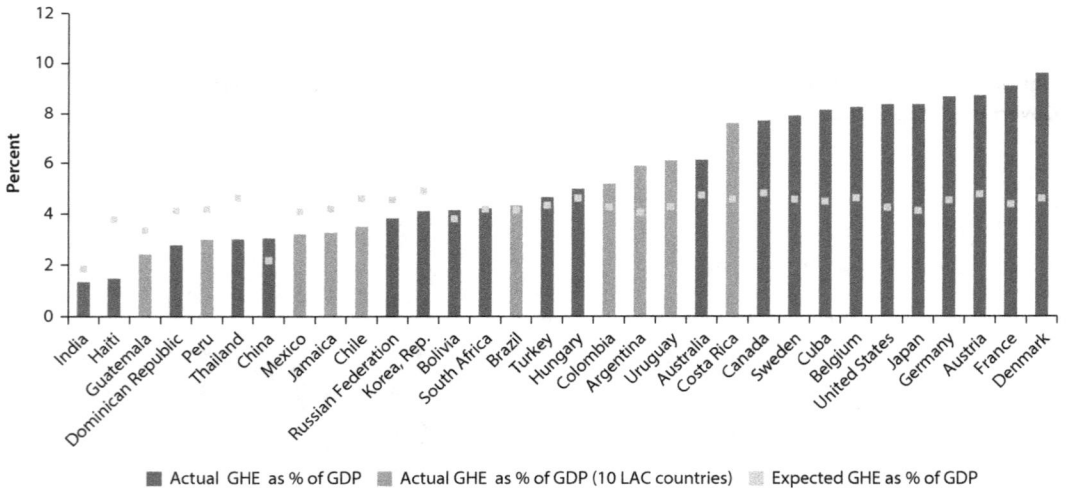

Source: World Bank calculations with data from World Bank World Development Indicators Data Bank 2012.
Note: GHE = government health expenditure; GDP = gross domestic product; LAC = Latin America and the Caribbean.

approaching the actual percentage spent by OECD countries. Furthermore, figure 2.18 also shows that the expected government expenditure as a percentage
of GDP falls around 4 percent for nearly all countries.

Though LAC countries lag behind the OECD in nearly every measure, they
outperform their expected values. Such success may be related—at least in

part—to policies and programs to advance UHC in the 10 LAC countries under study.

Moving Forward in LAC

Democratization, coupled with sustained, equitable economic growth and broad social reforms, has improved living conditions and increased demand for better health care. In this environment, health emerged as a fundamental human right and, in turn, UHC as a means to make this right a reality.

The exercise shows that the 10 countries under study generally fall behind the high-performing OECD countries but ahead of most less-developed countries. The LAC countries have also shown a tendency to perform better than expected, which can be partly attributed to sound public policies and increased public health expenditure. The region continues to show improved health outcomes and strengthening economies. Despite progress, however, inequality remains high. To counter inequality, countries must maintain macroeconomic stability and adapt to changing demographics, which fuel demands for more comprehensive health coverage. The region must find ways to expand fiscal space for health. Slowing population growth is almost certain to continue and countries will progressively age. This trend will challenge the region to become more creative in expanding financial protection and health care coverage in a sustainable manner to deal concurrently with NCDs and infectious diseases.

Notes

1. The term "government health expenditure" is the official National Health Accounts terminology. This variable includes funds from general revenues and social health insurance funds. This variable is sometimes referred to as "public health expenditure." They are used interchangeably in this report.

2. African heads of state approved the Abuja Declaration on HIV/AIDS, tuberculosis, malaria, and other infectious diseases (OAU 2001), which set a target of 15 percent of total government expenditure to be spent on health.

3. THE includes government health expenditure plus private health expenditure. The latter can be divided into out-of-pocket health expenditure and other private expenditures.

4. Several regressions were performed using THE per capita, government as percentage of government expenditure, out-of-pocket (OOP) health expenditure as percentage of THE, maternal mortality rate, life expectancy, infant mortality, and death rates as dependent variables. We controlled for level of development and demographics by using GDP, population size, and the dependency ratio as the independent variables. A single value for each variable was derived using 2012 data. Based on the controls, an expected value for each year could be calculated and then compared with the actual value to see if the country is performing at, above, or below its expected value.

5. The comparators were chosen to represent a broad spectrum ranging from government expenditure on health, private expenditure (as partially indicated by

out-of-pocket health expenditure) on health, and measurable health results. These indicators also had full data sets for the countries in question and provided a range of meaningful results.

6. The 4C countries were used by the Lancet Commission—that revised the case for investments in health on the occasion of the 20th anniversary of the 1993 World Development Report—as a reference because they achieve high levels of health status in 2011 despite having been classified as lower-middle income countries two decades earlier (Jamison and others 2013).

References

Anderson, T. P. 1988. *Politics in Central America: Guatemala, El Salvador, Honduras, and Nicaragua*. Westport, CT: Greenwood Publishing Group.

Bhutta, Zulfiqar A. 2004. *Maternal and Child Health in Pakistan: Challenges and Opportunities*. New York: Oxford University Press.

Bonilla-Chacín, María Eugenia, ed. 2014. *Promoting Healthy Living in Latin America and the Caribbean: Governance of Multisectoral Activities to Prevent Risk Factors for Noncommunicable Diseases*. Washington, DC: World Bank.

Carrión, Diego. 2001. "Democracy and Social Participation in Latin American Cities." *Development in Practice* 11 (2–3): 208–17.

Catoggio, Maria Soledad. 2014. "The Last Military Dictatorship in Argentina (1976–1983): The Mechanism of State Terrorism." Online Encyclopedia of Mass Violence. http://www.massviolence.org/IMG/pdf/AB_Case_Study_The_last_military_dictatorship_in_Argentina.pdf.

Cavagnero, E., B. Daelmans, N. Gupta, R. Scherpbier, and A. Shankar. 2008. "Assessment of the Health System and Policy Environment as a Critical Complement to Tracking Intervention Coverage for Maternal, Newborn, and Child Health." *The Lancet* 371: 1284–93.

Cepeda, Manuel José. 2004. "Judicial Activism in a Violent Context: The Origin, Role, and Impact of the Colombian Constitutional Court." *Washington University Global Studies Law Review* 3: 529–700.

Cetrangolo, O., G. Cruces, E. Fajnzlber, and M. Hopenhayn. 2006. *Shaping the Future of Social Protection: Access, Financing and Solidarity*. Montevideo, Uruguay: Economic Commission for Latin America and the Caribbean.

Conaghan, C. M., and R. Espinal. 1990. "Unlikely Transitions to Uncertain Regimes? Democracy without Compromise in the Dominican Republic and Ecuador." *Journal of Latin American Studies* 22 (3): 553–74.

Cord, L., L. Lucchetti, and C. Rodriquez-Castelan. 2013. *Shifting Gears to Accelerate Shared Prosperity in Latin America and Caribbean*. Washington, DC: World Bank.

Dangl, Benjamin. 2007. *The Price of Fire: Resource Wars and Social Movements in Bolivia*. AK Press.

De la Torre, A., and E. L. Yeyati. 2013. *Latin America and the Caribbean as Tailwinds Recede: In Search of Higher Growth*. Washington, DC: World Bank.

Doumerc, E. 2003. *Caribbean Civilisation: The English-Speaking Caribbean Since Independence*. Toulouse: Presses Universitaires du Mirail.

Draaisma, J., and N. Zamecnik. 2014. *Can LAC Afford Opportunities for All: The Distributional Impact of Fiscal Policy in LAC*. Washington, DC: World Bank.

Ferreira, F. H. G., J. Messina, J. Rigolini, L. F. López-Calva, M. A. Lugo, and R. Vakis. 2013. *Economic Mobility and the Rise of the Latin American Middle Class*. Washington, DC: World Bank.

Fiszbein, Ariel, Norbert Rudiger Schady, and Francisco H. G. Ferreira. 2009. *Conditional Cash Transfer: Reducing Present and Future Poverty*. Washington, DC: World Bank.

Flisser, Ana. 2009. "La medicina en México hacia el siglo XX." *Gaceta Médica de México* 145 (4): 353–356.

Garret, J., and M. Ruel. 2003. "Stunted Child–Overweight Mother Pairs: An Emerging Policy Concern." FCND Discussion Paper 148, IFPRI, Washington, DC.

Godinho, J. 2013. *Latin America: Making Sure Anti-Tobacco Efforts Don't Go Up in Smoke*. Washington, DC: World Bank. http://blogs.worldbank.org/latinamerica/latin -america-making-sure-anti-tobacco-efforts-don-t-go-smoke.

Grosh, M., A. Fruttero, and M. L. Oliveri. 2014. "The Role of Social Protection in the Crisis in Latin America and the Caribbean." In *Understanding the Poverty Impact of the Global Financial Crisis in Latin America and the Caribbean LCR Regional Study*, edited by M. Grosh, M. Bussolo, and S. Freije. Washington, DC: World Bank.

Harding, R. C. 2006. *The History of Panama*. Greenwood Publishing Group.

Huntington, Samuel P. 1991. *The Third Wave: Democratization in the Late Twentieth Century*. Norman: University of Oklahoma Press.

IMF (International Monetary Fund). 2013. *Regional Economic Outlook 2013: Western Hemisphere: Time to Rebuild Policy Space*. Washington, DC: IMF. http://www.imf.org /external/pubs/ft/reo/2013/whd/eng/pdf/wreo0513.pdf.

Iunes R., L. Cubillos-Turriago, and M. L. Escobar. 2012. "Universal Health Coverage and Litigation in Latin America." *En Breve* 178, World Bank, Washington, DC.

Jamison, Dean T., Lawrence H. Summers, George Alleyne, Kenneth J. Arrow, Seth Berkley, Agnes Binagwaho, Flávia Bustreo, David Evans, Richard G. A. Feachem, Julio Frenk, Gargee Ghosh, Sue J. Goldie, Yan Guo, Sanjeev Gupta, Richard Horton, Margaret E. Kruk, Adel Mahmoud, Linah K. Mohohlo, Mthuli Ncube, Ariel Pablos-Mendez, K. Srinath Reddy, Helen Saxenian, Agnes Soucat, Karen H. Ulltveit-Moe, and Gavin Yamey. 2013. "Global Health 2035: A World Converging within a Generation." *The Lancet* 382 (9908): 1898–955.

Kolb, G. L. 1974. *Democracy and Dictatorship in Venezuela, 1945–1958*. Connecticut College Monograph 10. Hamden, CT: Archon.

Lambert, P. 2000. "A Decade of Electoral Democracy: Continuity, Change and Crisis in Paraguay." *Bulletin of Latin American Research* 19 (3): 379–96.

Landivar, Jacinto. 2004. *Historia de la medicina*. Universidad de Cuenca, Facultad de Ciencias Médicas, Escuela de Medicina, Cuenca, Ecuador.

Le Gales-Camus, C., and J. Epping-Jorda. 2005. *Preventing Chronic Diseases: A Vital Investment*. Geneva: World Health Organization.

Maeda, Akiko. 2014. *Universal Health Coverage for Inclusive and Sustainable Development—A Synthesis of 11 Country Case Studies*. Washington, DC: World Bank.

Mainwaring, S., and A. Pérez-Liñan. 2005. "Latin American Democratization since 1978: Democratic Transitions, Breakdowns, and Erosions." In *The Third Wave of*

Democratization in Latin America: Advances and Setbacks, edited by F. Hagopian and S. Mainwaring. New York: Cambridge University Press.

Marinho, F., V. Gawryszewski, P. Soliz, and A. Gerger. 2013. *Region of the Americas: Changes and Challenges*. Washington, DC: Pan American Health Organization.

Miranda Canal, Néstor. 1984. "Apuntes para la historia de la medicina en Colombia." *Ciencia, Tecnología y Desarrollo* 3 (12).

OAU (Organization of African Unity). 2001. "Abuja Declaration on HIV/AIDS, Tuberculosis, and Other Related Infectious Diseases." African Summit on HIV/AIDS, Tuberculosis, and Other Related Infectious Diseases, Abuja, Nigeria, April 24–27. OAU/SPS/Abuja/3. http://www.un.org/ga/aids/pdf/abuja_declaration.pdf.

Omran, Abdel R. 1998. "The Epidemiologic Transition Theory Revisited Thirty Years Later." *World Health Statistics Quarterly* 51: 99–119.

PAHO (Pan American Health Organization). 2010. "Health and Human Rights." Concept Paper 50/12, 50th Directing Council, PAHO, Washington, DC.

———. 2014. "Strategy for Universal Access to Health and Universal Health Coverage." Document CD53/5, Rev 2, 53rd Directing Council, PAHO, Washington, DC.

Pogrebinschi, Thamy. 2013. "The Pragmatic Turn of Democracy in Latin America." Paper presented at the American Political Science Association Annual Meeting, Chicago, IL, August 29 to September 1.

Przeworski, Adam, ed. 2000. *Democracy and Development: Political Institutions and Well-Being in the World, 1950–1990*. Vol. 3. New York: Cambridge University Press.

Ravallion, M. 2013. *The Idea of Antipoverty Policy*. Cambridge, MA: National Bureau of Economic Research.

Rofman, Rafael. 2005. "Social Security Coverage in Latin America." Social Protection Unit and Human Development Network, World Bank, Washington, DC.

Rutgers, W., and S. Rollins. 1998. "Dutch Caribbean Literature." *Callaloo* 21 (3): 542–55.

Sáenz, María del Rocío, Juan Luis Bermúdez, and Mónica Acosta. 2010. "Universal Coverage in a Middle Income Country: Costa Rica." Background Paper, World Health Organization, Geneva.

Schiller, N. G. 2005. "Long-Distance Nationalism." In *Encyclopedia of Diasporas: Immigrant and Refugee Cultures Around the World. Part II*, edited by Melvin Ember, Carol R. Ember, and Ian Skoggard, 570–80. New York: Springer.

Shrimpton, Roger, and Claudia Rokx. 2012. *The Double Burden of Malnutrition: A Review of Global Evidence*. Washington, DC: World Bank.

Singh, Chaitram. 2008. "Re-democratization in Guyana and Suriname: Critical Comparisons." *European Review of Latin American and Caribbean Studies* 84 (April): 71–85.

Skidmore, Thomas E. 2009. *Brazil: Five Centuries of Change*. New York: Oxford University Press.

Sondrol, Paul C. 1992. "1984 Revisited? A Re-Examination of Uruguay's Military Dictatorship." *Bulletin of Latin American Research* 11 (2): 187–203.

The Economist. 2013. "The Latinobarómetro Poll. Listen to Me: A Slightly Brighter Picture for Democracy, But Not for Liberal Freedoms." http://www.economist.com/news/ame ricas/21588886-slightly-brighter-picture-democracy-not-liberal-freedoms-listen-me.

Tobar, Federico. 2001. *Breve historia de la prestación del servicio de salud en Argentina*. Buenos Aires: Ediciones Isalud.

United Nations. 1949. *Yearbook of the United Nations, 1948–49*. New York: United Nations.

———. 1976. "International Covenant on Economic, Social and Cultural Rights." Office of the High Commissioner for Human Rights. http://www.ohchr.org/EN /ProfessionalInterest/Pages/CESCR.aspx.

———. n.d. United Nations Treaties Collection Database (accessed November 11, 2014), https://treaties.un.org/pages/viewdetails.aspx?chapter=4&lang=en&mtdsg_no=iv -3&src=treaty#EndDec.

Valenzuela, Julio Samuel, and Arturo Valenzuela, eds. 1986. *Military Rule in Chile: Dictatorship and Oppositions*. Johns Hopkins University Press.

WHO (World Health Organization). 1946. *Constitution*. Geneva: WHO.

———. 2010. *The World Health Report 2010: Health System Financing—The Path to Universal Coverage*. Geneva: WHO.

———. 2014. Noncommunicable Diseases (NCD) Country Profiles. Geneva: WHO. http://www.who.int/nmh/countries/en/.

World Bank. 2011. "LAC's Decade: Ending or Beginning?" Presentation by the LAC Chief Economist, World Bank, Washington, DC, October 20.

———. 2012. *World Development Indicators*. Washington, DC: World Bank.

World Policy Forum. 2014. "Does the Constitution Guarantee Citizens the Right to Health?" http://worldpolicyforum.org/global-maps/do-citizens-have-a-specific -right-to-health/.

Yamin, A. E., and O. Parra-Vera. 2009. "How Do Courts Set Health Policy? The Case of the Colombian Constitutional Court." *PLoS Med* 6 (2). http://www.ncbi.nlm.nih.gov /pmc/articles/PMC2642877/pdf/pmed.1000032.pdf.

Youngers, C. 2000. *Peru: Democracy & Dictatorship*. Interhemispheric Resource Center.

Zuniga, J. M., S. P. Marks, and L. O. Gostin, eds. 2013. *Advancing the Human Right to Health*. New York: Oxford University Press.

CHAPTER 3

Universal Health Coverage Policies in Latin America and the Caribbean

Tania Dmytraczenko, Fernando Montenegro Torres, and Adam Aten

Abstract

During the past few decades, governments throughout Latin America and the Caribbean (LAC) have strengthened the performance of their health systems by developing new policies and interventions aimed at realizing the vision of universal health coverage (UHC). Governments have focused on reducing fragmentation in the financing and organization of health care systems, harmonizing the scope and quality of services across subsystems, leveraging public-sector financing in a more comprehensive and integrated manner, and creating incentives that promote improved health outcomes and financial protection. Health policies have emphasized making entitlements explicit, establishing enforceable guarantees, and instituting supply-side incentives to improve the quality of care and reduce geographical barriers to access. Efforts have also focused on enhancing governance and accountability. This chapter reviews these changes and identifies key trends in policies to advance UHC throughout the region in countries that have diverse health care systems and face distinct challenges.

Introduction

As discussed in the previous chapter, during the past two decades the LAC region experienced rapid changes in its demographic and epidemiological profiles while also generally enjoying a period of economic stability and expansion. A consolidation of democratic rights both increased demand for and facilitated the adoption of progressive social policies aimed at improving the welfare of the population. As the population's most elemental needs were increasingly being met—as evidenced by improvements in life expectancy and income, and by an expanding middle class—people directed their political influence toward demanding improvements in access to high-quality health care services and greater accountability from the public sector. In recent years, policy makers have attempted to respond to these demands by implementing a new set of inclusive health care reforms intended to extend coverage to affordable, better quality services to all who need them.

The quest to move toward UHC has been a central pillar of the reforms enacted in LAC, driving the design of policies to address rapidly changing population needs and epidemiological profiles (Baeza and Packard 2006). This is evident in the reforms in Chile that created FONASA (Fondo Nacional de Salud) in 1981 and the Universal Access with Explicit Guarantees (Acceso Universal con Garantías Explícitas—AUGE) plan in 2005; the special regime in Costa Rica in 1984 to cover the indigent and later, in the mid-1990s, the integration of the Ministry of Health primary-care providers into the social health insurance system; the Unified Health System (Sistema Único de Saúde—SUS) in Brazil in 1988, including the flagship Family Health Program that was scaled up starting in the late 1990s; the National Health Insurance System in Colombia through adoption of Law 100 in 1993; the Maternal and Child Health Insurance plan in Peru in 1999, which in 2002 was subsumed into the Comprehensive Health Insurance (Seguro Integral de Salud—SIS) plan; the Social Protection System in Health (Sistema de Protección Social en Salud—SPSS) plan, which includes the Seguro Popular as its main pillar, in Mexico in 2003; Plan Nacer in 2004 and its expanded version, Plan Sumar, in 2012 in Argentina; and the Integrated National Health System (Sistema Nacional Integrado de Salud—SNIS) in Uruguay in 2007. This list is not comprehensive, but covers key reforms to advance UHC.

Despite common historical links and similar economic challenges, LAC countries have found different ways to implement their aspirations to progressively deliver on the promise of UHC. Several countries enacted major reforms that encompass both the social health insurance subsystem financed by payroll taxes that covered mostly those who were employed in the formal sector and the subsystem financed by general revenue through ministries of health, which covered entire populations in theory but were often underfunded and ineffective in delivering on their mandate and by default became subsystems that served primarily the poor. Other countries opted for reforms that more directly tackled a single system.

The diversity of experience in the region reveals that there is no single method to achieve UHC and that whether or not a country has achieved or is on the "right" path toward UHC cannot be answered in a binary, simplistic way. The pursuit of UHC is shaped by social contracts, and each country has unique institutional arrangements and policy instruments at its disposal to implement reforms to advance UHC. In addition, policy makers confront country-specific challenges, and they must work to enhance the health of their populations within these constraints and available resources. Further, UHC is not static. Public policies need to be continuously updated as socioeconomic, epidemiological, and demographic realities change and innovations in public health measures, medical care, and diagnostic technologies broaden the scope of possible responses to the health care needs and demands of individual populations. Indeed, both the World Health Assembly (58.33) and PAHO Resolution CD53/5 noted that member states must strategically plan their paths and implied that attaining UHC should be viewed as an ongoing journey rather than a destination (PAHO 2014; WHO 2005).

Nonetheless, common traits emerge among key policies implemented to advance UHC during the past few decades in the region. As part of this study, background papers were produced under the Universal Health Coverage Studies Series (UNICO) for nine LAC countries: Argentina, Brazil, Chile, Colombia, Costa Rica, Guatemala, Jamaica, Mexico, and Peru. UNICO applies a structured protocol for reviewing policy implemented to (1) manage the benefits package, (2) manage inclusion of the poor and vulnerable groups, (3) improve efficiency in the provision of care, (4) address challenges in primary care, and (5) adjust financing mechanisms to better align incentives. The case studies reviewed policies aimed at expanding effective coverage for the poor and vulnerable. This chapter draws on those case studies to present a comparative analysis of the main coverage-expansion policies in the region and summarizes lessons learned in advancing UHC to yield insights for countries embarking down this path. Note, however, that the implemented reforms were shaped by contextual factors unique to each country, and therefore we generalize findings when possible while highlighting country-specific considerations.

A Conceptual Framework of Policies to Advance UHC in the Region

Achieving UHC has been a long-standing objective of health reforms in LAC; however, until recently much of the policy debate has focused intensely on financing, particularly on the merits of payroll-financed social insurance systems (the Bismarck model) compared to those financed by general tax revenues (the Beveridge model) and on single financing pools compared to multiple ones. Yet this dichotomy is an overly simplistic characterization of the reform agenda. "What really matters in achieving universal coverage is ensuring that the whole population has access to acceptable services (as defined by society) and financial protection" (Baeza and Packard 2006, 137). Moving people from one risk-pooling arrangement to the next may not be sufficient or necessary to achieve this goal. Indeed, a much broader array of policies have been implemented in the region to alleviate financial barriers to access and expand equitable health care to the population, particularly to the poor or those at risk of falling into poverty because of health care expenditures.

The framework proposed by Busse, Schreyögg, and Gericke (2007)—which appears in the World Health Report 2008 and in a slightly modified version in the 2010 report—is useful for analyzing the range of reforms to advance UHC that have taken place in LAC. The framework is colloquially referred to as the "WHO cube," and it proposes that the move to UHC should happen along three main dimensions: population coverage, benefits coverage, and financing.[1] This framework can be applied independent of a country's health system structure, model of care, or financing arrangements.

Population Coverage

Commonly referred to as the breadth of coverage, this dimension relates to expanding coverage to segments of the population that were previously not covered. In LAC, ministries of health ostensibly covered the entire population, but policies to advance UHC have made entitlements explicit and secured them with financing. Eligibility to these entitlements may be universal or restricted to certain population groups. It may or may not require enrolling beneficiaries, and enrollment may be mandatory or voluntary.

Benefits Coverage

Also called the depth of coverage, this dimension describes the package of services or benefits to which the population is entitled. To determine health care needs, a formal process is generally instituted that accounts for demand, expectations, and the resources society is willing and able to allocate to health care. Some countries have open-ended benefits that do not specify what is or is not covered, whereas other countries have adopted either positive or negative lists that itemize interventions that are either included or excluded. Scopes can vary considerably in the number of diseases and conditions treated as well as the complexity of care provided.

Financing

This dimension refers to the financial protection afforded—that is, the extent to which households can use the services they need without suffering financial hardship because of out-of-pocket payments. However, we contend that this perspective is too narrow, because the size of the overall resource envelope for the health sector as well as how efficiently those resources are used impact the ability to deliver UHC objectives. Therefore, the discussion that follows delves deeper into this dimension by considering three financing subfunctions: (1) mobilizing resources to generate sufficient and sustainable revenues, (2) pooling funds to ensure that the financial risks associated with accessing the health care system are shared, and (3) purchasing efficient and equitable services (Carrin, James, and Evans 2005; Kutzin 2001).

While the WHO cube is a useful construct for reviewing progress toward UHC, it is not a framework for analyzing health system performance. This report does not provide a comprehensive assessment of policies and programs to strengthen health systems. We recognize this as a limitation of the report.

Comparative Review of Policies to Advance UHC in LAC

The reforms being implemented in the region to advance UHC encompass a broad array of policies and interventions aimed at expanding access to health care services while protecting individuals from financial hardship. We review the experiences of Argentina, Brazil, Chile, Colombia, Costa Rica, Jamaica, Guatemala, Mexico, Peru, and Uruguay from the perspective of how the reforms have addressed population coverage, benefits coverage, and the financing of the system. Figure 3.1 shows a time line of the main reforms reviewed in this chapter. Although this is not a comprehensive review of UHC-related reforms

Figure 3.1 Timeline of Milestones on the Path to UHC in LAC

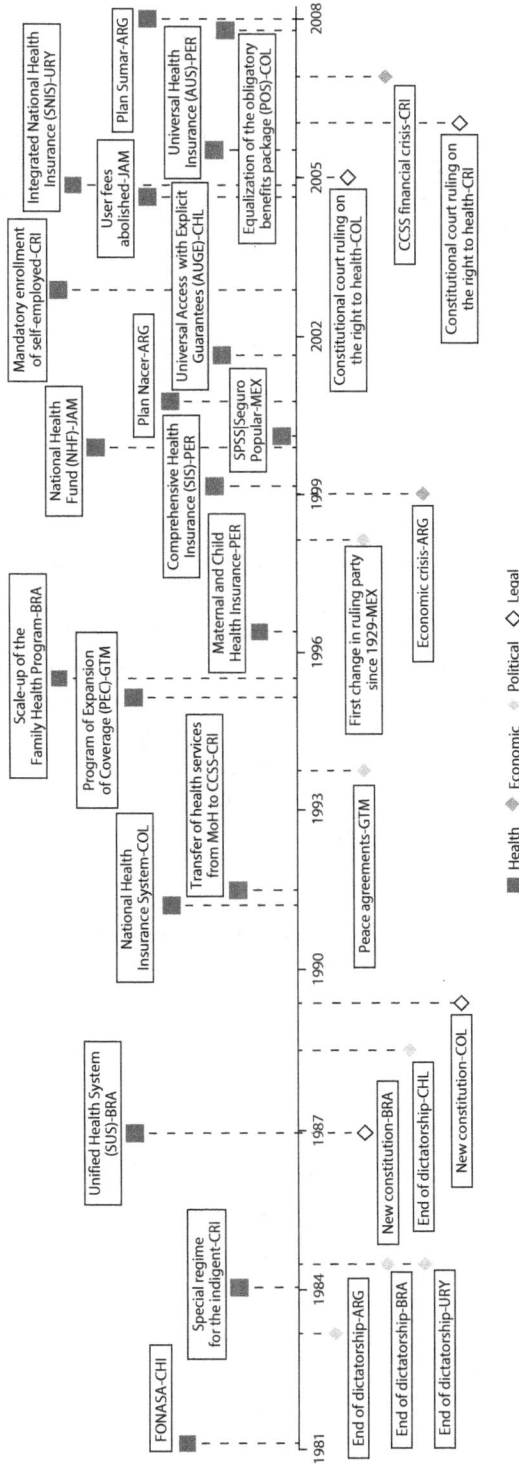

■ Health	◆ Economic	◆ Political	◇ Legal

Timeline milestones:

- FONASA-CHI
- Special regime for the indigent-CRI
- End of dictatorship-ARG
- End of dictatorship-BRA
- End of dictatorship-URY
- Unified Health System (SUS)-BRA
- New constitution-BRA
- End of dictatorship-CHL
- New constitution-COL
- National Health Insurance System-COL
- Peace agreements-GTM
- Transfer of health services from MoH to CCSS-CRI
- Scale-up of the Family Health Program-BRA
- Program of Expansion of Coverage (PEC)-GTM
- Maternal and Child Health Insurance-PER
- First change in ruling party since 1929-MEX
- Economic crisis-ARG
- National Health Fund (NHF)-JAM
- Plan Nacer-ARG
- Comprehensive Health Insurance (SIS)-PER
- SPSS|Seguro Popular-MEX
- Universal Access with Explicit Guarantees (AUGE)-CHL
- Constitutional court ruling on the right to health-COL
- Mandatory enrollment of self-employed-CRI
- Integrated National Health Insurance (SNIS)-URY
- User fees abolished-JAM
- Plan Sumar-ARG
- Universal Health Insurance (AUS)-PER
- Equalization of the obligatory benefits package (POS)-COL
- CCSS financial crisis-CRI
- Constitutional court ruling on the right to health-CRI

Years: 1981, 1984, 1987, 1990, 1993, 1996, 1999, 2002, 2005, 2008 throughout the region, these policies are emblematic of positive changes occurring elsewhere.

As discussed in the previous chapter, reforms to advance UHC in LAC took place within an economic, political, and legal context that gave rise to and shaped the policies implemented in the health sector; some key events are shown in the lower half of figure 3.1. In addition, it bears highlighting that the reforms were not drawn on a blank slate but rather addressed specific fragilities within existing health systems. Although each country in the LAC region has its own particularities, they share a common history in the evolution of health policies during the last century that created two separate and unequal subsystems according to employment and socioeconomic strata: better financed social health insurance subsystems, to which access is restricted to contributing members and their families, and a tax-financed Ministry of Health for the seeming benefit of the entire population but which in practice serves primarily those not covered by social health insurance (Atun and others 2015; Cotlear and others 2014; Kurowski and Walker 2010; Ribe, Robalino, and Walker 2010).[2] Reforms to advance UHC have used various approaches to reduce this segmentation. Brazil and Costa Rica have each opted for an integrated system, albeit through different models. Costa Rica gradually extended the population covered under a single social health insurance scheme, the Costa Rican Social Security System (Caja Costarricense de Seguro Social—CCSS, commonly referred to as the Caja), financed primarily through payroll contributions. Brazil created the SUS, which replaced the former social health insurance system and is financed through national and subnational health funds, which, in turn, are financed from general tax revenues at levels legislated by the constitution (Couttolenc and Dmytraczenko 2013). Most of the countries analyzed chose a path to UHC that involved creating or expanding subsidized insurance while maintaining a pluralistic system in which contributory schemes coexist with parallel pooling arrangements that use general tax revenues to subsidize enrollment of the poor; we call these semi-integrated systems. Those who are not yet formally insured through one of these schemes can continue to access Ministry of Health services, as can the entire population. Chile, Colombia, and Uruguay have achieved high levels of health system integration. Chile and Colombia have made progress in equalizing benefits packages across subsystems. In Uruguay, the SNIS offers a single benefits package for both publicly funded and contributory beneficiaries. In each country, however, a per-beneficiary funding gap between subsystems remains, and subsidized beneficiaries access primarily or exclusively public facilities.[3] Reforms in Argentina, Mexico, and Peru have not directly addressed contributory regimes, but they have created subsidized schemes that aim to reduce disparities between the two. A third group of countries have segmented systems that maintain the social health insurance schemes financed by payroll contributions while making efforts to supplement Ministry of Health services in ways other than by creating an insurance mechanism for the poor. Guatemala is one example, where reforms include contracting private providers to deliver care in areas not reached by the public network. Table 3.1 summarizes key characteristics of health systems in the LAC countries

Table 3.1 Key Characteristics of Health System Financing and Service Delivery

Country	Degree of segmentation	Primary sources of revenue	Primary service delivery network
Brazil	Integrated	SUS—fiscal resources	Public or private facilities financed by SUS
Costa Rica	Integrated	Contributory insurance (CCSS)—payroll taxes and fiscal resources (subsidies for vulnerable groups)	CCSS (own) facilities
Chile	Advanced semi-integrated	Contributory insurance (ISAPRES)—payroll taxes and voluntary premiums; subsidized insurance (FONASA)—payroll taxes and fiscal resources (subsidies for vulnerable groups)	Private facilities (ISAPRES); private facilities (contributory members of FONASA) and public facilities (subsidized and contributory members of FONASA)
Colombia	Advanced semi-integrated	Contributory insurance (Régimen Contributivo)—payroll taxes; subsidized insurance (Régimen Subsidiado)—fiscal resources and cross-subsidies from the Régimen Contributivo	Private facilities (Régimen Contributivo); public facilities (Régimen Subsidiado)
Uruguay	Advanced semi-integrated	Contributory insurance (FONASA)—payroll taxes; separately managed subsidies for vulnerable groups—fiscal resources	Nonprofit private facilities (IAMC); public facilities (ASSE)
Argentina	Semi-integrated	Contributory insurance (Obras Sociales)—payroll taxes; subsidized insurance (Plan Nacer/Plan Sumar)—fiscal resources	Contributory insurance (own) facilities; Ministry of Health facilities (Plan Nacer/Plan Sumar)
Mexico	Semi-integrated	Contributory insurance (IMSS, ISSSTE)—payroll taxes; subsidized insurance (SPSS-Seguro Popular)—fiscal resources	Contributory insurance (own) facilities; Ministry of Health facilities (SPSS-Seguro Popular)
Peru	Semi-integrated	Contributory insurance (EsSalud)—payroll taxes; subsidized insurance (SIS)—fiscal resources	Contributory insurance (own) facilities; Ministry of Health facilities (SIS)
Guatemala	Segmented	Contributory insurance (IGSS)—payroll taxes	Contributory insurance (own) facilities; Ministry of Health and publicly contracted nongovernmental organization facilities

Sources: Brazil—Couttolenc and Dmytraczenko 2013; Gragnolati, Lindelow, and Couttolenc 2013; Costa Rica—Montenegro 2013, Cercone and others 2010; Chile—Bitran 2013; Paraje and Vásquez 2012; Colombia—Montenegro and Bernal-Acevedo 2013; Uruguay—Aran and Laca 2011; World Bank 2012a; Argentina—Cortez and Romero 2013; Belló and Mecerril-Montekio 2011; Mexico—Bonilla-Chacín and Aguilera 2013, Gómez Dantés and others 2011, Scott and Diaz 2013; Peru—Francke 2013; Alcalde-Rabanal, Lazo-González, and Nigenda 2011; Guatemala—Lao Pena 2013; Becerril-Montekio and López-Dávila 2011.

analyzed and highlights relevant fragmentation in financing and service delivery.

Figure 3.2 shows the relative coverage of various schemes. In several countries, some people are covered by more than one scheme, which leads to overall coverage rates in excess of 100 percent.[4] This is most notable in Brazil, where approximately one-quarter of the population, mostly those employed in the formal sector, has supplemental private insurance. The implication is that although the SUS eliminated the social health insurance scheme financed by the payroll tax, it did

Figure 3.2 Population Coverage by Type of Scheme, 2000–10 (or Nearest Year)

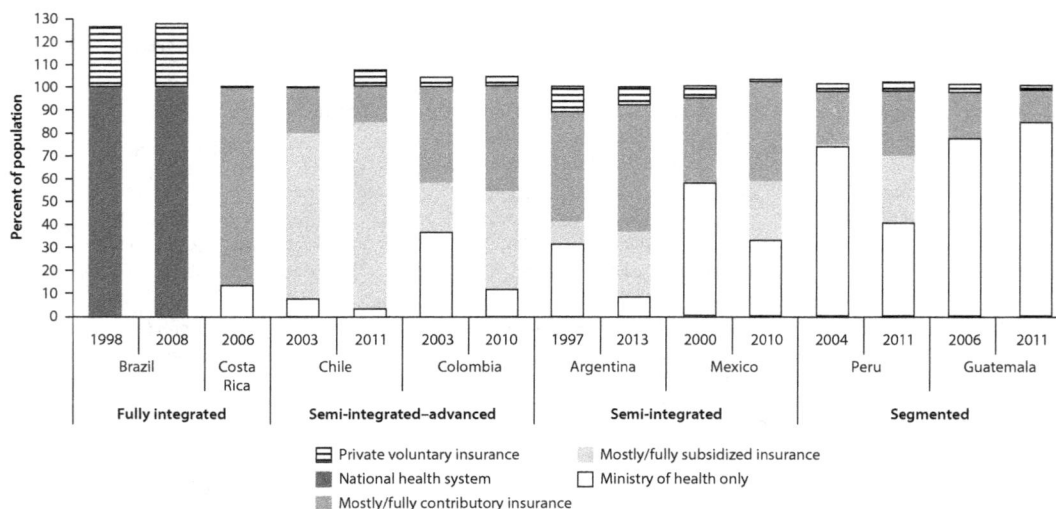

Sources: Study estimates based on Argentina—ECV 1997; SUMAR Memorias 1997; PAMI Memorias 2012; EPH 2013; ENGH 2013; Brazil—PNAD 1998, 2008; Chile—CASEN 2003, 2011; Colombia—ECV 2003, 2010; Costa Rica—ENSA 2006; Guatemala—ENCOVI 2006, 2011; Mexico—ENIGH 2000, 2010; Peru—ENAHO 2004, 2011.
Note: Data about private voluntary insurance in Chile is not comparable across time periods, because the 2003 CASEN did not collect data on this indicator. Also, Uruguay is not included, because the authors did not have access to this survey data.

not eliminate segmentation, which persists through private insurance offered as an employment fringe benefit. Also, this practice is incentivized through tax breaks. This points to a limitation of the categories utilized in figure 3.2. The distinction between contributory and subsidized schemes is not absolute. Employee and/or employer contributions can be tax deductible, as in the case of private insurance in Brazil; or contributory schemes may receive direct subsidies, which applies to the CCSS and the Mexican Institute of Social Security. In addition, because contributions are often based on income rather than actuarially defined costs, insurance funds on occasion run deficits and benefit from tax-financed bailouts (Ribe, Robalino, and Walker 2010). Likewise, subsidized schemes can be partially financed by contributions. This is most notable in Colombia, where there are cross-subsidies from the Régimen Contributivo to the Régimen Subsidiado of the National Health Insurance System; and in Chile, where four funds comprise FONASA, and members pay contributions and receive subsidies to varying degrees according to their capacity to pay, with the poorest members being fully subsidized. Seguro Popular and SIS are open to the entire population, and only those with capacity are required to make a contribution; however, in practice there are relatively few contributory members. A feature that distinguishes the subsidized schemes and the Brazilian SUS from a traditional ministry of health is that the former has defined financing, generally on a capitation basis or as a legally stipulated share of revenues; whereas the funding level for the latter is determined through the government budget planning process.

Population Coverage

LAC countries have implemented diverse models to expand population coverage. Some opted for programs that target specific population groups, and others chose programs that are universal in nature. Regardless, health care reforms have prioritized the use of public subsidies to cover vulnerable populations. Most health care reforms require explicit enrollment of beneficiaries, either on a mandatory or voluntary basis.

Some reforms to advance UHC are designed to be universal, and their legal frameworks overhauled services for the entire population. These include reforms in Brazil, Chile, Colombia, Costa Rica, and Uruguay. Other programs are narrower in scope and target specific health conditions or population subgroups, as in Jamaica, where the National Health Fund (NHF) subsidizes patients suffering from the most prevalent noncommunicable diseases. (Later, the government abolished user fees for public facilities, which affected everyone who uses these services.) Programs in Guatemala and Argentina, at least initially under Plan Nacer, targeted mainly women and children, whereas programs in Mexico and Peru aim to reach those who are not covered by social health insurance and tend to be poor. Table 3.2 provides a summary of the main characteristics of reforms to advance UHC in the studied countries, including the target beneficiaries.

Table 3.2 Key Characteristics of Population Coverage under Selected Reforms to Advance UHC

Country	Programs/policies to advance UHC	Target population	Enrollment
Argentina	Plan Nacer/Plan Sumar	Mothers and children not covered by contributory insurance/women <65, adolescents and children	Voluntary
Brazil	Unified Health System (SUS)/Family Health Program	Entire population	No enrollment
Chile	FONASA/Universal Access with Explicit Guarantees (AUGE)	Entire population	Mandatory
Colombia	National Health Insurance System/ Subsidized Regime	Entire population through the separately managed Régimen Subsidiado and Régimen Contributivo	Mandatory
Costa Rica	Costa Rican Social Security System (CCSS)/ expansion of population covered and integration of primary care	Entire population	Mandatory
Guatemala	Program of Expansion of Coverage (PEC)	Population in rural and low-density areas	No enrollment
Jamaica	National Health Fund (NHF)	Individuals diagnosed with chronic conditions	Voluntary
Mexico	Social Protection System in Health (SPSS)/ Seguro Popular	Those not covered by contributory insurance	Voluntary
Peru	Comprehensive Health Insurance (SIS)	Those not covered by contributory insurance	Voluntary
Uruguay	Integrated National Health System (SNIS)	Entire population through a contributory fund (FONASA) and separately managed fiscal funds for vulnerable groups	Mandatory

Sources: Argentina—Cortez and Romero 2013; Brazil—Couttolenc and Dmytraczenko 2013; Chile—Bitran 2013; Colombia—Montenegro and Bernal-Acevedo 2013; Costa Rica—Montenegro 2013; Guatemala—Lao Pena 2013; Jamaica—Chao 2013; Mexico—Bonilla-Chacín and Aguilera 2013; Peru—Francke 2013; Uruguay—Aran and Laca 2011; World Bank 2012a.

Irrespective of the scope of the programs aimed at advancing UHC, reforms tend to define explicit entitlements through legal and regulatory frameworks. These programs differ from traditional ministries of health, which, as noted above, in theory cover the population. Most coverage expansion programs often require the formal and individual enrollment of beneficiaries (see table 3.2). Also, either by design or in the manner in which they are implemented, most programs place particular emphasis on including the poor. For example, Brazil's SUS is explicitly universal in nature and has no explicit enrollment, yet its flagship program, the Family Health Program, was initiated as a pilot in the country's poorest region and its scale-up prioritized poorer, rural communities (Couttolenc and Dmytraczenko 2013). Likewise, Costa Rica's single social health insurance program gradually brought into the fold informal-sector workers and vulnerable groups, and service delivery reforms in the mid-1990s formally incorporated the Ministry of Health primary health care infrastructure, which served primarily the poor, into the common umbrella of the vertically integrated social health insurance institution (Montenegro 2013).[5] Mexico's Seguro Popular targeted those who were not insured under existing social health insurance schemes, and who were mostly from the lower end of the income distribution (Bonilla-Chacín and Aguilera 2013). In Chile, FONASA now covers 82 percent of the population, and beneficiaries are from across the income spectrum; the poor are almost exclusively covered under this scheme. (Chapter 4 has a lengthier discussion on this issue.)

These programs exemplify the evolving nature of reforms to advance UHC, which expand the sphere of beneficiaries through various mechanisms. Sometimes this is done by increasingly capturing the eligible population within an existing program, as in Chile, Colombia, Costa Rica, and Mexico. Other times, the programs are modified. For example, in Argentina Plan Sumar built on Plan Nacer by extending eligibility to adolescents and women up to age 65. The SIS in Peru was preceded by two narrower insurance programs for mothers, young children, and school-age children.

Policies to advance UHC also build upon the health systems that were already in place. In some countries, the reforms have expanded population coverage by reducing or eliminating segmentation across the tax- and payroll-financed subsystems. This is the case in Costa Rica and Brazil, which have a single integrated system that covers the entire population (or most of it). Chile and Colombia reduced their uninsured populations through enrollment in one of two subsystems, but cross-subsidization and the equalization of benefits between the two (through AUGE in Chile and a constitutional court ruling in Colombia) have contributed to fairly advanced levels of integration. Uruguay has also equalized benefits between subsystems, although for the most part contributory and subsidized groups access different providers. In addition, there is no cross-subsidization from payroll contributions. These aspects are discussed further in the Benefits Coverage and Financing sections below. In contrast, reforms in Argentina, Mexico, and Peru expanded the subsidized subsystem without tackling the contributory regimes.

Benefits Coverage

All reforms analyzed have moved to make entitlements explicit, and most countries opt to define a positive benefits list instead of having open-ended benefits. Countries that have integrated systems or more advanced stages of integration tend to offer comprehensive benefits that cover the range from primary care to high-complexity care. Reforms in all countries place particular emphasis on strengthening primary care. Chile, Colombia, and Uruguay have tackled the difficult issue of equalizing benefits across subsystems.

Most countries in the region have enacted entitlement-based policies that attempt to explicitly define the set of benefits to which the population has rights. Some countries, including Brazil, Colombia, and Costa Rica, have open-ended benefits—that is, the specific interventions covered are not identified. Most countries offer more circumscribed packages; however, the scope varies considerably (see table 3.3). In Chile and Uruguay, the list of services is comprehensive and includes preventive, curative, rehabilitative, and palliative care across all

Table 3.3 Key Characteristics of Benefits under Selected Reforms to Advance UHC

Country	Programs/policies to advance UHC	Benefits covered	Service delivery
Argentina	Plan Nacer/Plan Sumar	Positive list Primary care for pregnant women, children and adolescents, plus some specialized and high-complexity interventions (for example, high-risk pregnancy, neonatal care)	Ministry of Health facilities at the federal and state level
Brazil	Unified Health System (SUS)/Family Health Program	Open-ended Comprehensive benefits from primary to high-complexity care	Ministry of Health facilities at the federal, state, and municipal levels, plus publicly financed contracted private facilities
Chile	FONASA/Universal Access with Explicit Guarantees (AUGE)	Positive list Comprehensive benefits from primary to high-complexity care, with explicit quality and maximum copay guarantees for 80 conditions that apply to both FONASA and ISAPRES beneficiaries	Private and Ministry of Health facilities, though FONASA members without capacity to pay (who have zero copay) access primarily public facilities
Colombia	National Health Insurance System/Régimen Subsidiado	Open-ended with few exclusions Comprehensive benefits from primary to high-complexity care, with equal benefits for the Régimen Subsidiado and Régimen Contributivo (Plan Obligatorio de Salud—POS)	Private and Ministry of Health facilities, though Régimen Subsidiado beneficiaries access primarily public facilities
Costa Rica	Costa Rican Social Security System (CCSS)/expansion of population covered and integration of primary care	Open-ended with formulary for medicines Comprehensive benefits from primary to high-complexity care	CCSS facilities

table continues next page

Table 3.3 Key Characteristics of Benefits under Selected Reforms to Advance UHC *(continued)*

Country	Programs/policies to advance UHC	Benefits covered	Service delivery
Guatemala	Program of Expansion of Coverage (PEC)	Positive list Basic primary health care interventions	Publicly financed contracted nongovernmental organizations
Jamaica	National Health Fund (NHF)	Positive list Prescribed medicines for 15 chronic conditions	Accredited public or private pharmacies
Mexico	Social Protection System in Health (SPSS)/ Seguro Popular	Positive list The Universal Health Services Catalog (CAUSES) covers 284 primary- and secondary-care interventions and associated medicines The Catastrophic Health Expenditures Fund covers 57 high-complexity interventions	Mostly Ministry of Health providers at the federal and state levels
Peru	Comprehensive Health Insurance (SIS)	Positive list The Essential Health Insurance Plan (PEAS) of the free SIS Gratuito covers 140 conditions, including maternal and neonatal care, some obstetric conditions, cancers, communicable diseases, and acute care, as well as a few noncommunicable diseases and chronic conditions Three additional packages, with varying premiums, include higher-cost interventions	Ministry of Health facilities at the central and regional levels; participation of non–Ministry of Health providers is limited, because SIS fees do not cover the full cost of intervention
Uruguay	Integrated National Health System (SNIS)	Positive list Comprehensive benefits with a single Integrated Health Care Plan (PIAS) for the entire population that covers preventive, curative, rehabilitative, and palliative care	Nonprofit facilities (IAMC); private and decentralized public facilities (ASSE) for FONASA members; ASSE for subsidized vulnerable groups

Sources: Argentina—Cortez and Romero 2013, Plan Sumar website: http://www.msal.gov.ar/vamosacrecer/index.php?option=com_content &view=category&layout=blog&id=340&Itemid=290; Brazil—Gragnolati, Lindelow, and Couttolenc 2013; Chile—Bitran 2013; Paraje and Vásquez 2012, AUGE 80 website: http://web.minsal.cl/AUGE_introduccion; Colombia—Montenegro and Bernal-Acevedo 2013; Costa Rica— Montenegro 2013; Guatemala—Lao Pena 2013; Jamaica—Chao 2013, NHF website: http://www.nhf.org.jm; Mexico—Bonilla-Chacín and Aguilera 2013; Scott and Diaz 2013; Peru—Francke 2013, SIS website: http://www.sis.gob.pe/Portal/index.html; Uruguay—World Bank 2012a; Ministerio de Salud Pública.

levels of the service delivery network. Mexico's Seguro Popular and Peru's SIS also cover a wide range of conditions, but mostly for care provided at the primary and secondary levels, with few exceptions; in Mexico (and also Uruguay), for example, a separate fund finances high complexity care for listed low-incidence but high-cost conditions that can put affected households at risk of impoverishment. Elsewhere, packages address specific health priorities. For example, in Jamaica the NHF benefits are limited to subsidies for noncommunicable disease medicines, and user fees were abolished in public health facilities. Both policies implemented in Jamaica address the problem of high out-of-pocket payments for health. Guatemala's Expansion of Coverage Program

(Programa de Extensión de Cobertura—PEC) contracts nongovernmental organizations to deliver primary-care interventions free of charge, and it has a heavy focus on maternal and child health care services. Similarly, Argentina's Plan Sumar covers maternal and child health care services, but its benefits also extend to adolescents and women under age 65, and it includes some specialized and high-complexity care, particularly for newborns (for example, those with congenital heart conditions or pneumonia), childbirth deliveries, and nutritional disorders.

With the exception of Jamaica's NHF, packages generally offer at least ambulatory health care services, particularly primary care. Indeed, strengthening primary care was a focus of programs throughout the region, even in countries that have broader reforms and comprehensive benefits. That is, the emphasis on primary care was not only an issue of including services in the benefits packages; in many instances it also entailed reorienting the care model toward promotion, prevention, and community outreach. Costa Rica transferred ownership of primary-care facilities from the Ministry of Health to the CCSS, further integrating the service delivery network and providing improved access to better and safer management of chronic diseases to the formerly uninsured, hence reducing the higher use of inpatient and emergency care by this group (Cercone and others 2010). Under the Family Health Program, a flagship of Brazilian reforms to advance UHC, multidisciplinary health teams are responsible for delivering facility- and community-based primary care within their ascribed catchment area and serve as a point of entry into the SUS (Couttolenc and Dmytraczenko 2013). The Integrated Health Care Plan (Plan Integral de Atención en Salud—PIAS) of the Uruguayan SNIS reorients the care model away from a focus on curative services toward an integrated care model that eliminates or greatly reduces copayments for the management of diabetes and hypertension, maternal health interventions, and preventive services for children and adolescents (Sollazzo and Berterretche 2011; World Bank 2012a).

As mentioned previously, programs and benefits packages evolve over time to increasingly correspond to a country's epidemiological needs. Peru's SIS includes the Essential Health Insurance Plan (PEAS), an extensive primary-care package with some specialized services to address noncommunicable diseases and chronic conditions. The SIS was a consolidation of two existing, more targeted schemes— one for school-age children and another for mothers and young children—that offered more limited benefits (Francke 2013). Plan Nacer has been expanded into Plan Sumar, which extends benefits beyond the original maternal and child health care packages. Chile's AUGE plan also defined an essential package to be covered by its two social health insurance subsystems, which started with 25 priority health conditions in 2005 and was expanded to 69 in 2010 and 80 in 2014 (Bitran 2013; http://web.minsal.cl/AUGE_introduccion). Similarly, Seguro Popular's package has been extended over time, from 78 interventions to the current 284 interventions. However, often these expansions entailed policy revisions, because countries in the region generally lack or have weak institutionalized arrangements for systematically reviewing and modifying the conditions and services included in benefits packages or assessing the adoption of new technologies to deliver current benefits on an ongoing basis.

Although enacting an entitlement-based reform is a major policy change, translating de jure benefits into de facto services often requires instituting a series of policies, rules, and regulations governing the financing and provision of services. Entitlement does not automatically translate into availability of services, nor does it necessarily convert into higher utilization or improvements in quality. This is discussed in subsequent chapters.

For the most part, the reforms to advance UHC in LAC have not discarded existing structures but have adapted them to new challenges. In most cases, the same providers that delivered services to poor segments of the population in the period preceding the entitlement reforms, usually Ministry of Health providers, continue to do so but under modified arrangements. Although services not included in the benefits packages continue to be financed and provided in the traditional way, new management models are being implemented that place the patient at the center and create incentives to deliver measurable results. In several cases, this entails formal contracts between financiers and providers of health care services. For example, in Uruguay the reform that created FONASA in 2007 also made it possible for its beneficiaries to elect a public provider that would then establish a management contract with the purchasing agent and receive FONASA-financed capitation payments. Reforms in Colombia included provisions for public providers to establish contracts with private and public insurance. However, in most countries (including Colombia and Uruguay), beneficiaries of contributory schemes continue to have access to private-sector and/or the social health insurance's own providers; in contrast, beneficiaries of subsidized regimes access only or mostly public providers. Shortfalls persist in terms of equitable access to quality services because of vast differences among services delivered under different subsystems.

A few countries are attempting to address these issues by equalizing benefits or setting quality-of-care standards that apply across the social health insurance subsystems. The landmark Constitutional Court ruling T-760/2008 in Colombia mandated unifying the obligatory benefits package covered under the contributory and subsidized regimes (Plan Obligatorio de Salud—POS), and subsequent regulations operationalized the ruling by gradually extending the POS of the contributory regime to different age groups until all beneficiaries of the subsidized regime were covered in 2012 (Tsai 2010, *Comisión de Regulación en Salud* Agreements 04/2009, 011/2010, 027/2011, and 032/2012). The AUGE reform in Chile and SNIS reform in Uruguay each created a single explicit benefits package. They also specified the treatments covered, established quality standards for their delivery, and instituted guarantees for key aspects of effective coverage, such as maximum waiting times, which addressed known weakness of the public system. Brazil has done the same, but on a much smaller scale, by defining maximum waiting times for SUS patients to receive treatment following a cancer diagnosis.[6] Mexico has been monitoring effective coverage, a measure of the likelihood that individuals will actually experience health gains from receiving needed interventions (Lozano and others 2006), but the reforms implemented thus far have concentrated on improving quality in the public subsystem rather than equalizing benefits across subsystems. Similarly, the SIS in Peru instituted protocol requirements, quality audits, and explicit guarantees under PEAS for services that are provided primarily but not exclusively in public facilities.

Financing

Public funding for health has increased, with financing for programs aimed at advancing UHC coming primarily from general taxation, often with specific earmarks for health. Some countries have opted for a single pool that captures the entire population, whereas others have instituted arrangements that increase the diversity of risks within pools and have reduced disparities in benefits and per capita spending across pools. Others have attempted to reduce these disparities by reforming only the publicly subsidized subsystem through changes in the way resources are mobilized, allocated, and/or used to pay providers. Although few countries have fully split the financing and provision functions, they have .universally embraced payment methods in which the money follows the patient and that, unlike historic line-item budgets, promote efficiency in the delivery of cost-effective interventions. However, the extent to which these mechanisms replace line-item financing varies considerably. Reforms have also extended financial protection by eliminating user fees or capping copays, in some cases including those for high-cost interventions.

Following the flow-of-funds structure of the system of health accounts (OECD 2000; WHO 2003) and the health financing framework proposed by Kutzin (2001), we examine aspects of the reforms related to resource mobilization, pooling arrangements, and mechanisms to purchase services or pay and manage providers. An important aspect in assessing whether reforms have had a major impact on resource mobilization is to determine whether the overall level of public revenue for the health sector increased (Kutzin 2008). Rising income also spurs demand for improved access to health care and typically translates into increased public expenditures on health and a reduction in the share of health financed through household out-of-pocket payments (Savedoff and others 2012; Schieber and Maeda 1999). LAC is no exception. As highlighted in the previous chapter, the region has generally experienced stable growth during the last two decades, barring the dips associated with the financial crisis. Rising incomes and social programs have lifted millions out of poverty and enlarged the middle class. Public financing for health increased as a share of gross domestic product (GDP) in all 10 countries during the last decade (World Bank 2012b), though only Costa Rica and Uruguay surpassed the 6 percent threshold proposed by the Pan American Health Organization (PAHO 2014, 94). Public spending on health accounts for more than 15 percent of total government expenditures, the average for high-income countries of the Organisation for Economic Co-operation and Development (OECD), except in Brazil (7.6 percent) and Jamaica (10.7 percent). This raises concerns that some countries may be reaching the upper limit of their ability to capture a larger share of the budget for the sector, particularly where health already absorbs one-fifth or more of the public revenues,[7] as in Argentina (22.5 percent), Uruguay (25.2 percent), and Costa Rica (27.7 percent).

Public resources are being used to finance programs to advance UHC, which are heavily subsidized if not entirely funded through general government revenues. By defining per-beneficiary amounts to be financed from the budget, setting legal minimum allocations for health, labeling taxes as being for health or earmarking payroll taxes or other levies, several reforms ring-fenced public revenues for health to finance extensions of coverage and prioritize those without capacity to pay (table 3.4). A number of reforms also sought to reduce the burden of out-of-pocket payments for health by eliminating or capping user fees and copays or by creating special funds to finance care for high-cost, low-frequency conditions that can drive affected families into poverty (for example, Mexico's Catastrophic Health Expenditure Fund and Uruguay's National Resource Fund). Brazil's 1988 constitution eliminated user fees for publicly financed services and decentralized the administration of health care services, and a subsequent constitutional amendment codified the share of revenues to be allocated for health at each level of government (Couttolenc and Dmytraczenko 2013). Mexico's Social Protection System in Health (Sistema de Protección Social en Salud—SPSS), which launched Seguro Popular, increased stability in public funding by statutorily defining a social contribution per family that is linked to an inflation-indexed minimum wage and is to be financed by the federal government and states (Bonilla-Chacín and Aguilera 2013). By replacing historical budgets with actuarially calculated premiums to determine state transfers, the reform also reduced disparities in federal spending across states and eliminated user fees in public facilities. Argentina created a capitation system based on actuarial calculations and risk assessment paid to provinces on top of historical budgets (Cortez and Romero 2013). Colombia increased public funding for the Régimen Subsidiado, and, along with Costa Rica, it has the highest share of public spending in total health expenditures among the study countries (World Bank 2012b). The Régimen Subsidiado is financed by a solidarity levy on formal-sector payrolls as well as legally defined national and local fiscal transfers. Costa Rica finances noncontributory CCSS enrollees through earmarked taxes on luxury goods, alcohol, soda, and imports (Montenegro 2013). Similarly, Jamaica's NHF is financed through earmarks on alcohol, petroleum, and motor vehicle levies. The AUGE plan in Chile was accompanied by a substantial hike in public spending on FONASA financed through general taxation with a one percentage-point increase in the value-added tax and other sources (Bitran 2013). Even in countries where the reforms did not greatly increase the overall level of financing (such as in Argentina) nor create specific resource mobilization mechanisms (such as in Guatemala and Peru), they did leverage existing funding to improve access to services for marginalized populations. However, funding for the largely budget-financed PEC in Guatemala is highly volatile and subject to ebbs and flows in political support (Lao Pena 2013), and in Peru the SIS has not had a significant budget nor has it improved public financing (Francke 2013).

Table 3.4 Key Characteristics of Financing under Selected Reforms to Advance UHC

Country	Programs/policies to advance UHC	Resource mobilization	Pooling	Purchasing	Cost-effectiveness and financial protection
Argentina	Plan Nacer/Plan Sumar	Defined per-beneficiary amount financed through general taxation	Ministry of Health program paid from general budget to provinces and from provinces to providers	Actuarially defined capitation payment adjusted for performance (for transfer from national level to provinces) and on a fee-for-service basis from provinces to providers	Prioritized cost-effective primary health care interventions Increased public financing reduced disparity in per-beneficiary spending between social health insurance and the public subsystem
Brazil	Unified Health System (SUS)/Family Health Program (FHP)	Minimum expenditure financed from general taxation (constitutionally defined share of revenues at the federal, state, and municipal levels)	Health funds at each level of government (federal, state, municipal) National funds are used to pay federal providers and are transferred to state and municipal funds to pay providers at those levels	SUS: a mix of budget financing, capitation, performance-based payments, case-based payments, and fee-for-service FHP (and other priority programs): capitation and performance-based payments (for transfers from the federal level to state and municipal funds)	Prioritized cost-effective primary health care interventions Increased public financing Eliminated user fees
Chile	FONASA/Universal Access with Explicit Guarantees (AUGE)	Payroll tax and a general taxation-financed subsidy for those without capacity to pay	FONASA collects contributions and subsidies and pays public and private providers	Capitation, adjusted for age and socioeconomic level of the municipality, with some fee-for-service for municipal primary health care Historic budgets, fee-for-service, and prospective payments to public hospitals Fee-for-service and case-based payments to private providers Copay from FONASA contributory members only	Prioritized cost-effective interventions Improved referrals and counter-referrals across levels of care for AUGE conditions Set maximum deductible for AUGE conditions

table continues next page

Table 3.4 Key Characteristics of Financing under Selected Reforms to Advance UHC *(continued)*

Country	Programs/policies to advance UHC	Resource mobilization	Pooling	Purchasing	Cost-effectiveness and financial protection
Colombia	National Health Insurance System/Régimen Subsidiado	Per-beneficiary amount financed through general taxation and earmarked taxes at the national, state, and municipal levels plus cross-subsidies financed through earmarked payroll taxes	Payroll tax cross-subsidies and national and municipal funds are pooled at the municipal level to pay for health plans for beneficiaries of the Régimen Subsidiado and to pay providers for services outside the benefits package	Capitation payments for Régimen Subsidiado health plans Health plans have discretion over selection of provider payment methods and utilize a diverse range Capitation payments for public hospitals	Increased public financing
Costa Rica	Costa Rican Social Security System (CCSS)/expansion of population covered and integration of primary care	Payroll tax and a defined per-beneficiary amount financed through earmarked taxes (on luxury goods, alcohol, soda, and imports) for those without capacity to pay	Single pool managed by CCSS used to pay own providers	CCSS (own) facilities paid through a historical global budget	Prioritized cost-effective primary health care interventions
Guatemala	Program of Expansion of Coverage (PEC)	General taxation through the budget	Ministry of Health program paid from general budget	Capitation payments for contracted nongovernmental organizations	Prioritized cost-effective primary health care interventions No user fees in contracted providers (or public facilities)
Jamaica	National Health Fund (NHF)	Tobacco tax, payroll tax, and special consumption tax (on alcohol, petroleum, and motor vehicles)	NHF	Grants to the Health Promotion Fund and Health Support Fund (for infrastructure development) Fee-for-service for approved medicines (cover 45–75 percent of retail price)	Prioritized cost-effective promotion of healthy lifestyles and medicines for management of NCDs Reduced out-of-pocket payment for medicines A separate policy eliminated users in public facilities

table continues next page

Table 3.4 Key Characteristics of Financing under Selected Reforms to Advance UHC *(continued)*

Country	Programs/policies to advance UHC	Resource mobilization	Pooling	Purchasing	Cost-effectiveness and financial protection
Mexico	Social Protection System in Health (SPSS)/Seguro Popular	Defined per-beneficiary amount linked to the minimum wage financed through general taxation (federal and state levels) and, in theory, contributions of families with capacity to pay	Federal contributions for Seguro Popular are pooled at the federal level and transferred to states, which use these funds plus state contributions to pay state-level providers Catastrophic Health Expenditure Fund (federal level)	Actuarially defined capitation payment (for transfer from federal level to states) Budget financing for CAUSES services Fee-for-service for benefits covered by the Catastrophic Health Expenditure Fund	Prioritized cost-effective interventions Increased public financing and reduced disparity in per-beneficiary spending between the contributory and subsidized subsystem and across states Eliminated user fees
Peru	Comprehensive Health Insurance (SIS)	General taxation through the budget and, in theory, premiums from members with capacity to pay Runs arrears if fee-for-service payments exceed budget	SIS is an autonomous entity with a direct budget allocation from the Ministry of Finance	Fee-for-service for PEAS services rendered Providers have greater flexibility in use of SIS funds than Ministry of Health budget	Prioritized cost-effective primary health care interventions Eliminated user fees for PEAS services
Uruguay	Integrated National Health System (SNIS)	Payroll tax and a defined per-beneficiary amount financed through general taxation for those without capacity to pay	Payroll contributions pooled into FONASA and used to pay public and private insurers; for those without capacity to pay, financing from general budget is used to pay public providers The National Resource Fund (FNR) pools funds to finance high-complexity/high-cost interventions	Contracted public and private providers paid on a risk-adjusted (by age and gender) capitation basis plus a performance-based payment Fee-for-services for benefits covered by the FNR	Reduced copay for prioritized cost-effective interventions and eliminated copay in public facilities (ASSE) Increased public financing and reduced disparity in per-beneficiary spending between social health insurance and public subsystem

Sources: Argentina—Cortez and Romero 2013; Brazil—Couttolenc and Dmytraczenko 2013; Chile—Bitran 2013; Colombia—Montenegro and Bernal-Acevedo 2013; Costa Rica—Montenegro 2013; Guatemala—Lao Pena 2013; Jamaica—Chao 2013; Mexico—Bonilla-Chacín and Aguilera 2013; Peru—Francke 2013; Uruguay—Aran and Laca 2011; World Bank 2012a.

As previously discussed, the LAC region has long been characterized by frag-
mented health care systems in which a tax-financed public subsystem coexists
with social health insurance financed by payroll taxes, as well as a private subsystem financed primarily through direct out-of-pocket payments, and in some
countries nonnegligible private insurance market. The experiences of various
OECD countries suggest that pooling arrangements can reduce this segmentation
and foster equity and efficiency in managing health care funds. Pooling arrangements facilitate cross-subsidies from the rich to the poor and spread risk across
younger and older segments of the population and from the healthy to the ill.

Brazil opted for a national health system financed by revenue taxes that
replaced the previous contributory social health insurance. One-quarter of the
population has supplemental private insurance, mostly obtained as an employment fringe benefit and subsidized by tax exemptions (figure 3.2). The elimination of the payroll-financed subsystem sets Brazil apart. Mandatory general
taxation allocations are transferred to funds at the national, state, and municipal
levels and are used for intergovernmental transfers and to pay providers at each
level of the system.

Outside Brazil and the Caribbean, social health insurance financed by mandatory contributions from employers and employees continues to be predominant
in the region. Over time, Costa Rica, which has an integrated system like Brazil,
expanded coverage of the payroll tax–financed CCSS by gradually extending
mandatory enrollment beyond formal-sector workers and by using public subsidies to incentivize enrollment of the self-employed (the state pays a little more
than half of the individual's total contribution) and to fully finance enrollment
of the population that seeks care but does not have the capacity to pay. Subsidies
account for approximately one-quarter of total funding, and these are pooled
with payroll contributions into the CCSS to finance its own network of providers
(Cercone and others 2010). In 2007, Uruguay created FONASA, a single pool
that unifies mandatory payroll contributions from civil servants as well as those
employed in the private sector and pensioners. Although the vision of the reform
is to eventually extend this coverage to all, for now most of the population without the capacity to pay is financed through the general budget and those
resources are not currently pooled with contributory funds, as they are in Costa
Rica (Sollazzo and Berterretche 2011).

Chile and Colombia have maintained payroll-financed systems, but they
have made significant strides in reducing segmentation by creating a separate
pool funded primarily through tax revenues and payroll contributions. This
allows coverage to be greatly expanded for those previously not captured under
social health insurance and hence increases the diversity of risk in the pool
(figure 3.2). In Chile, FONASA covers over four-fifths of the population and,
in 2011, 58 percent of its funds was financed through tax revenues and the
remainder was financed through payroll contributions from members with the
capacity to pay. There is also the option to use mandatory contributions to
purchase plans from for-profit private insurers (Instituciones de Salud
Previsional—ISAPRES), which cover mostly the wealthy, healthy, and young

(i.e., "cream skimming" the low-risk population). In addition, enrollees may also have the option of paying voluntary premiums for supplemental coverage. There is no formal cross-subsidization between the two subsystems, yet ISAPRES members are known to revert to the public system for treatment of catastrophic illnesses.[8] In contrast, in Colombia payroll taxes are pooled into a single fund, a portion of which is earmarked to subsidize the population without the capacity to pay. This population is covered under the Régimen Subsidiado, which is financed primarily through general tax revenues from the federal government and to a lesser extent municipalities. Cross-subsidies from contributory members account for approximately one-third of the Régimen Subsidiado's total financing (Montenegro 2013). In Chile, FONASA is also the insurer and uses funds to pay providers, whereas in Colombia funds are transferred to health plans (Empresas Promotoras de Salud—EPS) that in turn pay providers. In both countries and in Uruguay as well, services financed by the subsidized subsystem are mostly provided through the public delivery network. Also, as previously mentioned, recent reforms such as AUGE in Chile, PIAS in Uruguay, and regulations operationalizing constitutional court ruling T-760 in Colombia aim to equalize benefits packages and reduce disparities in the quality of care available to beneficiaries of the two subsystems. The reforms have also reduced inequalities in financing. In Colombia, capitation payments are now almost the same in both regimes (Montenegro and Bernal-Acevedo 2013). In Uruguay, the per capita spending gap between the public providers serving primarily the subsidized population (ASSE) and those serving contributory FONASA members (IAMC) was reduced from 1:1.8 in 2007 to 1:1.3 in 2010 through increased public financing (World Bank 2012a).

Most reforms to advance UHC have entailed changes to purchasing and provider payment and management mechanisms, though the arrangements are diverse. There is broad acknowledgement that historical line-item budgets and weak accountability of providers contributed to poor performance of health systems in terms of responsiveness to changing health care needs and emerging demands. A trend in the region is the introduction of formal and informal performance agreements, and in some cases legally enforceable contracts, with public and private entities. A few countries, notably Chile and Colombia and more recently Uruguay, implemented managed competition models whereby social health insurance contributions can be used to finance health plans from public or private insurers that in turn purchase services from public or private providers. Private insurers contract entirely or mostly private providers—that is, there is a complete separation of purchasing and provider functions, at least in the nonsubsidized subsystems (Chile's ISAPRES, Colombia's Régimen Contributivo, and Uruguay's FONASA). A variety of methods are used to pay providers, whether public or private, usually involving a combination of capitation, fee-for-service and case-based payments depending on the level of care. However, in most cases the public delivery network that serves primarily the subsidized portion of the system continues to be financed in part through historical budgets, though to a much lesser extent than prior to the reforms.

To improve effectiveness and accountability, even countries that have not formally split the financing and provider functions have modified resource allocation mechanisms in the public sector by instituting financial and nonfinancial incentives for public providers. By transferring federal funds to the subnational level on the basis of actuarially defined capitation payments, Argentina and Mexico provide incentives for the identification, enrollment, and monitoring of beneficiaries. Both Argentina and Brazil created a system whereby explicit agreements that define performance targets govern the transfer of funds to subnational governments and/or providers. In Brazil, actual transfers are not conditional on meeting targets, but in Argentina 40 percent of the transfer is contingent on achieving tracer indicators, and fee-for-service payments to providers incentivize them to reach out to the population in their catchment area to deliver priority interventions. Under SIS, Peru pays providers of on a fee-for-service basis. In Guatemala, PEC introduced results-based financing contracts with nongovernmental organizations to provide publicly financed services. Increasingly, countries are incentivizing quality improvements—for example, Argentina's Plan Sumar and, more recently, Brazil's National Program for Improvement in Primary Care Access and Quality launched in 2011.

Reforms aimed at achieving UHC in these countries have also provided greater autonomy in the use of public funds. For example, in Argentina under Plan Sumar facilities can invest a portion of public resources to finance priorities defined at the local level. Some facilities allow a small portion of the performance-based payment to be used to pay incentives to staff, albeit this is a minority. The SIS in Peru also offers greater flexibility in managing funds relative to the regular Ministry of Health budget, though there is not as much leeway as there was in the funds derived from the collection of user fees (Francke 2013). It is relevant to point out that in many countries the changes introduced to the allocation of financial resources were amounts that were marginal and parallel to traditional budget mechanisms—that is, many providers still rely on budget financing for the bulk of their expenditures, such as in Argentina, Brazil, Guatemala, Jamaica, Mexico, and Peru.

Lessons Learned from Policies and Programs to Advance UHC

The policies and programs to advance UHC in LAC have expanded coverage along the three dimensions of the WHO cube, filling the box to a greater or lesser extent. Although each country fills the space in its own way, some key themes emerge about how countries balanced the tensions that arise from making choices in a resource-constrained environment to prioritize the UHC dimensions.

Leveraging Public Financing to Reach the Poor

Although most of the debate surrounding the health reforms in the 1980s and 1990s in LAC focused on reducing segmentation in financing by expanding or creating a virtual or de facto single pool, another core aspect of the reforms was the establishment of mechanisms to reach the poor. This focus on the poor is even more apparent in the recent wave of reforms. Irrespective of whether countries opted for national health systems financed through general revenue, social health insurance financed through payroll taxes, or a mix of both, reaching the poor requires a commitment to mobilize public subsidies. In all countries studied, schemes that aimed to expand coverage for the poor were publicly financed primarily though general revenues. Some countries set minimum levels of health spending or labeled taxes for health, whereas others earmarked levies on luxury goods or alcohol and tobacco. Few countries leverage cross-subsidies from the contributory subsystem to the subsidized one.

The majority of countries increased public financing for health care—in absolute terms, as a share of GDP and as a share of total expenditures on health. Note that although the share of out-of-pocket payments has generally been reduced, in absolute terms this type of spending has been rising. As families in the region enjoy higher incomes, they consume more goods and services, and health care seems to be no exception. This is not in itself a problem if households are not experiencing financial hardship to access needed health care services; although not all reforms had an explicit objective of expanding financial protection, this was the result in many countries. This is discussed in greater detail in the next chapter.

Defining (or Not Defining) the Benefits Package

In the 1980s and 1990s in LAC, a considerable amount of energy was devoted to defining a benefits package of cost-effective interventions. Our review reveals a rather pragmatic approach to this issue in the countries studied. Some define a detailed benefits package, whereas others adopt an approach closer to that of the OECD countries in which a positive list is defined in broad terms, such as in Israel and the Netherlands, which focus on adopting new technologies at the margin. When defined, the packages can be comprehensive or limited; when limited, they tend to focus on ambulatory, primary care, and they often start with services for mothers and children. However, in at least one country, Jamaica, the subsidy program covered medicines for conditions that accounted for the largest share of the burden of disease.

Packages are not static and tend to expand over time to cover more complex treatments and services that benefit a wider range of the population and respond to the changing demographics and to epidemiological conditions of the country. Although we did not delve into how decisions are made about what is covered or not, we speculate that they are based on a combination of affordability, technical consideration regarding service effectiveness and costs, public demand and normative choices, and lobbying by interested parties. What is clear is that the absence of explicit and transparent processes to determine the expansion of benefits and adoption of new technologies can be costly and lead to suboptimal outcomes. Judicialization of the right to health care for all in LAC can have the adverse effect of increasing inequality in access if those with deeper pockets are better able to mount lawsuits to obligate the state to provide the services they require or desire (Iunes, Cubillos-Turriago, and Escobar 2012).

Paying and Managing Providers

Few countries tackled the behemoth task of fully separating purchaser and provider functions, whereby public funds would be used to buy services from whichever provider, public or private, offers the best quality-price combination. In purchasing, as in defining the benefits package, most countries took a rather pragmatic approach. In large part, publicly financed services continue to be delivered through public providers, and in many countries these are still largely paid through the government budget. However, the way in which providers are paid or managed has changed. Some countries switched to paying providers through capitation (often with monitoring of priority interventions), whereas others built mechanisms on top of regular budget transfers to incentivize results either through capitation for enrollment of beneficiaries or fee-for-service payments for services delivered. Countries that have decentralized systems also use federal transfers based on enrollment of beneficiaries, achievement of coverage, or other targets to reduce disparities in financing at the subnational level and promote priority programs. In some cases, the funds transferred were substantial, but not in all. Reforms also generally increased provider autonomy to manage funds with the scope coverage-expansion program and instituted greater accountability by establishing explicit agreements that outline roles, responsibilities, and expected results.

Prioritizing Primary Care

Many countries emphasized delivering primary care to improve access for the poor who lacked basic services while also managing health care costs. (Primary care is typically cost-effective and helps prevent diseases and conditions that can be costly to treat.) Many countries began by focusing on maternal and child health care services and expanded to cover prevention of noncommunicable diseases and more specialized services. However, lack of integration across the levels of the health care networks becomes a bottleneck to delivering effective care. Some countries are implementing regulations and policies to amplify and strengthen integrated networks, though efforts in many cases are still incipient (for example, Brazil, Colombia, Costa Rica, and Uruguay). These initiatives often entail innovations in digital and electronic clinical information systems (for example, eHealth) that systematically collect, integrate, and electronically exchange information across the care continuum, facilitating referral and counter-referral. For example, electronic medical records allow patients who would ideally enter the system at the primary-care level, to be followed as they access more specialized secondary or tertiary care and require diagnostic services that may not be available at the lower level. Recent surveys suggest that a majority of countries in the region are implementing or intending to implement eHealth policies or plans (OSILAC 2007; WHO 2006). These sometimes include a Telehealth component, which involves delivering health care services using information and communication technologies. Some countries use these to alleviate human resource constraints in remote or low-density areas and improve the quality of care at the primary level.

Equalizing Subsystems

The persistence of two-tiered systems (tax-financed ministries of health and payroll-financed social health insurance) has meant that considerable inequalities remain in the timely access to high-quality services. Countries in more advanced stages of reform—that is, those that have achieved high levels of overall coverage—are starting to implement policies to harmonize benefits across subsystems, including by instituting explicit guarantees. This sequencing of reforms seems to indicate that countries tend to first improve access to and raise the quality of care available for large segments of the population, including the poor and vulnerable groups, then address the more difficult issue of reducing disparities in the benefits available to different segments of the population.

Notes

1. Though the WHO cube does not explicitly include quality as a dimension, we consider it an essential aspect of UHC. We discuss it to some extent under benefit coverage in this chapter and devote chapter 5 to a more in-depth discussion of the issue.

2. The Caribbean countries do not generally share the same history of employment-based social health insurance, and therefore these observations regarding segmentation do not apply to Jamaica.

3. The term *public* refers to Ministry of Health facilities at the national or subnational level. It excludes facilities that belong to the social health insurance system, even though in some countries these are public entities. The distinction is that access to the latter is often restricted to beneficiaries of the schemes, whereas access to the former is unrestricted.

4. No inferences should be made about changes in private insurance coverage in Chile because the 2003 survey did not collect data on this indicator.

5. Vertical integration refers to financing and provision of services by the same institution.

6. The issue of waiting time is discussed at length in chapter 5.

7. Only two OECD countries exceed this threshold: New Zealand (20.3 percent) and Switzerland (20.6 percent).

8. Though not well documented, migration from private to public services is known to occur in other countries in the region.

References

Alcalde-Rabanal, Jacqueline Elizabeth, Oswaldo Lazo-González, and Gustavo Nigenda. 2011. "Sistema de salud de Perú." *Salud Pública de México* 53 (Suppl. 2): 243–54.

Aran, D., and H. Laca. 2011. "Sistema de salud de Uruguay." *Salud Pública de México* 53 (Suppl. 2): 197–207.

Atun, Rifat, Luiz Odorico Monteiro de Andrade, Gisele Almeida, Daniel Cotlear, Tania. Dmytraczenko, Patricia Frenz, Patrícia Garcia, Octavio Gómez-Dantés, Felicia M. Knaul, Carles Muntaner, Juliana Braga de Paula, Felix Rígoli, Pastor Castell-Florit Serrate, and Adam Wagstaff. 2015. "Health-System Reform and Universal Health Coverage in Latin America." Series on Universal Health Coverage in Latin America. *The Lancet* 385: 1230–47.

Baeza, C., and T. Packard. 2006. *Beyond Survival: Protecting Households from Health Shocks in Latin America*. Washington, DC: World Bank.

Becerril-Montekio, Víctor, and Luis López-Dávila. 2011. "Sistema de salud de Guatemala." *Salud Pública de México* 53 (Suppl. 2): 243–54.

Belló, Mariana, and Víctor M. Mecerril-Montekio. 2011. "Sistema de salud de Argentina." *Salud Pública de Mexico* 53: s96–109.

Bitran, Ricardo. 2013. *Explicit Health Guarantees for Chileans: The AUGE Benefits Packages*. UNICO Study Series 21, World Bank, Washington, DC.

Bonilla-Chacín, Maria Eugenia, and Nelly Aguilera. 2013. "The Mexican Social Protection System in Health." UNICO Study Series 1, World Bank, Washington, DC.

Borda, O. 2001. "Comentarios sobre la diversidad de los movimientos sociales." In *Movimientos sociales, Estado y democracia en Colombia*, edited by M. Archila and M. Pardo. Bogota: Universidad Nacional de Colombia.

Busse R., J. Schreyögg, and C. Gericke. 2007. "Analyzing Changes in Health Financing Arrangements in High-Income Countries: A Comprehensive Framework Approach." HNP Discussion Paper, World Bank, Washington, DC.

Carrin G., C. James, and D.B. Evans. 2005. "Achieving Universal Health Coverage: Developing the Health Financing System." Technical Briefs for Policy-Makers, Number 1, WHO/EIP/HSF/PB/05.01, World Health Organization, Geneva.

Cercone, J., E. Pinder, J. P. Jimenez, and R. Briceno. 2010. "Impact of Health Insurance on Access, Use and Health Status in Costa Rica." In *The Impact of Health Insurance in Low- and Middle-Income Countries*, edited by Maria-Luisa Escobar, Charles C. Griffin, and R. Paul Shaw. Washington, DC: Brookings Institution Press.

Chao, Shiyan. 2013. "Jamaica's Effort in Improving Universal Access within Fiscal Constraints." UNICO Study Series 6, World Bank, Washington, DC.

Cortez, Rafael, and Daniela Romero. 2013. "Increasing Utilization of Health Care Services among the Uninsured Population: The Plan Nacer Program." UNICO Study Series 12, World Bank, Washington, DC.

Cotlear, Daniel, Octavio Gómez-Dantés, Felicia Knaul, Rifat Atun, Ivana C. H. C. Barreto, Oscar Cetrángolo, Marcos Cueto, Pedro Francke, Patricia Frenz, Ramiro Guerrero, Rafael Lozano, Robert Marten, and Rocío Sáenz. 2015. "Overcoming Social Segregation in Health Care in Latin America." Series on Universal Health Coverage in Latin America 2. *The Lancet* 385: 1248–59.

Couttolenc, Bernard, and Tania Dmytraczenko. 2013. "Brazil's Primary Care Strategy." UNICO Study Series 2, World Bank, Washington, DC.

Francke, Pedro. 2013. "Peru's Comprehensive Health Insurance and New Challenges for Universal Coverage." UNICO Study Series 11, World Bank, Washington, DC.

Gómez Dantés, O., S. Sesma, V. M. Becerril, F. M. Knaul, H. Arreola, and J. Frenk. 2011. "The Health System of Mexico." *Salud Pública de México* 53 (Suppl. 2): s220–32.

Gragnolati, Michele, Magnus Lindelow, and Bernard Couttolenc. 2013. *Twenty Years of Health System Reform in Brazil: An Assessment of the Sistema Único de Saúde*. Washington, DC: World Bank.

Iunes R., L. Cubillos-Turriago, and M. L. Escobar. 2012. "Universal Health Coverage and Litigation in Latin America." *En Breve* 178, World Bank, Washington, DC.

Kurowski, Christoph, and Ian Walker. 2010. "Financing for Universal Health Coverage in Latin America and the Caribbean." Background paper, Human Development Department, Latin America and the Caribbean Region, World Bank, Washington, DC.

Kutzin, Joseph. 2001. "A Descriptive Framework for Country-Level Analysis of Health Care Financing Arrangements." *Health Policy* 56: 171–204. http://www.equinetafrica.org/bibl/docs/KUTequity01022007.pdf.

———. 2008. "Health Financing Policy: A Guide for Decision-Makers." Health Financing Policy Paper, Regional Office for Europe of the World Health Organization, Barcelona.

Lao Pena, Christine. 2013. "Improving Access to Health Care Services through the Expansion of Coverage Program (PEC): The Case of Guatemala." UNICO Study Series 19, World Bank, Washington, DC.

Lozano, R., P. Soliz, E. Gakidou, J. Abbot-Klafter, D. M. Feehan, C. Vidal, J. P. Ortiz, and C. J. Murray. 2006. "Benchmarking of Performance of Mexican States with Effective Coverage." *The Lancet* 368: 1729–41.

Ministerio de Salud Pública. *La Construcción del Sistema Nacional Integrado de Salud 2005–2009.* http://www.psico.edu.uy/sites/default/files/cursos/nas_la_construccion.pdf.

Montenegro Torres, Fernando. 2013. "Costa Rica Case Study: Primary Health Care Achievements and Challenges with the Framework of the Social Health Insurance." UNICO Study Series 14, World Bank, Washington, DC.

Montenegro Torres, Fernando, and Oscar Bernal-Acevedo. 2013. "The Subsidized Regime of Colombia's National Health Insurance System." UNICO Study Series 15, World Bank, Washington, DC.

OECD (Organisation for Economic Co-operation and Development). 2000. *A System of Health Accounts.* Paris: OECD.

OSILAC (Observatory for the Information Society in Latin America and the Caribbean). 2007. *Monitoring eLAC2007: Progress and Current State of Development of Latin American and Caribbean Information Societies.* Santiago, Chile: United Nations.

PAHO (Pan American Health Organization). 2014. "Strategy and Plan of Action on eHealth." 51st Directing Council, 63rd Session of the Regional Committee, CD51/13 (Eng.), PAHO, Washington, DC.

Paraje, Guillermo, and Felipe Vásquez. 2012. "Toward Universal Health Coverage: The Case of Chile." World Bank, Washington, DC.

Ribe, Helena, David A. Robalino, and Ian Walker. 2010. *Achieving Effective Social Protection for All in Latin America and the Caribbean: From Right to Reality.* Washington, DC: World Bank.

Savedoff, William, David de Ferranti, Amy L. Smith, and Victoria Fan. 2012. "Political and Economic Aspects of the Transition to Universal Health Coverage." *The Lancet* 380: 924–32.

Schieber, George, and Akiko Maeda. 1999. "Health Care Financing and Delivery in Developing Countries." *Health Affairs* 18 (3): 193–205.

Scott, Ewan, and Karl Theodore. 2013. "Measuring and Explaining Health and Health Care Inequalities in Jamaica, 2004 and 2007." *Pan American Journal of Public Health* 33 (2): 116–21.

Scott, John, and Beatriz Yadira Diaz. 2013. "Health Inequalities in Mexico: 2000–2010." World Bank, Washington, DC.

Sollazzo, Ana, and Rosario Berterretche. 2011. "El Sistema Nacional Integrado de Salud en Uruguay y los desafíos para la Atención Primaria." *Ciência & Saúde-Coletiva* 16 (6): 2829–40.

Tsai, Thomas C. 2010. "Second Chance for Health Reform in Colombia." *The Lancet* 375: 109–10.

WHO (World Health Organization). 2003. *Guide to Producing National Health Accounts: with Special Applications for Low-Income and Middle-Income Countries.* Geneva: WHO.

———. 2005. "Sustainable Health Financing, Universal Coverage and Social Health Insurance." Resolution WHA58.33, Fifty-eighth World Health Assembly, Geneva, May 16–25.

———. 2006. *Building Foundations for eHealth: Progress of Member States: Report of the Global Observatory for eHealth.* Geneva: WHO.

———. 2010. *The World Health Report 2010: Health System Financing—The Path to Universal Coverage.* Geneva: WHO.

World Bank. 2012a. "Republic of Uruguay Integrated National Health System Analysis of the Governability of the SNIS Benefit Plan (PIAS)." Report 80084-UY, World Bank, Washington, DC.

———. 2012b. "World Development Indicators." http://data.worldbank.org/data-catalog/world-development-indicators.

Progress toward Universal Health Coverage in Latin America and the Caribbean: Outcomes, Utilization, and Financial Protection

Tania Dmytraczenko, Gisele Almeida, Heitor Werneck,
James Cercone, Yadira Díaz, Daniel Maceira, Silvia Molina,
Guillermo Paraje, Fernando Ruiz, Flávia Mori Sarti, Ewan Scott,
John Scott, and Martín Valdivia

Abstract

The region has made considerable progress implementing schemes aimed at expanding universal health coverage in the past quarter-century. Measureable improvements in equity have been identified during the same period. Socioeconomic gradients are clearly present in health status, with the poor having worse observed health outcomes than the rich, but disparities have narrowed, particularly for early stages of the life course. Countries have reached high levels of coverage for maternal and child health services but, despite narrowing inequality, services remain pro-rich. Coverage of noncommunicable disease interventions is not as high as maternal and child health services and service utilization is skewed toward the better off, though these disparities continue to narrow as well. Primary care services are in general more equally distributed across income groups than is specialized care. Prevalence of noncommunicable diseases has not declined as expected given drops in mortality across these groups. Greater access to services, and hence diagnosis, among wealthier individuals may be masking differences in actual prevalence between income groups. Catastrophic health expenditures have declined in most countries, though the picture regarding equity is mixed due to measurement limitations.

Introduction

The previous chapter showed the diverse paths that Latin American and Caribbean countries have taken in moving toward universal health coverage (UHC). In this chapter we attempt to measure their progress along these diverse paths. A number of studies have assessed the health reforms in specific countries (Bitrán, Muñoz, and Prieto 2010; Cercone and others 2010; Giedion and

Uribe 2009; Gragnolati, Lindelow, and Couttolenc 2013). This chapter complements the foregoing work by applying common metrics across all the study countries to gauge their individual progress toward UHC and compare them to other countries engaged in similar efforts.

But first we must identify quantifiable, meaningful measures for assessing the broad range of reforms aimed at advancing UHC in Latin American and Caribbean countries. And these broad assessment tools must also capture data specific to any given country, whose reforms were designed, after all, to address particular national challenges. We draw on proposed definitions of UHC to identify indicators that measure progress along the three dimensions of the World Health Organization (WHO) cube. These can be derived from existing data sources available over multiple periods for at least a subset of countries. We then investigate changes along the major dimensions of UHC among socioeconomic subgroups over a period spanning the policies and programs described in the previous chapter. We want to see whether improvements are occurring across income groups. The analysis builds on previous work on income-related inequalities in health status and health care utilization in six Latin American and Caribbean countries (Almeida and Sarti 2013). Original data analysis was carried out for 9 of the 10 countries whose health policies were reviewed in the previous chapter.[1] We broadened the discussion to include other countries in the region when comparable data was available.

It is worth noting that this study is not attempting to establish causality between reforms and the changes witnessed. Other studies have done this and their main findings are summarized in Giedion, Alfonso, and Díaz (2013).

Breadth of Coverage

Over the past decade, most countries have seen a rapid expansion of population coverage, mostly through scale-up of general tax-subsidized insurance schemes that target the poor and finance services delivered primarily in the public health care network. As envisioned, when first rolled out, these schemes are highly pro-poor. At a high level of overall population coverage, subsidized scheme enrollment becomes more evenly distributed across income groups while coverage of employment-based schemes becomes even more skewed toward the rich than it had already been.

Breadth is one dimension of UHC, and it refers to the proportion of the population covered by a scheme that pools funds enabling beneficiaries to access health services without incurring financial hardship (OECD 2004; WHO 2008, 2010). Coverage through pooling mechanisms is generally high in the region; some countries reach levels equivalent to OECD countries (OECD 2011; figure 4.1). Though coverage levels correlate strongly with income, outliers exist: Colombia's population coverage, for example, is considerably higher than Peru's, though the two countries have similar per capita incomes, adjusted for differences in purchasing power.

As discussed in the previous chapter, countries in the region have implemented diverse coverage models. Costa Rica chose to expand coverage of a single,

Figure 4.1 Population Coverage of Pooling Mechanisms with Ring-Fenced Financing, Relative to GDP per Capita (PPP in Current International $, 2013)

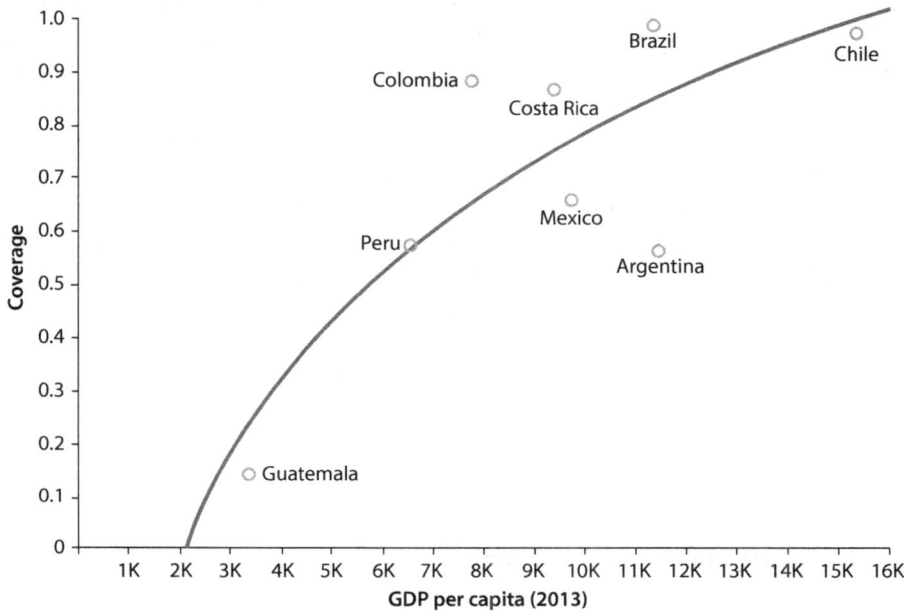

Sources: World Development Indicators and study estimates based on Argentina—ECV 1997; SUMAR Memorias 1997; PAMI Memorias 2012, EPH 2013; ENGH 2013; Brazil—PNAD 2008; Chile—CASEN 2011; Colombia—ECV 2010; Costa Rica—ENSA 2006; Guatemala—ENCOVI 2011; Mexico—ENIGH 2010; Peru—ENAHO 2011.
Note: Ring-fenced financing refers to setting legal minimum levels of spending on health, labeling taxes as being for health, or earmarking payroll taxes or other levies for health. GDP = gross domestic product.

mostly contributory social health insurance scheme, the Costa Rican Social Security System (CCSS). Brazil created a national health system—the Unified Health System (SUS, *Sistema Único de Saúde*)—that replaced the previous social health insurance model. Most countries—Argentina, Chile, Colombia, Mexico, Peru, and Uruguay—have chosen to maintain contributory schemes financed mostly from payroll taxes and to create separate pooling arrangements that subsidize, from general tax revenues, enrollment of the poor. Within this group, Chile, Colombia, and Uruguay have achieved a high level of integration between the two subsystems. In contrast, Guatemala and Jamaica have made efforts to supplement budget-financed ministry of health services in ways other than through the creation of an insurance mechanism for the poor. In Guatemala, this includes contracting private providers to deliver care in areas not reached by the public network. In Jamaica, it has entailed eliminating user fees and creating a fund, financed mostly through earmarked taxes, that subsidizes medicines for those suffering from noncommunicable diseases (NCDs).

Except in Brazil and Jamaica, private voluntary insurance has remained low and strongly pro-rich. Changes, if any, in the share of the population having this type of coverage have been modest (one or two percentage points in either direction), though the decline in Mexico and rise in Jamaica were more significant. The growth of private insurance in Brazil occurred entirely in the bottom 40 percent of the population, and the proliferation of low-premium policies has led to heightened enforcement of regulations designed to weed out junk policies (box 4.1).

Total enrollment in social health insurance has increased steadily over the past decade. In Costa Rica as well as in countries with semi-integrated systems—a subsidized regime and a contributory subsystem comprised of one or more schemes—overall coverage is distributed fairly equally across income groups.[2] This can be illustrated by the concentration curve, which plots the cumulative distribution of the variable in question against the cumulative distribution of individuals ranked in ascending order of standard of living, income in this case (Wagstaff and others 2011). In figure 4.2, the distribution of total health insurance coverage (contributory plus subsidized schemes) corresponds closely with the line of equality, along which the distribution of the variable being measured is unrelated to the living-standards measurement; this is most pronounced in countries with high levels of coverage such as Chile and Colombia. This equality is achieved by faster expansion of the subsidized regime, which is pro-poor in nature (i.e., the

---

Box 4.1 Private Health Insurance Coverage in Brazil, 1998–2008

Coverage of voluntary private medical[a] insurance decreased slightly, 1.7 percent, in Brazil from 1998 to 2008, but with notable differences across income groups (figure B4.1.1). Though private insurance coverage is positively correlated with income, the share of the population in the top two quintiles enrolled in private plans is shrinking (a 5.3 percent drop between 1998 and 2008), while the opposite is true for the bottom 40 percent (a 23.3 percent rise). Voluntary private health insurance in Brazil, particularly among adults,[b] is mostly obtained as an employment fringe benefit (nearly three-quarters of policies were employment-based in 2008, according to data from the National Regulatory Agency for Private Health Insurance and Plans); changes in private coverage are largely attributable to shifts in the labor market. Unemployment declined sharply, from 12.4 in 2003 to 7.9 percent in 2008, and the share of formal sector employment increased from 39.7 to 44.0 percent in the same period, with benefits accruing to the poor who were overrepresented among the informally employed.

Figure B4.1.1 Private Medical Insurance Coverage by Quintile

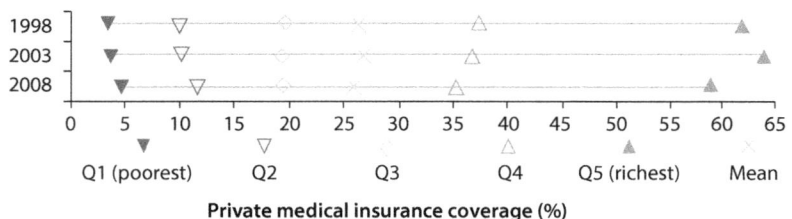

Private medical insurance coverage (%)

Sources: PNAD 1998, 2003, and 2008.
a. This analysis excludes dental-only plans.
b. This analysis was done for the adult population. Population coverage of private medical insurance including children is slightly lower, 24 percent compared to 26 percent for the adult population in 2008.

Figure 4.2 Distribution of Social Health Insurance Coverage across Income Groups

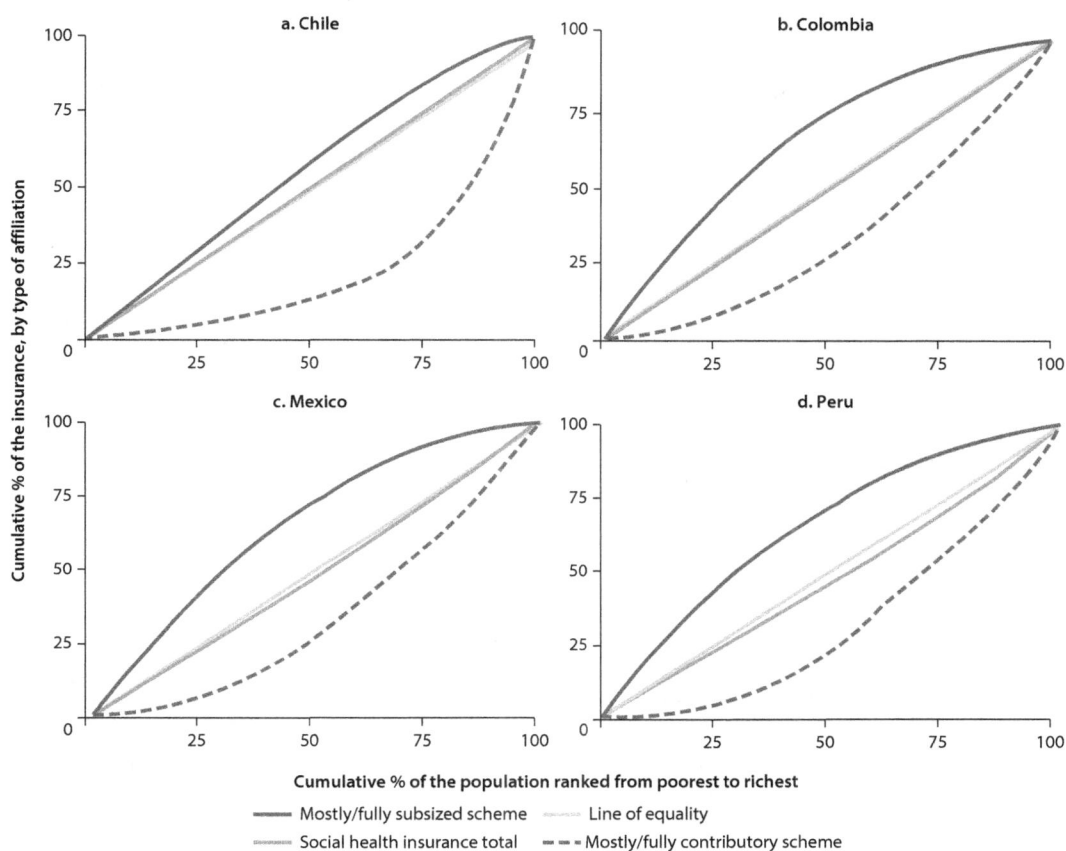

Sources: Study estimates based on Chile—CASEN 2011; Colombia—ECV 2010; Mexico—ENIGH 2010; Peru—ENAHO 2011.
Note: Subsidized: Chile—FONASA; Colombia—Régimen Subsidiado; Mexico—Seguro Popular; Peru—Sistema Integral de Salud. Contributory: Chile—ISAPRES; Colombia—Régimen Contributivo; Mexico—IMSS, ISSSTE, PEMEX. Social health insurance total is the sum of the subsidized and contributory regimes.

concentration curve lies above the line of equality) and counterbalances the contributory subsystem, whose enrollees tend to comprise the better off.

An interesting pattern emerges in enrollment in the two schemes as overall social health insurance expands within and across countries. At low levels of overall coverage (for example, Peru at 24–57 percent), the subsidized regime is increasingly pro-poor because it captures mostly those who are poor and uninsured. The negative and rising (in absolute value) concentration index reflects this—a summary statistic derived from the concentration curve that ranges between 1 and negative 1: it is positive when the variable of interest is concentrated among the wealthy, and negative when the opposite is true (figure 4.3). In Peru and Mexico, the contributory regimes also become less pro-rich owing to growth in middle-class enrollments.

In countries with high levels of total coverage, however, such as Colombia (64–88 percent) and Chile (92–97 percent), expansion is occurring from growth

Figure 4.3 Trend in Concentration of Social Health Insurance Subsystems across Income Groups, by Levels of Coverage

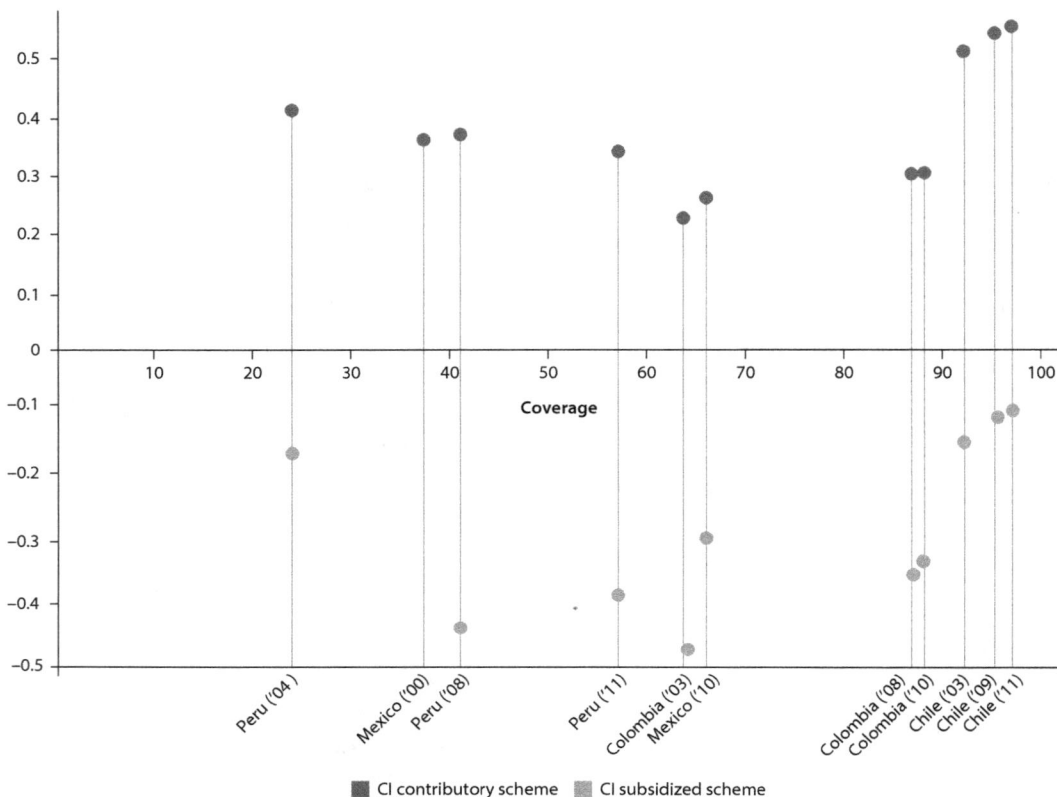

Sources: Study estimates based on Chile—CASEN 2003, 2009, and 2011; Colombia—ECV 2003, 2008, and 2010; Mexico—ENIGH 2000 and 2010; Peru—ENAHO 2004, 2008, and 2011.
Note: CI = concentration index.

in the mostly subsidized regimes. As middle-class enrollment ramps up, these regimes become less pro-poor. As illustrated in figure 4.4, the subsidized regime expands in part because the better off migrate to this subsystem from the contributory one. In turn, the contributory subsystem comprises ever-greater concentrations of the rich beyond a certain level of overall coverage. In Chile, where near-universal insurance coverage has been attained, the share of the population as well as the number of people enrolled in the fully contributory scheme actually declined in the study period. As the uninsured population dwindles, overrepresentation of the poor in this group declines; in Chile, the situation is reversed: 4 percent of the population in the top two quintiles is uninsured compared with 2 percent in the bottom three quintiles.

These broad categories—insured/uninsured, contributory/subsidized—mask a more nuanced reality. For instance, the subsidized regimes in Mexico and Peru

Figure 4.4 Population Distribution (by Quintile) across Health Insurance Subsystems

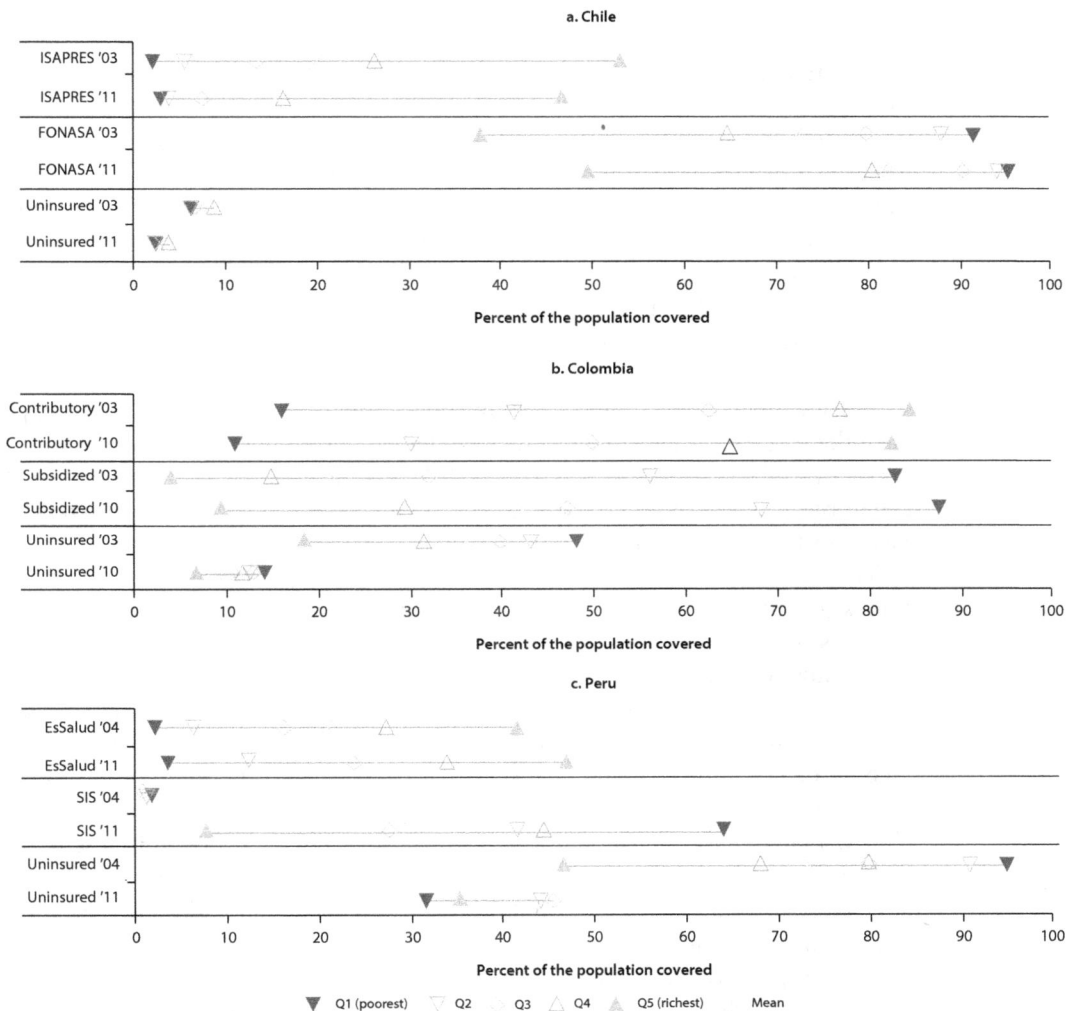

a. Chile

b. Colombia

c. Peru

Percent of the population covered

▼ Q1 (poorest)　▽ Q2　◇ Q3　△ Q4　▲ Q5 (richest)　Mean

Sources: Study estimates based on Chile—CASEN 2003 and 2011; Colombia—ECV 2003 and 2010; Peru—ENAHO 2004 and 2011.
Note: Uninsured refers to those who are not enrolled in a formal insurance scheme, although they may still have access to the public health system.

allow in theory for premiums to be collected from enrollees who have capacity to pay, though in practice this is not happening; in Chile, over a third of the budget of the subsidized regime is financed from member contributions. Similarly, in several countries, the contributory regimes are to some extent subsidized. This is true in Costa Rica, which expanded coverage to the poor and vulnerable populations by financing their enrollment in the CCSS through tax-financed subsidies. It is also true in Mexico, where the contributory schemes receive public subsidies. Even in countries where some people do not belong to a specific scheme, they can still receive services free of charge in public facilities if they are deemed to be poor. Even prior to the reforms of the 1990s, health ministries in most countries were responsible, at least on paper, for delivering care to the population. This was particularly the case for those not covered by employment-based or other insurance schemes or those who were unable to afford private care. And, to this day, health ministries continue to provide care to the so-called uninsured. For instance, Guatemala and Peru still report substantial coverage by their health ministries, 70 and 58 percent respectively (see table 5.1 in PAHO 2012). Further, even those insured under contributory or private schemes revert to tertiary teaching hospitals, which are generally tax-funded public facilities, when they need highly specialized (and expensive) care. So what has changed in practice?

This discussion points to the limitations of defining UHC according to who is entitled to certain programs or what benefits people receive in theory. In the next sections, we will delve more deeply into the dimensions of UHC by looking at both the scope (services covered) and the depth of coverage (proportion of direct costs covered; WHO 2008, 2010). We will assess service utilization and its financial implications as opposed to de jure entitlements. We also examine progress in health outcomes across population groups.

Throughout the analysis, we will ask whether gains are seen across all population segments. This effort takes us beyond the measurement of population averages—as with tracking the Millennium Development Goals (MDGs)—to measuring how benefits are distributed across the population. Our methods for measuring health inequality are summarized in boxes 4.2 and 4.3. For cross-country comparability, we elected to use socioeconomic groupings measured by income or consumption. In exceptional cases, when income and consumption data were unavailable, we used a wealth index. This is but one dimension of equity. Depending on the country context, for policy purposes, it might be relevant to look at variations across national territory, ethnic groups, gender, education, or other social determinants of health. These should all be analyzed to build a comprehensive picture of equity in the region (CSDH 2008).

In addition, we postulate that a comprehensive measure of UHC should extend into areas related to public health and primary care, essential components of health policy. As highlighted in the previous chapter, a common thread of reforms in the region has been a renewed focus on public health interventions aimed at reducing the likelihood of people falling sick in the first place, and primary care, including preventive services. Our living-standard measures rely on individual or household rankings. Health promotion and disease-prevention interventions are generally population based. So it is more challenging to analyze disparities in access than is the case with disparities in personal services accessed by specific individuals. We propose, instead, to measure changes in risk behaviors and lifestyles that have an impact on health and can be modified through health (and other) policies and interventions.

Finally, we realize countries in the region are in different stages of the demographic and epidemiological transition. We attempt to assess progress by measuring relevant indicators for the different stages of the life course and that

Box 4.2 Summary of the Methodology

For the analysis of population and services coverage and financial protection over time, we examined 56 nationally representative household surveys from nine countries: Argentina, Brazil, Chile, Colombia, Costa Rica, Guatemala, Jamaica, Mexico, and Peru (see table 4.2). In addition, we included data from the Demographic and Health Surveys (DHS) reported in the Health Equity and Financial Protection Datasheets (World Bank 2012), adding variables for LAC countries with data for the time period under study (Bolivia, the Dominican Republic, and Haiti).

To measure progress in the three UHC dimensions and health outcomes, change over time is analyzed across the population distribution, using the same set of questions for multiple variables, which are investigated at two or more points in time. Given the heterogeneity of the surveys across countries in Latin America and the Caribbean in terms of type, frequency, and data collection, it is a challenging undertaking to assess service coverage and financial protections among countries. To meet this challenge and ensure reliable results, we were careful to revise and select comparable variables across surveys. We also employed techniques to adjust the recall period and normalize binary variables for the study countries.

Our methodology expands and complements techniques previously used to measure inequality in service coverage for adults in selected LAC countries (Almeida and Sarti 2013) and is fully described in O'Donnell and Wagstaff (2008) and Wagstaff and others (2011). Appendix A provides further details of the methodology. We used the ADePT software to ensure comparability. Comparisons of health and utilization variables in two or more countries are important for assessments of UHC-related public policy and its impact on equity. Nevertheless, different populations and population groups may have justifiable differences in health outcomes and service utilization—for example, the elderly will have more health problems than adolescents and will therefore use more health services. So it is necessary to standardize for the characteristics responsible for justified variations in health and health care utilization. Age and sex have been used for the standardization of most variables, with the exception of child, maternal, and reproductive outcomes and services. In addition to age and sex, health-utilization variables require standardizing variables that describe need because those with greater health needs are expected to use more health services. The methodology calls for comparing the actual and the need-expected distribution to assess inequalities. To calculate need-expected distribution, need is proxied with health-status measures such as self-assessed health (SAH) status, chronic conditions, physical limitations, and/or difficulty with daily activities, when available. Our calculations are based on the indirect-standardization method. This method is preferred to direct standardization because it is more accurate for individual-level data analysis and it corrects the actual distribution of the variable of interest. It does this by comparing the actual distribution with the distribution that would be observed if individuals had their own characteristics, but with the same mean effects of those characteristics on the variable of interest as the entire population (Wagstaff and others 2011).

For the analysis, we used measures describing inequality across population groups and between the extreme categories. Their results have distinct characteristics and may suggest different actions. Measures used include concentration indices, concentration curves, and quintile distributions in their absolute and relative forms (see box 4.3).

Box 4.3 Measures of Inequality

Measures	Description
Quintile distributions	Distribution of the population by a living-standards measure (income, consumption, or wealth) into five groups of 20 percent, ranked from the worst off (Q1) to the better off (Q5). Rate ratio (Q5/Q1) is a relative measure of the socioeconomic-related inequality between two extremes, calculated as the mean value of the variable of interest for the 20 percent of the population with the highest living standards (Q5) divided by the mean value of the same variable for the 20 percent of the population with the lowest living standards (Q1). Rate difference (Q5-Q1) is an absolute measure of the socioeconomic-related inequality between two extremes, calculated as the mean variable of interest for the 20 percent of the population with the highest living standards (Q5) minus the mean of the variable of interest for the 20 percent of the population with the lowest living standards (Q1).
Concentration curve	The concentration curve is a measure of inequality across the entire population distribution that plots the cumulative share of the variable of interest against the cumulative population, ranked by socioeconomic position (income, consumption, or wealth) or any other variable that can be rank-ordered.
Concentration index	The concentration index (CI) is a summary measure of the information contained in the concentration curve, calculated as twice the area between the concentration curve and the line of equality. Its value ranges from −1 to 1 and is equal to zero when there is no inequality. By convention, when the variable of interest is disproportionately concentrated among the poor (the rich) the value of the CI is negative (positive) and the greater the inequality, the greater the CI in absolute terms. The CI measures relative inequality, i.e., the cumulative fraction of the variable of interest. The absolute CI is obtained by multiplying the CI by the population mean of the variable of interest; it measures the cumulative amount of the variable or interest.
Horizontal index	The horizontal inequity index (HI) is the need-standardized concentration index, calculated as the difference between the concentration index of the actual and need-predicted health care utilization.

relate to various health conditions, particularly maternal and neonatal health, and nutritional disorders, in addition to communicable and noncommunicable diseases (table 4.1).

Health Outcomes, Risk Factors, and Service Utilization across Different Segments of the Population

The Early Years

Child mortality rates have dropped significantly, as have disparities across wealth groups, though rates remain higher among the poor. Utilization of child health services has risen but is still generally pro-rich despite lessening inequality. Disease prevalence, which is concentrated among the poor, has not behaved as expected given the drop in mortality. Better access to services, and hence diagnosis, among wealthier individuals may be masking changes in actual prevalence.

Table 4.1 Indicators According to Relevance to Stages of the Life Course

	Early years	*Youth to middle years*	*Middle years and beyond*

Outcome	Under-five mortality rate
	Acute respiratory
	  infection
	Diarrhea
	Stunting
		Intimate partner violence
		  (women)
		Traffic accidents and injuries
			Self-assessed health status
			Asthma
			Depression
			Diabetes
			Heart disease

Risk factor		Alcohol consumption Tobacco use (women)	Diagnosed hypertension Obesity

Utilization	Full immunization
	Medical treatment of
	  acute respiratory
	  infection
	Treatment of diarrhea
	  (oral rehydration)
		Contraceptive prevalence rate
		Antenatal care
		Skilled birth attendance
		Cervical cancer screening
			Breast cancer screening
			
			Preventive care visit
			Curative care visit
			Outpatient care visit
			Inpatient admission

Financial protection		Catastrophic health expenditures Impoverishment	

Table 4.2 Surveys Analyzed

Country	*Survey*	*Year*
Argentina	National Risk Factor Survey (ENFR)	2005 and 2009
	National Utilization and Expenditure Survey (ENUG)	2003, 2005, and 2010
	National Household Expenditure Survey (ENGH)	1997 and 2005
Brazil	National Household Sampling Survey (PNAD)	1998, 2003, and 2008
	Pesquisa Nacional de Demografia e Saúde da Criança e da Mulher (PNDS)	1996 and 2006
	Household Budget Survey (POF)	2003 and 2008
Chile	National Socioeconomic Characterization Survey (CASEN)	2003, 2009, and 2011
	National Health Survey (ENS)	2009
	Health and Quality of Life National Survey (ENCAVI)	2006
	Survey of Satisfaction and Health Expenditures (ESGS)	2006
Colombia	Quality of Life Survey (ECV)	2003, 2008, and 2010
	Demographic and Health Survey (ENDS)	1995, 2000, 2005, and 2010
	National Nutrition Survey (ENSIN)	2005 and 2010
	National Health Survey (ENS)	2007
Costa Rica	Sexual and Reproductive Health Survey (ENSSR)	1999
	National Nutrition Survey (ENN)	2008
	National Health Survey (ENSA)	2006
	National Income and Expenditure Survey (ENIG)	2004 and 2013
Guatemala	Maternal and Infant Health Survey (ENSMI)	1995, 1998, 2002, and 2008–09
	National Survey on Life Conditions (ENCOVI)	2006 and 2011
Jamaica	Jamaica Survey of Living Conditions (JSLC)	2004, 2007, and 2009
Mexico	National Health Survey (ENSA)	2000
	National Health and Nutrition Survey (ENSANUT)	2006 and 2012
	National Income and Expenditure Survey (ENIGH)	2000, 2006, and 2010
Peru	Demographic and Health Survey (DHS)	1996, 2000, and 2004–08
	National Household Survey (ENAHO)	2004, 2008, and 2012

Note: To supplement DHS–Equity Datasheet results, we analyzed the Haiti DHS 2012. We also reestimated the contraceptive prevalence indicator for all LAC countries using the WHO definition (http://apps.who.int/gho/indicatorregistry).

Figure 4.5 Under-Five Mortality Rates, 1995–2012

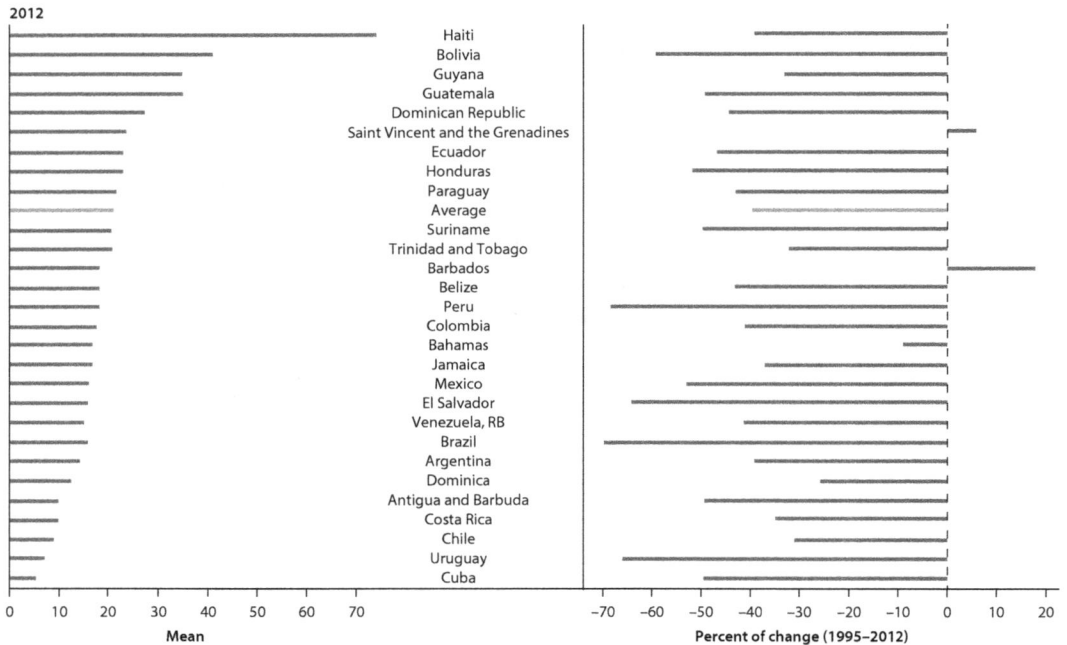

Haiti
Bolivia
Guyana
Guatemala
Dominican Republic
Saint Vincent and the Grenadines
Ecuador
Honduras
Paraguay
Average
Suriname
Trinidad and Tobago
Barbados
Belize
Peru
Colombia
Bahamas
Jamaica
Mexico
El Salvador
Venezuela, RB
Brazil
Argentina
Dominica
Antigua and Barbuda
Costa Rica
Chile
Uruguay
Cuba

Mean

Percent of change (1995–2012)

Source: UNICEF and others 2013.

The region has seen substantial improvements in infant and child mortality since 1990; by 2012 it had nearly reached the MDG target of reducing the under-five child mortality rate by two-thirds from 1990 to 2015 (figure 4.5). The rate of progress in Latin America for this MDG has outpaced that of most other regions (Liu and others 2012; UNICEF and others 2013). Improvements were seen in almost every country (the few exceptions are likely due to data quality), though there was considerable variation across the region. The strongest declines were seen in Brazil, Peru, Uruguay, and El Salvador—all of which have met the MDG goal ahead of schedule; progress in the Caribbean, however, is lagging.

Although overall trends in child mortality are unambiguously positive, the picture is mixed when it comes to differentials in mortality rates across wealth groups. Children today, irrespective of their place in the socioeconomic distribution, have a lower probability of dying than they did in 1995, and the gap between the poorest and the wealthiest has been reduced in all countries studied (figure 4.6). Yet poor children still die at a much higher rate than their rich age-mates; the probability of children in the poorest quintile dying before age five can be between 1.5 and 6 times higher than those in the top wealth tier. Whether measured as the simple ratio of the mortality rate in the top and bottom quintiles or through the concentration index that accounts for the

Figure 4.6 Under-Five Mortality Rates: Averages and Quintile Distribution, 1995–2012 (or Nearest Year)

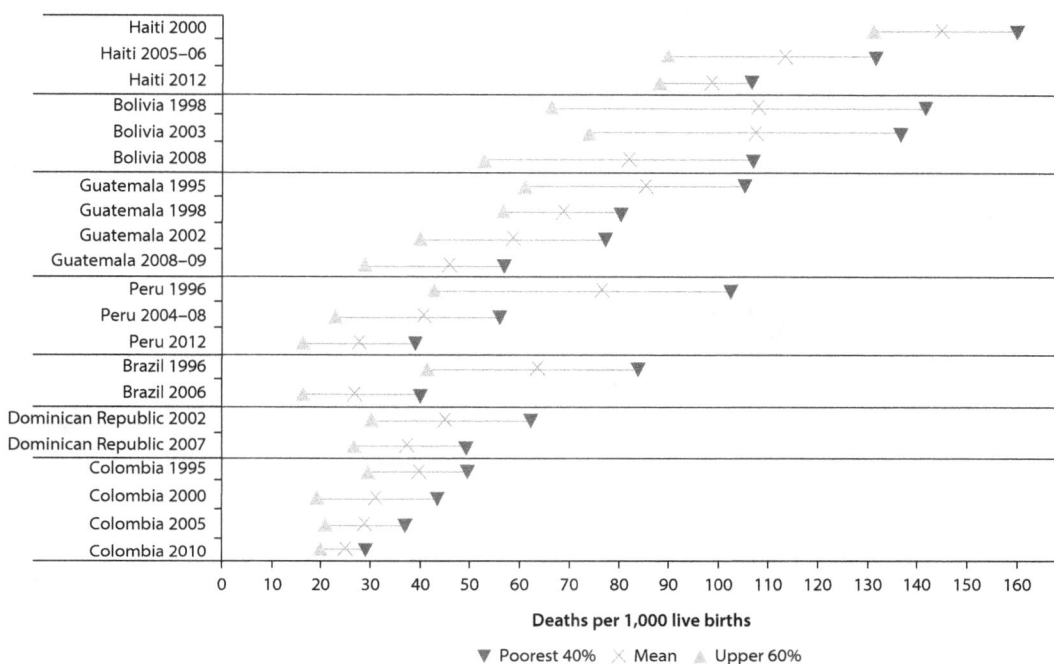

Sources: DHS–Equity Datasheet. Otherwise, study estimates based on Brazil—PNDS 2006; Guatemala—ENSMI 1998, 2002, and 2008–09; Haiti—DHS 2012; Peru—DHS 2012.
Note: Wealth quintiles were used for this analysis.

distribution of mortality across the population, relative inequality is highest in Guatemala, and Bolivia. Furthermore, relative inequality has risen in Guatemala between 1998 and 2002. This indicates that the drop in the national under-five mortality rate was driven by improvements among the better off. Colombia has the lowest mortality rate and most equitable distribution among the sampled countries.

The data are sparse on mortality disaggregated by socioeconomic status. This is the case in Latin America more so than elsewhere in the developing world because vital-statistic systems—which generally do not collect information on living standards—are replacing occasional surveys as the source of mortality data. Equity analysis is feasible when vital-statistic systems accurately and reliably record information on place of residence (Gonzalez and others 2009). But that is not yet the case in many Latin American and Caribbean countries, where systems still need to improve. An analysis of infant mortality rates by place of residence in Mexico, for example, shows a strong correlation between marginality and infant mortality, as well as a wide (as much as tenfold) gap in rates between the better- and worst-off localities (figure 4.7).

Figure 4.7　Municipalities Ordered by Infant Mortality Rate and Marginality Index—Mexico, 2005

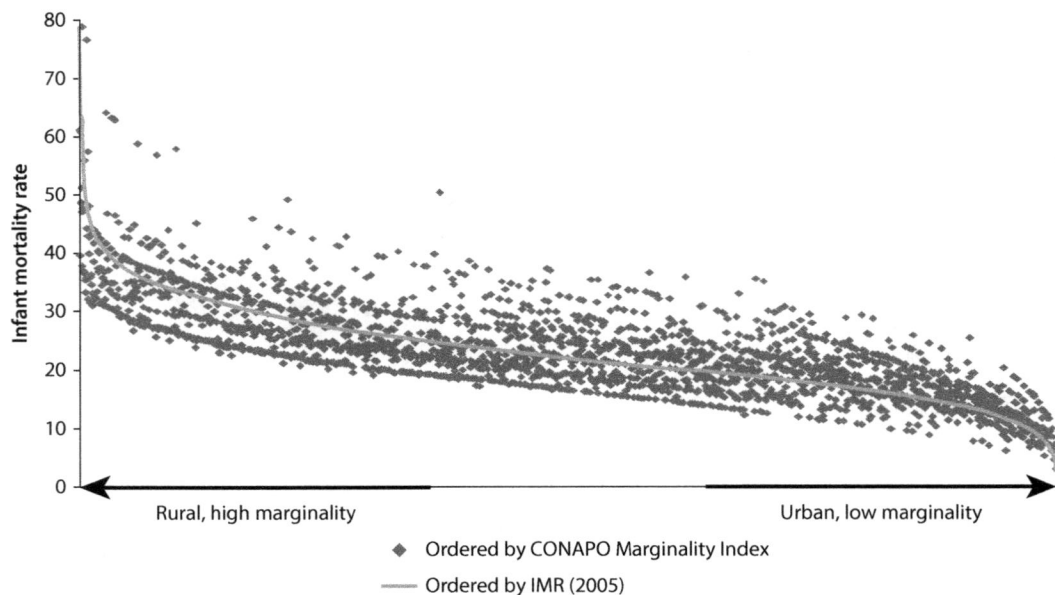

Source: Elaboration by John Scott based on the CONAPO Municipal Infant Mortality Rates database for 2005 (http://www.conapo.gob.mx/es/CONAPO/Estimacion_de_la_mortalidad_infantil_para_Mexico_las_entidades_federativas_y_los_municipios_2005) and the CONAPO Marginality Index for municipalities (CONAPO 2011).

Childhood Illnesses

Improvements in child health can be attributed in large part to a reduction in the burden of disease associated with diarrhea, respiratory infections, meningitis, and other infectious diseases. In 1995 these conditions were the single largest contributor to loss of healthy life in children under 5, accounting for 41 percent of disability-adjusted life years in Latin America and the Caribbean (LAC). A decade and a half later their share had dropped to 21 percent (IHME 2010). Reduction in deaths from pneumonia, measles, and diarrhea contributed most to lessening the global burden of disease in children younger than five years. In the years from 2000 to 2010, the fastest annual rate of decline in cause-specific mortality in the Americas came from reduced neonatal mortalities due to diarrhea, tetanus, and pneumonia; among children aged 1–59 months, similar reductions were seen in mortalities from diarrhea, meningitis, AIDS, and pneumonia (Liu and others 2012). Among these, diarrhea and pneumonia account for the highest burden of disease at the outset of this 10-year period. With the strong decline in mortality from diarrhea, pneumonia is today the principal cause of death in children under age five (Rudan and others 2008). Figure 4.8 shows the incidence of diarrhea and acute respiratory infections in the 0–5 age group across socioeconomic quintiles. Because these illnesses are fairly common, they don't require large-sample population surveys to collect data disaggregated by socioeconomic strata (in contrast, for example, to meningitis or AIDS). The prevalence of acute respiratory infections has fallen in all countries, except Haiti from 2005

Figure 4.8 Prevalence of Childhood Illnesses: Averages and Quintile Distribution, 1995–2012 (or Nearest Year)

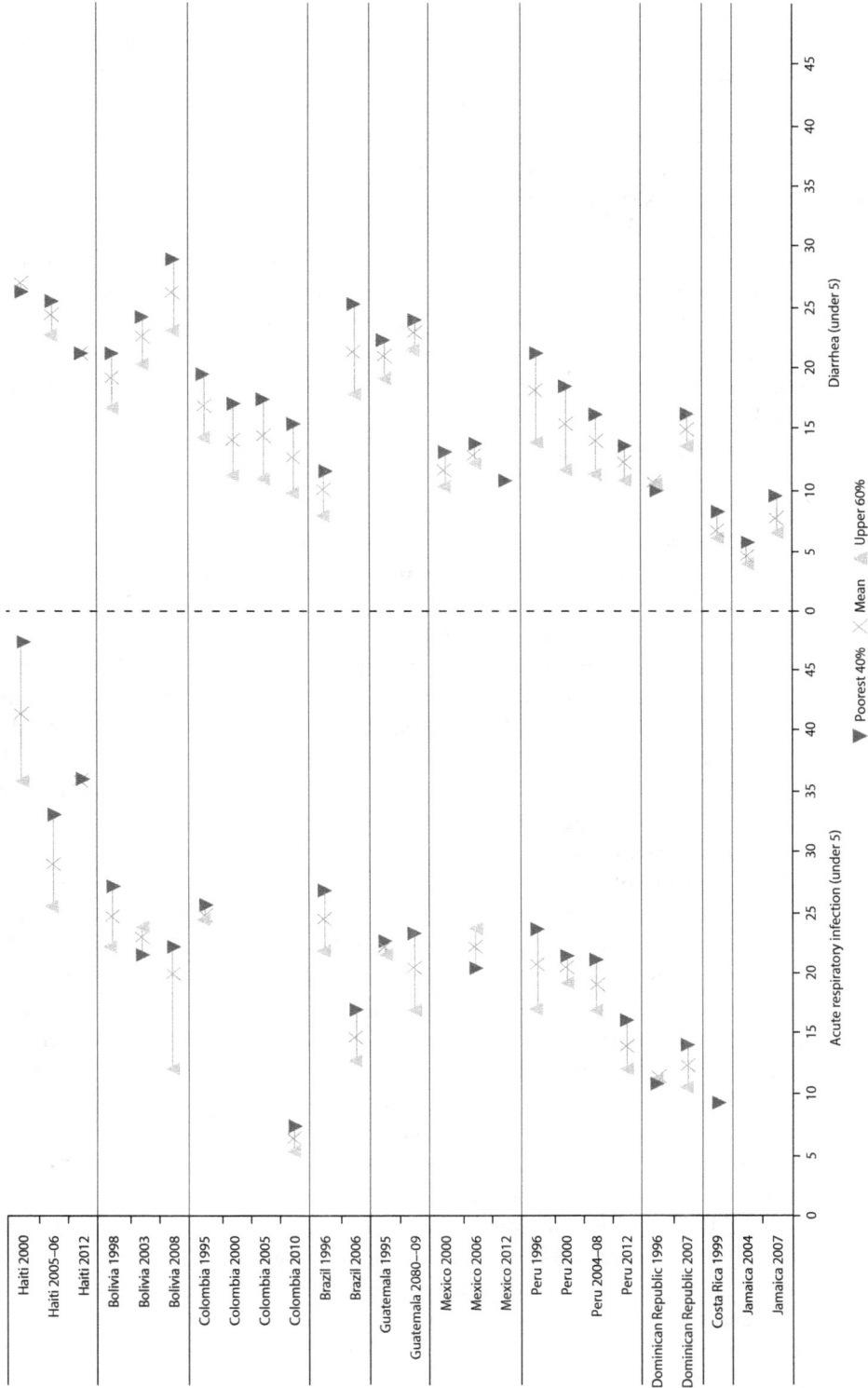

Sources: DHS—Equity Datasheet. Otherwise, study estimates based on Brazil—PNDS 2006; Costa Rica—ENSSR 1999; Guatemala—ENSMI 2008–09; Haiti—DHS 2012; Jamaica—JSLC 2004 and 2007; Mexico—ENSA 2000, ENSANUT 2006 and 2012; Peru—DHS 2012.

Note: Wealth quintiles, were used for this analysis except for Jamaica and Mexico.

to 2012 (and the Dominican Republic, where the increase was marginal). Given the decline in mortality due to the disease, one would expect a similar decline in diarrhea prevalence. This is not reflected in the data, however, perhaps because of better access to diagnoses. Unlike acute respiratory infections, diarrhea is not necessarily an acute condition and is therefore more likely to go undetected.

This discussion highlights a challenge with prevalence data: it is difficult to separate the existence of the condition from its detection. Although the condition itself may be more prevalent among the poor, more cases are probably diagnosed (and treated) among the better off. This explains why the inequality gradient is not as severe for disease prevalence as for mortality. Still, the results in figure 4.8 show that in all cases diarrhea is more prevalent among the poor. Acute respiratory infections are also more prevalent among the poor in most countries, except for Mexico; independent of the measure used, equity has worsened everywhere except Haiti. This may reflect the equity improvements in access to care discussed below.

Child Health Services

Immunization. Vaccinating children against major childhood diseases and preventing and treating diarrhea and pneumonia (in addition to malaria) were the top two best buys in health based on averted cost per disability-adjusted life year (Laxminarayan and Ashford 2008). Figure 4.9 presents data on coverage of these services disaggregated by socioeconomic strata. Note the distinctions among the three health-intervention indicators. There is a clear protocol for basic immunization and a known target: before age two all children should receive at least one dose of the anti-tuberculosis vaccine, BCG, three doses of polio vaccine, three doses of diphtheria-tetanus-pertussis (DTP3) vaccine, and one dose of measles vaccine.[3] Oral rehydration is also a specific treatment known to reduce dehydration and deaths from diarrheal diseases. But, unlike vaccination, the target illness is not as clear: not all children who have diarrhea need oral rehydration salts or homemade rehydration solution. The indicator on percentage of children receiving medical treatment for acute respiratory infection has an even greater shortcoming because it does indicate whether children received specific, effective interventions such as oral antimicrobials and antipyretics, for example, in the case of mild pneumonia. Crude coverage—the percentage of the population with a health need (children with cough and rapid breathing) that sought medical treatment—is reported, but not whether the interventions are highly likely to produce health gains. This limitation is common to many utilization measures. The concept of effective coverage (Shengelia and others 2005) and other metrics that measure the quality of services are discussed in greater detail in the next chapter.

With the exception of Jamaica, immunization rates have increased throughout the region, although levels remain well below the target of 100 percent, particularly in Haiti and the Dominican Republic (45 and 55 percent respectively).[4] The largest gains were seen in Bolivia and Guatemala, which started at fairly low levels but have caught up to their neighbors. Although immunization rates are generally higher among the better off, some countries, such as Bolivia, Colombia,

Figure 4.9 Full Immunization, Medical Treatment of Acute Respiratory Infections, and Treatment of Diarrhea: Averages and Quintile Distribution, 1995–2012 (or Nearest Year)

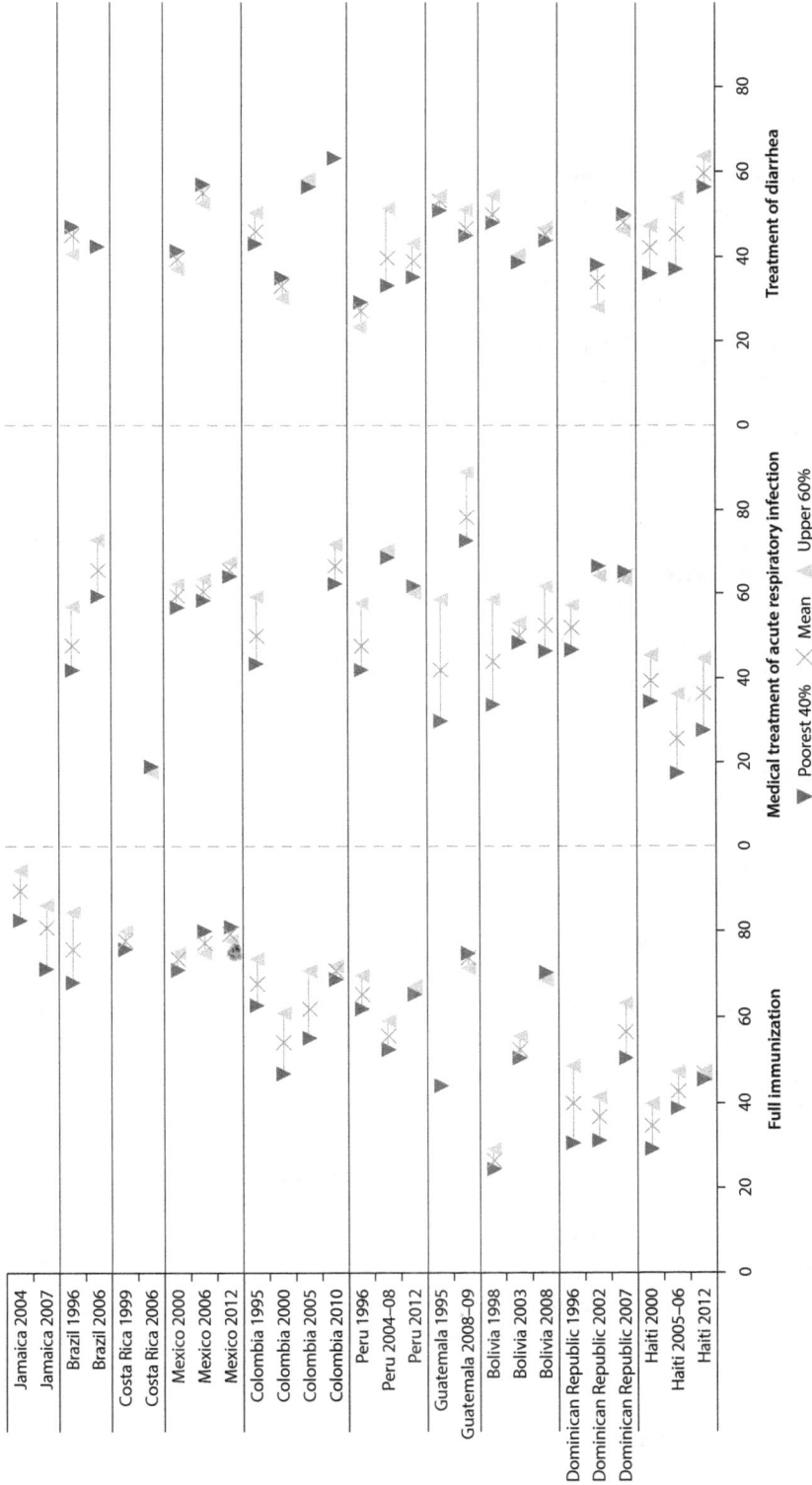

Sources: DHS—Equity Datasheet. Otherwise, study estimates based on Brazil—PNDS 2006; Costa Rica—ENSSR 1999; Guatemala—ENSMI 2008–09; Haiti—DHS 2012; Jamaica—JSLC 2004 and 2007; Mexico—ENSA 2000, ENSANUT 2006 and 2012; Peru—DHS 2012.

Note: Wealth quintiles, were used in the analysis except for Jamaica and Mexico.

and Mexico, have reduced disparities by raising rates particularly among the poor. The drop in vaccination rates among the very rich in Colombia and Mexico is worrisome,[5] especially if it signals a backlash to vaccines like those seen in Europe and the United States and leads to disease outbreaks (Omer and others 2009). Relative inequality has fallen, either across the entire distribution or between the poorest and richest. Jamaica is an exception: distribution has worsened and the gap has grown between the bottom and top tiers of the population.

Treatment of Acute Respiratory Infections. Health care use has increased for acute respiratory infections. It stands above 60 percent in most countries, except for Haiti and Peru. The rate in Haiti remains below 40 percent, although the population average is inching upward. In Peru, advances made since the mid-1990s have been partially reversed. Although disparities have eased, services remain generally pro-rich, whether measured in absolute or relative terms, between the socioeconomic extremes or across the entire population distribution.

Treatment of Diarrhea. A more mixed picture emerges with treatment of diarrhea. As with immunization and medical treatment of respiratory infections, rates of utilization (via oral rehydration salts and homemade solutions) have increased, except in Bolivia and Guatemala. In contrast to services delivered by health professionals, the use of rehydration treatment is concentrated among the better off in some countries (Bolivia, Guatemala, Haiti, and Peru), while the situation is reversed in Brazil, the Dominican Republic, and Mexico. Disparities are generally small, though Guatemala has seen a sizable increase in the absolute-rate difference between the poorest and wealthiest in society.

Improvements in child health were the result of mass public health campaigns and vertical programs for immunization and oral rehydration, as well as other interventions such as growth monitoring and breast-feeding (Jimenez and Romero 2007; Richardson and others 2010; Victora and others 2011). These programs were ramped up in the 1980s but were gradually replaced by strengthened primary-care programs in the 1990s and 2000s, which have also been effective in improving health outcomes for children, especially among the poorest segments of society (Macinko and others 2006; Rasella, Aquino, and Barreto 2010). In addition to direct health interventions, other factors known to contribute to improved health outcomes for children include educational attainment, particularly of the mother (Gakidou and others 2010) and sanitation (Fink, Günther, and Hill 2011); the region has seen significant improvements in both these factors. Fink and others find that access to improved sanitation affected not only mortality but also diarrhea and mild or severe stunting. Nutritional deficiencies are not a major contributor to the burden of disease in the region (accounting for approximately 7 percent of the overall burden) and stunting rates are generally low. Nonetheless, some countries, particularly in Central America and the Andean region, report relatively high rates of stunting. It is clear from figure 4.10 that poor outcomes are strongly negatively correlated with wealth and disparities

Figure 4.10 Stunting: Averages and Quintile Distribution, 1995–2010 (or Nearest Year)

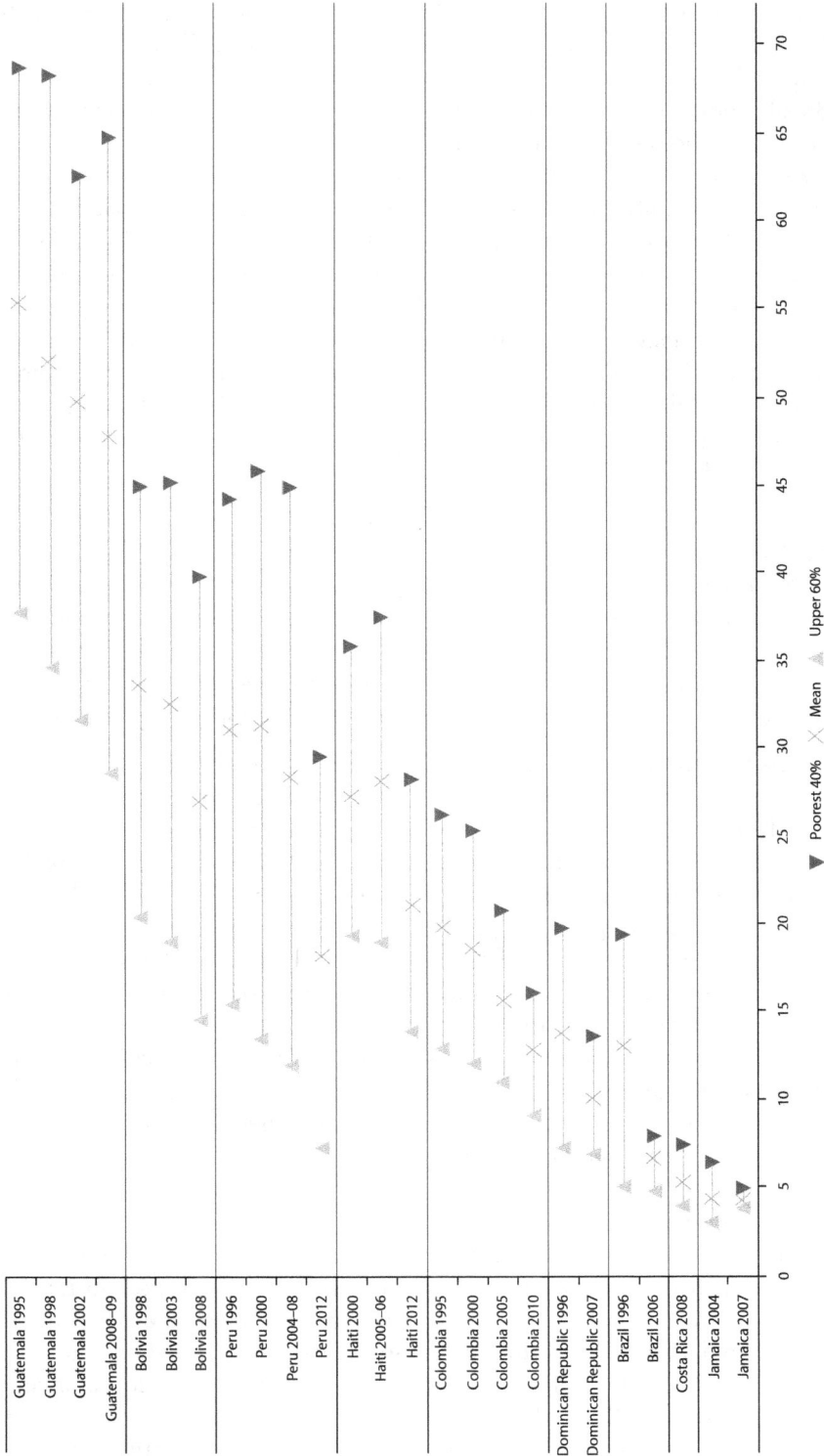

Sources: DHS—Equity Datasheet. Otherwise, study estimates are based on Brazil—PNDS 2006; Costa Rica—ENANU 2008; Guatemala—ENSMI 1998, 2002, and 2008–09; Haiti—DHS 2012; Jamaica—JSLC 2004 and 2007; Peru—DHS 2012.

Note: Wealth quintiles, were used in the analysis except for Jamaica.

have not narrowed uniformly. Indeed, inequalities remain large precisely in some of the countries most affected by malnutrition (Bolivia, Guatemala, Peru, and Haiti), whereas countries that have made strong gains in national stunting levels (Brazil, Colombia, the Dominican Republic) have done so by reducing malnutrition among the poorest segment of their populations.

As we noted in chapter 2, several LAC countries expanded social-protection services, specifically, programs that make cash transfers to poor families contingent on their use of education and health services (Brazil, Chile, Colombia, Jamaica, and Mexico). Evidence is mixed on the impact of conditional cash transfers on child health outcomes. But there are some positive results. The Mexico *Oportunidades* program has been shown to have reduced infant mortality, lowered the incidence of illness, and increased height-for-age in some age groups; Colombia's *Familias en Acción* has also had a demonstrated impact on height-for-age in children under two years and reduced incidence of diarrhea in rural areas (Fiszbein, Schady, and Ferreira 2009).

Youth to the Middle Years

The surveys analyzed are weak instruments for tracking health outcomes and risk factors associated with the principal causes for injury and poor health among young adults (violence, traffic accidents, alcohol and tobacco use). The exceptions are the reproductive health surveys, which show improvements in level of care and equitable use of services. Disparity is narrowest for services that are less dependent on well-functioning health systems.

Adolescents and young adults are a vulnerable group in the region. Indeed, males 15–19 years old were the only group for which mortality increased (by 1 percent) from 1990 to 2010 (PAHO 2012); this in a region that saw a six-year gain in overall life expectancy in the same period (IHME and World Bank 2013). Accidents and injuries are the principal cause of mortality in the 15–24-year-old age group, accounting for 57 percent of all deaths, compared with less than 7 percent in the general population. Homicides make up 30 percent of deaths among adolescents and young adults, followed by road accidents (18 percent). Pregnancy-related complications are the third most important cause of mortality for young women (7 percent). In this section, we review the distribution across socioeconomic groups of health outcomes and risk factors associated with the principal causes of mortality among young adults; where feasible, we also present evidence on related health services.

Accidents and Injuries

Violence. Violence is pervasive in the region, which is home to 42 out of the top 50 cities with the highest homicide rates worldwide (Seguridad, Justicia y Paz 2013). Violence is clustered in poor and marginalized areas of urban centers and concentrated among the bottom of the social gradient, defined by adult literacy (PAHO 2012). By way of some contrast, intimate-partner violence affects the middle wealth quintiles, where women tend to have more education and job opportunities outside the home than those in the lowest quintile (figure 4.11);

Figure 4.11 Gradient in Prevalence of Intimate Partner Violence in the Past 12 Months, 2009 (or Nearest Year)

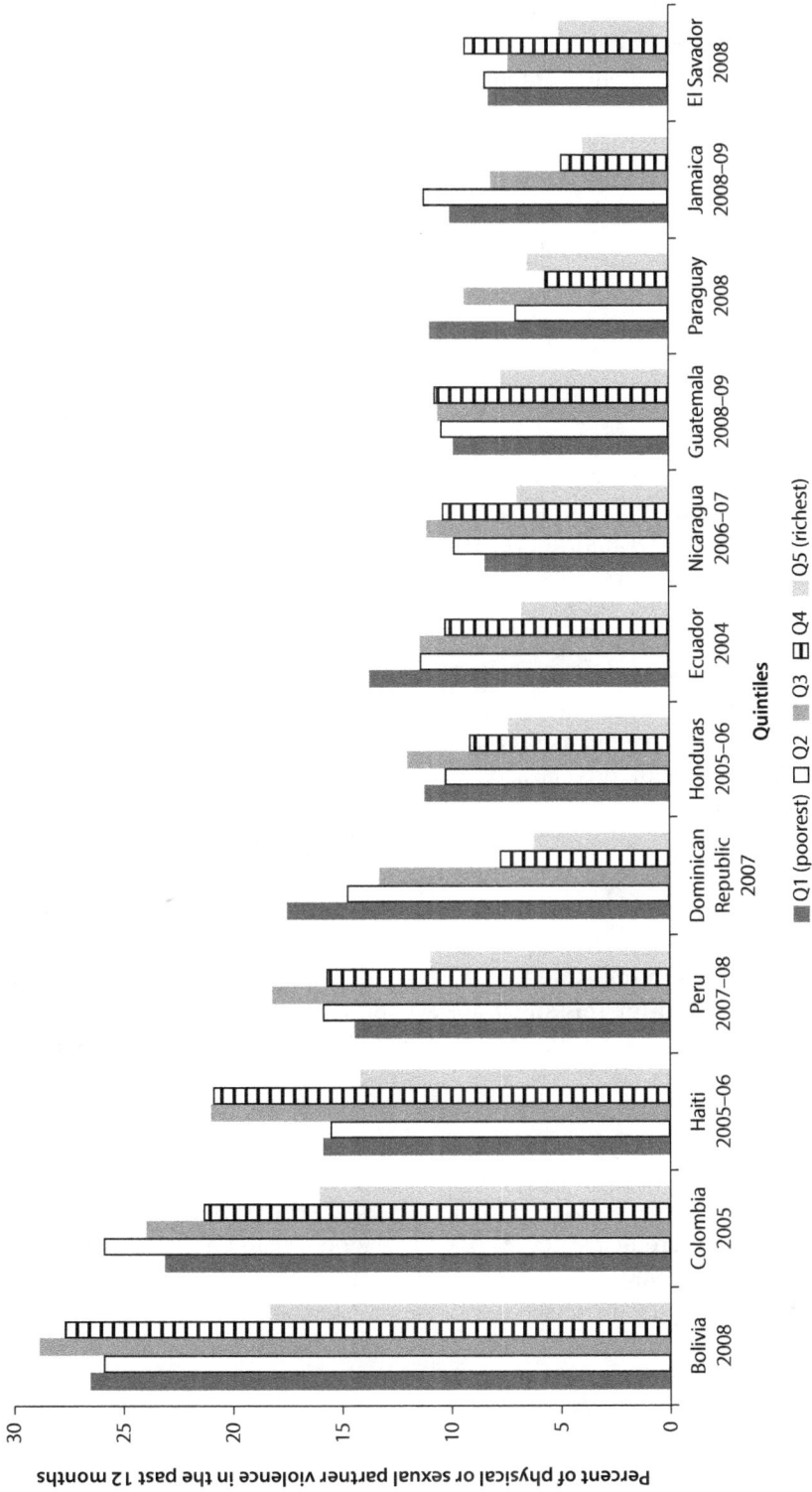

Source: World Bank calculations based on data in Bott and others 2012.

101

women who challenge traditional gender roles are at greater risk for domestic violence (Bott and others 2012). Prevalence of intimate-partner violence in the past 12 months is highest among women aged 15–19.

Road Accidents. The surveys of road accidents in the regions are so heterogeneous that it's difficult to make comparisons across countries. Only surveys from Mexico (2006, 2012) and Jamaica ask if an injury resulted from a road accident, and the concentration index is statistically significant only for Mexico (see appendix C), where both accidents and traffic injuries are more concentrated among the better off (for accidents: $CI_{2006}=0.1546$ and $CI_{2012}=0.1001$; injuries: $CI_{2000}=0.1246$). Accidents in Brazil are also positively correlated with income $(CI_{2008}=0.2027)$. Age-adjusted mortality rates show, however, that males in the lower spectrum of the literacy gradient have a higher risk of dying from traffic accidents (PAHO 2012); one possible explanation meriting further investigation is that lack of access to quality emergency care may be contributing to higher mortality among the poor, even though they have fewer traffic accidents and fewer injuries. For the most part, the surveys reviewed do not ask about emergency care.

Risk Factors

Alcohol Consumption. Certain behaviors, such as alcohol consumption, put youths at greater risk of injury. Teenagers who drive after drinking have a greater risk of being involved in a crash than older adults, and most alcohol-related road crashes occur with drivers aged 16–24 (Council on Scientific Affairs 1986; Mayhew and others 1986). Globally, 9 percent of all deaths among 15–29-year-olds are related to alcohol, compared with 4 percent in the general population (WHO 2011). Lack of standardization makes comparability across countries difficult for one of the leading risk factors for premature death and disability in the region—ranked fourth in the region overall, but first in the Andean subregion and second in Central America (IHME and World Bank 2013). The household surveys reviewed for this study are a poor source on the topic. There is wide variation in how questions are formulated. For example, some surveys ask whether the respondent has "ever consumed alcohol" (Argentina, Costa Rica), has "consumed in the past 12 months" (Costa Rica), has a relative who "consumes in excess" (Chile), or how much was "consumed in the last episode of drinking" (Guatemala). Yet another shortcoming of the surveys we analyzed: they capture alcohol consumption in adults 18 years and older, missing younger teenagers who are at particular risk for alcohol-related accidents and violence. The Mexican survey is the only one that defines, from 2006 onwards, a specific threshold of five (four for women) or more standard drinks on at least one day during the last 30 days, a pattern of drinking that can bring the blood alcohol concentration level to 0.08 percent or more (http://www.cdc.gov/alcohol/faqs .htm#heavyDrinking) (figure 4.12). Interestingly, the change in question formulation reveals that while drinking is more prevalent among the poor, the opposite is true for heavy drinking. The amount of drinking doesn't vary much for the

Figure 4.12 Alcohol Consumption in Mexico, 2000–12

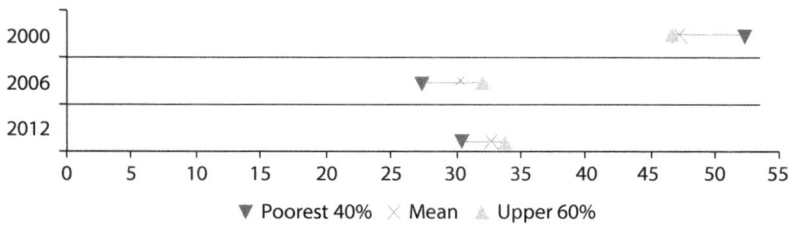

Sources: Study estimates based on ENSA 2000, ENSANUT 2006 and 2012.

middle class; the increased rate between 2006 and 2012 was driven by a rise in drinking at the very high and the very low ends of the income distribution.

Tobacco Use. Youth are also more susceptible to certain behaviors, such as smoking, which are risk factors for NCDs later in life. Ninety percent of smokers take up the habit before the age of 18 and 98 percent before age 26; those who take up the habit early are more likely to become regular smokers and less likely to quit (Breslau and Peterson 1996; HHS 2014). Evidence is sufficient to infer a causal relationship between smoking and a range of NCDs, including lung, liver, and colorectal cancers among others, obstructive pulmonary disease, diabetes, and rheumatoid arthritis (HHS 2014). The surveys we looked at have better coverage of smoking among women than men. Figure 4.13 shows a decline in the percentage of women who are current smokers in the region (with the exception of Haiti), though compared with other regions, LAC countries still have a high rate of women smokers (Bonilla-Chacín 2014); rates are particularly high in the Southern Cone countries. A similar downward trend is seen among men, though their rates of smoking are higher. The analysis of equity, however, reveals a gender difference: women smokers tend to be rich (except in Brazil, the Dominican Republic, and Haiti), whereas smoking is more prevalent among poor men.

Whether behavioral (such as alcohol and tobacco use) or environmental (such as unsafe roads and vehicles), risk factors need to be addressed with population-based interventions that go beyond the health sector. These interventions include taxation, legislation, regulation, and access to better information (Jamison and others 2013). A number of countries in the region have implemented effective multisectoral preventive measures, particularly to reduce tobacco use (Bonilla-Chacín 2014). Smoking among adults has dropped. So these policies are working. As with alcohol use, tobacco interventions need to target youths and young adults. It is alarming, for instance, that tobacco smoking among 13–15 year-olds increased in Brazil and six Caribbean countries, including Jamaica, between 2008 and 2010 (Bonilla-Chacín 2014). Policies that target youth need to be monitored. The surveys we analyzed are inadequate instruments to track health outcomes and risk factors among the young because, for the most part, the questions capture answers only for adults 18 years and older; reproductive health surveys, by way of some contrast, cover women 15–49 years of age.

Figure 4.13 Tobacco Use among Women Age 15–49: Averages and Quintile Distribution, 2000–12 (or Nearest Year)

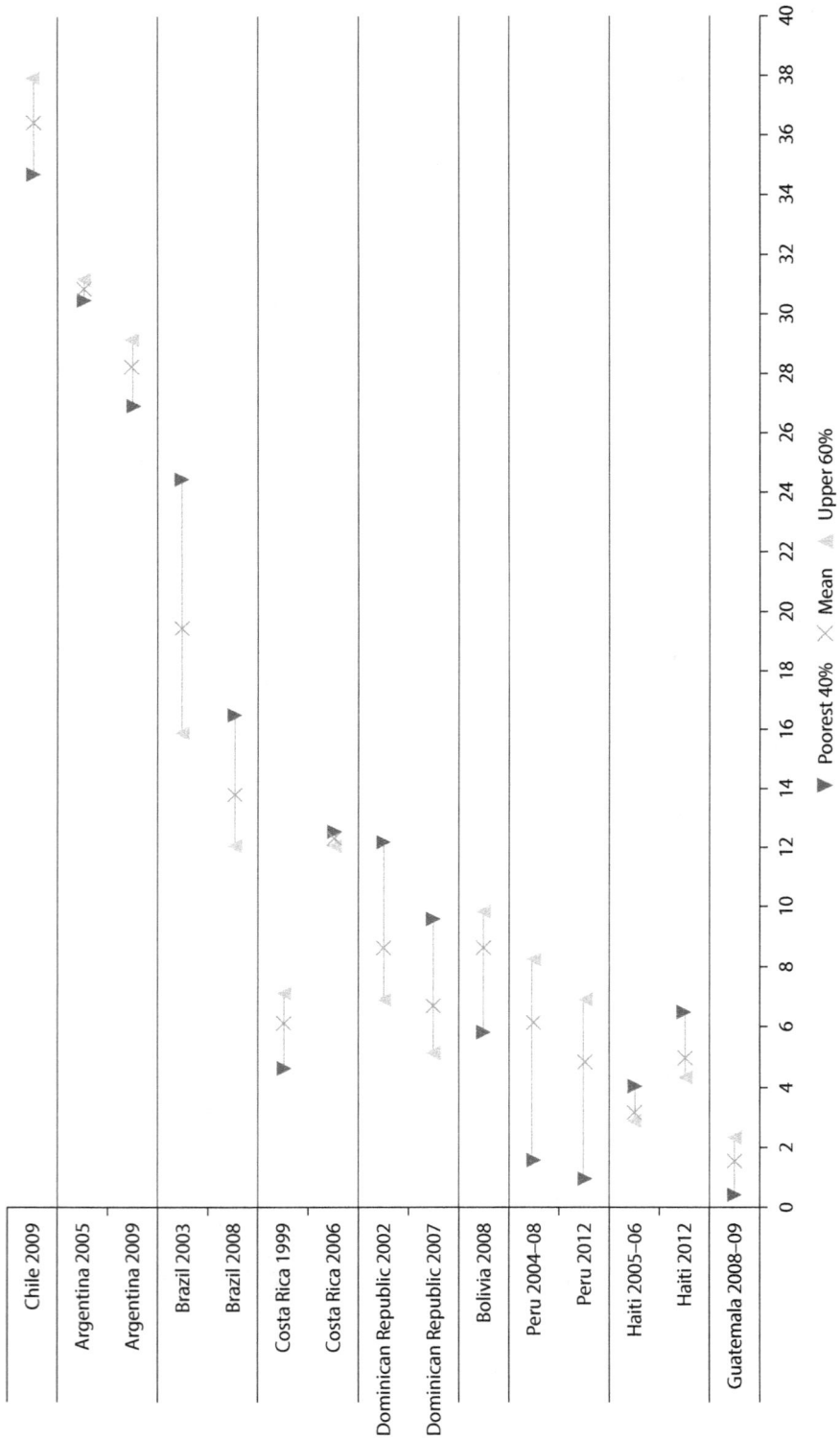

Chile 2009

Argentina 2005

Argentina 2009

Brazil 2003

Brazil 2008

Costa Rica 1999

Costa Rica 2006

Dominican Republic 2002

Dominican Republic 2007

Bolivia 2008

Peru 2004–08

Peru 2012

Haiti 2005–06

Haiti 2012

Guatemala 2008–09

0 2 4 6 8 10 12 14 16 18 20 22 24 26 28 30 32 34 36 38 40

▼ Poorest 40% ✕ Mean ▲ Upper 60%

Sources: DHS—Equity Datasheet. Otherwise, study estimates based on Argentina—ENFR 2005 and 2009; Brazil—WHS 2003, PNAD 2008; Chile—ENS 2009; Costa Rica—ENSSR 1999, ENSA 2006; Guatemala—ENSMI 2008–09; Haiti—DHS 2012; Peru—DHS 2012.

Note: Wealth quintiles, were used in the analysis except Argentina and Chile (income quintiles). Age group was women 18–49 for Brazil, Chile, and Costa Rica due to age group of survey population sample.

Maternal and Reproductive Health Services

As noted earlier, complication related to pregnancy is a top-three cause of mortality and the single highest clinical cause (i.e., excluding accidents and injuries) among women in the 15–34 age group in all LAC countries. Maternal mortality is nevertheless a rare event, making it difficult to evaluate mortality differentials across a wealth or income gradient constructed from survey data because a large sample size would be required. Analysis of maternal mortality by years of schooling (an oft-used measure of social inequality that highly correlates with income and poverty and for which information is generally available in death certificates) reveals a strong negative association. In 1990, the population quintile with the lowest level of education accounted for more than half of maternal deaths in the Americas. This share dropped to 35 percent by 2010, but is still three times greater than the number of deaths occurring in the most educated group (PAHO 2012).

Contraceptive Prevalence, Antenatal Care, and Delivery. Contraceptive use, antenatal care, and delivery by a skilled birth attendant are all considered best-buy interventions to reduce the disease burden associated with pregnancy; they also improve neonatal health outcomes (Jamison and others 2006). The region has generally reached high levels of coverage across these services, though Haiti, Guatemala, and Bolivia—the poorest countries studied—lag behind their wealthier neighbors (figure 4.14). Although still pro-rich, reproductive health services are becoming more equitable. Colombia and Peru have made the largest gains, particularly in maternal services. It is notable that women in the upper end of the income distribution had already attained high levels of coverage; the rise in national averages was achieved by expanding coverage to the poorest 40 percent of the population. Also noteworthy: disparities are wider for deliveries, a hospital-based service, than for antenatal care, which is mostly delivered in outpatient settings. In turn, there are greater disparities in use of antenatal care than contraceptives, where differences across population subgroups are small. In short, higher levels of equity have been attained for services that are not as dependent on a well-functioning health system.

Cervical-Cancer Screening. Cervical cancer is a leading cause of mortality in women 15 years and older. It killed 29,100 women in Latin America and the Caribbean in 2010, of which a third were between the ages of 15 and 49 years (Forouzanfar and others 2011). Fortunately, both the probability of cervical cancer death and its incidence have been declining since 1980; nevertheless, Paraguay, Bolivia, and Nicaragua are still reporting high incidences of cervical cancer. Regular Pap smear tests help to identify precancerous cervical lesions so they may be treated to prevent cervical cancer and early-stage asymptomatic invasive cervical cancer (USPSTF 2012). Cervical-cancer screening guidelines are available in all countries studied. Guidelines vary by age and frequency, but in most countries the recommendation is for women aged 25–64 years to be screened by means of a Pap smear cytology every three years. Average levels of cervical-cancer screening

Figure 4.14 Maternal and Reproductive Health Services: Averages and Quintile Distribution, 1995–2012 (or Nearest Year)

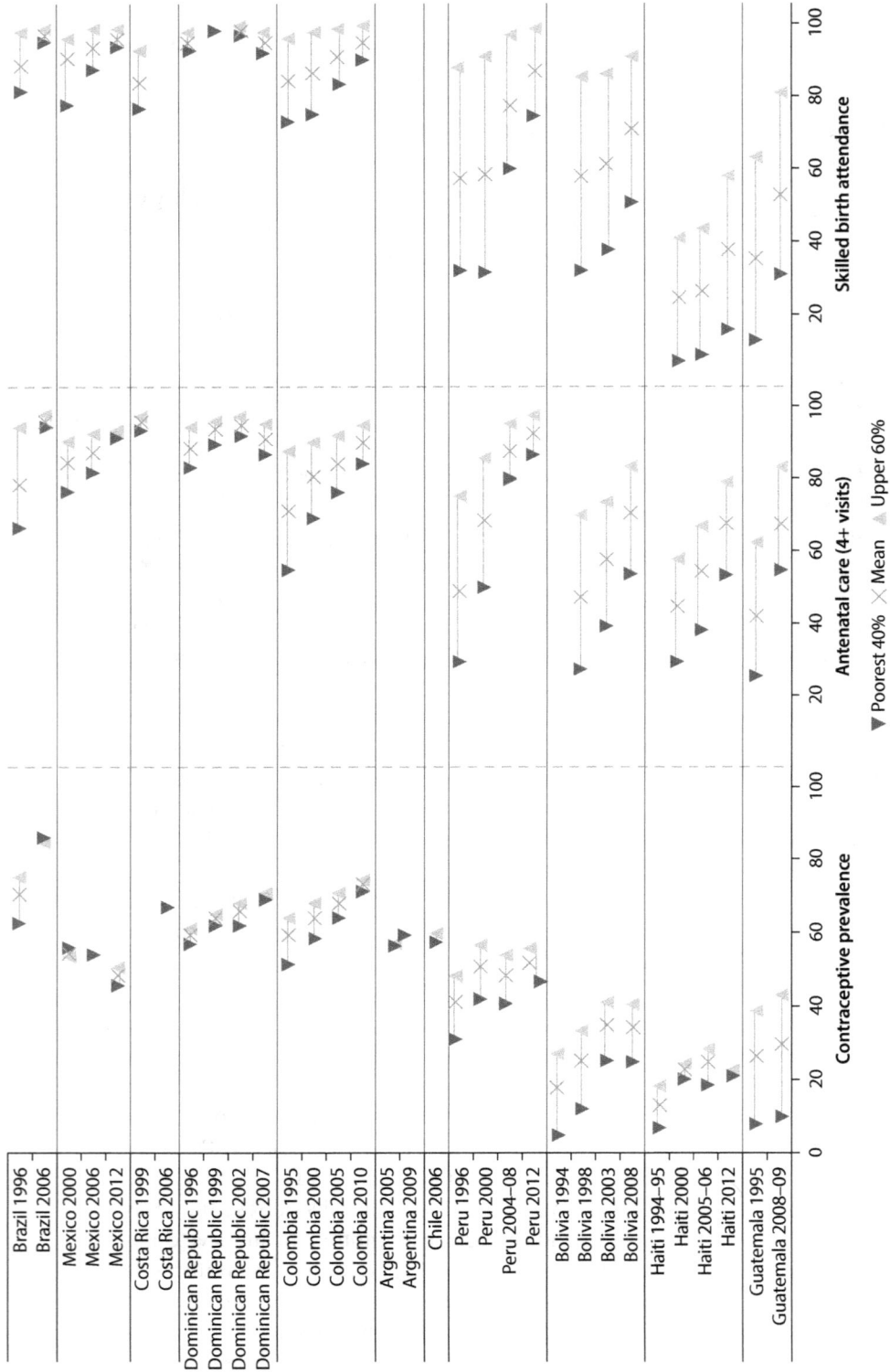

▼ Poorest 40% ✕ Mean ◢ Upper 60%

Contraceptive prevalence   Antenatal care (4+ visits)   Skilled birth attendance

Sources: DHS—Equity Datasheet for skilled antenatal care and birth attendance. Study estimates for contraceptive prevalence rate and all variables for Argentina—ENFR 2005 and 2009; Brazil—PNDS 2006; Chile—ENCAVI 2006; Costa Rica—ENSSR 1999, ENSA 2006; Guatemala—ENSMI 2008–09; Haiti—DHS 2012; Mexico—ENSA 2000, ENSANUT 2006 and 2012; Peru—DHS 2012.
Note: Wealth quintiles were used in the analysis, except Argentina, Chile, and Mexico (income quintiles).

have been increasing in all eight countries (no data is available for Jamaica) (figure 4.15). Screening is pro-poor in Mexico and pro-rich, to varying degrees, elsewhere. Mexico also has the highest overall level and has made the largest gain, although all countries are closing the gap between the rich and the poor in cervical-cancer screening. Mexico and Costa Rica, which have high coverage rates and little inequality, are, along with Chile, precisely the countries that have seen the steepest drops in mortality from cervical cancer between 1980 and 2010. However, the results must be interpreted with caution, as the Mexico figures have been adjusted to account for a shorter recall period relative to other countries and figures for Colombia and Guatemala are for a younger age group.

The Middle Years and Beyond

Progress in increased service coverage has coincided with greater and more equitable access to health services among adults, although significant socioeconomic inequities remain for most services in the majority of countries. A troublesome fact: average levels of NCDs and their risk factors have been consistently increasing over time and across countries, providing health systems with the opportunity to concentrate efforts and resources to timely diagnosis and treatment of NCDs and risk factors and to leverage campaigns on health promotion and disease prevention.

The indicators presented in this section measure health conditions that are more prevalent in middle-aged adults and the elderly. Health-outcome indicators for these age groups include self-assessed health (SAH), arthritis, asthma, diabetes, and heart disease and their risk factors—hypertension and obesity. Service-utilization measures include mammography and curative, preventive, outpatient, and hospital services. Surveys used for the analysis under this study are heterogeneous for all age groups across countries; therefore, only individuals 18 years of age or older were included in the analysis of variables for the middle years and beyond. We do not have data on indicators specific to the elderly, a limitation given the aging demographic profile of the region. In addition, other than breast cancer screening, the service-utilization variables that we can measure with available household survey data cannot be directly tied to a specific health condition. In this regard, we lose the logical chain between services and outcomes that we were able to establish with the indicators for the earlier stages of the life course.

Health measurements involve more, of course, than life expectancy and mortality. They include other crucial dimensions such as morbidity (illness/injury), functional and physical limitations, and SAH status and/or perception, among others. SAH is a good predictor of other health outcomes and mortality (Ider and Benyamini 1997; Mossey and Shapiro 1982), a useful measure of health and health inequalities within countries (Lora 2012), and a widely used measure of health needs in equity studies (Almeida and Sarti 2013; O'Donnell and Wagstaff 2008; van Doorslaer and Masseria 2004; Wagstaff and van Doorslaer 2000). Nevertheless, SAH status is subjective. It also has a weak association with

Figure 4.15 Cervical Cancer Screening: Averages and Quintile Distribution, 2000–12 (or Nearest Year)

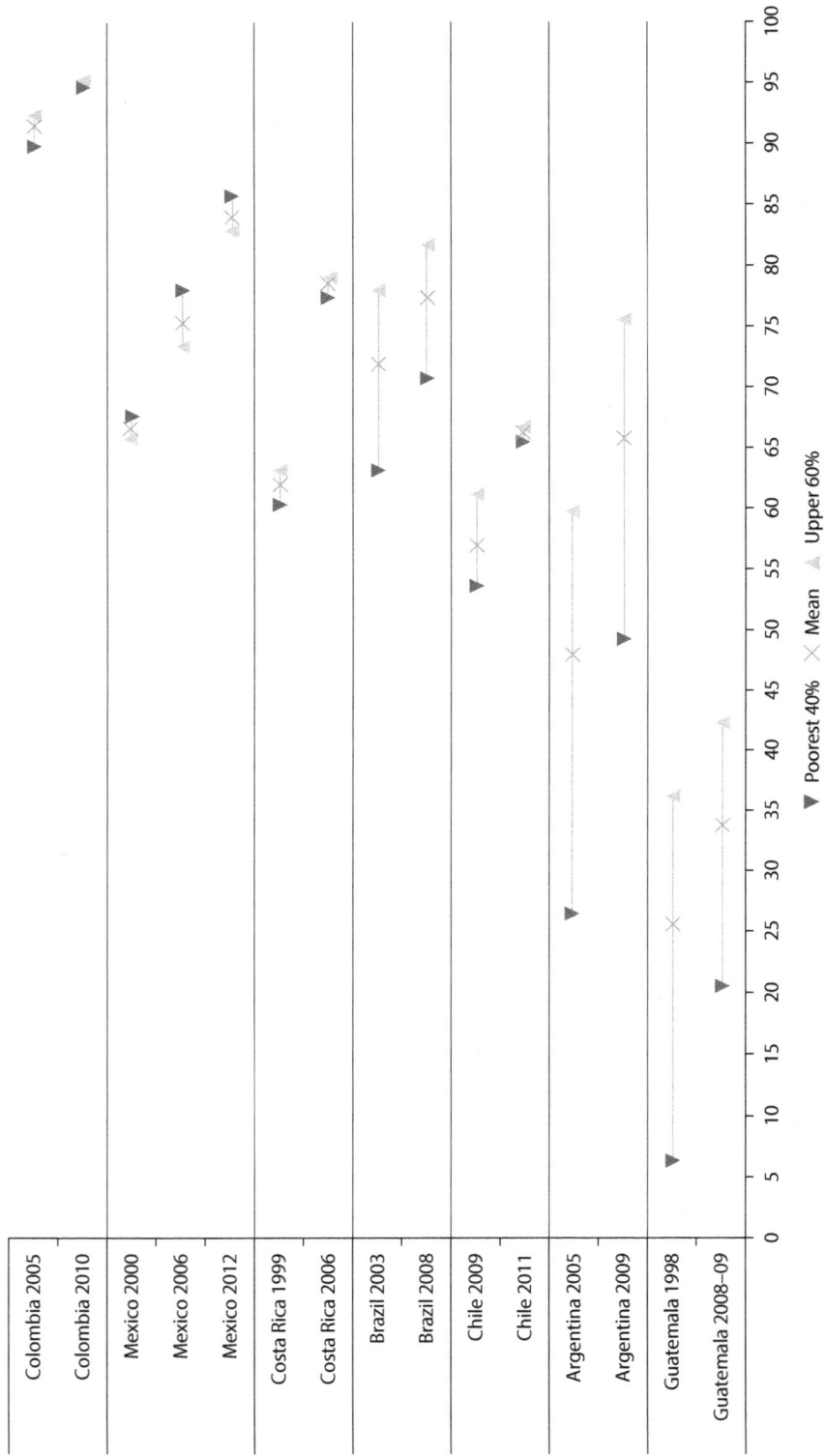

Legend: ▼ Poorest 40% ✕ Mean ◢ Upper 60%

Sources: Study estimates based on Argentina—ENFR 2005 and 2009; Brazil—PNAD 2003 and 2008; Chile—ENS 2009, CASEN 2011; Costa Rica—ENSSR 1999, ENSA 2006; Colombia—ENDS 2005 and 2010; Guatemala—ENSMI 1998 and 2008–09; Mexico—ENSA 2000, ENSANUT 2006 and 2012.

Note: Proportion of women age 18–69 who had a Pap smear in the last three years, unless restricted by the age group of survey population sample. Brazil (25–69); Mexico (20–69); Colombia, Costa Rica, and Guatemala (18–49).

self-reported health conditions probably owing to differences across cultures in health values and expectations, which render its comparability across countries difficult, especially for Latin American countries (Lora 2012).

Poor SAH status was analyzed for Argentina, Brazil, Chile, Colombia, Costa Rica, Jamaica, and Mexico. Respondents were asked to rate their health status using a Likert-scale response (very bad, bad, fair, good, or very good). Those who reported their health status to be anything other than good, that is, who had "less-than-good" SAH, were analyzed. Average levels for this variable indicate that, for the latest year reported, about 20 percent of the population in Argentina and Jamaica, 30 percent in Brazil, 25 percent in Colombia, and 36 percent in Mexico report less-than-good health status.

We expect that the average level of less-than-good SAH will gradually decline for the region over time. When baseline data is compared with the latest available data (figure 4.16), Argentina, Brazil, and Colombia show slight increases in the average level of less-than-good SAH among those reporting a worsening health status. This situation is reversed for Jamaica and Mexico. Quintile distribution for this variable shows a huge and persistent gap between the SAH status reported by the rich and by the poor, those in the upper quintiles reporting considerably fewer problems with their health than those in the poorest quintile, across all countries and all years. Figure 4.17 shows a clear social gradient in less-than-good SAH status for all quintiles.

Figure 4.16 Less-Than-Good Self-Assessed Health Status: Averages and Quintile Distribution, 2000–12 (or Nearest Year)

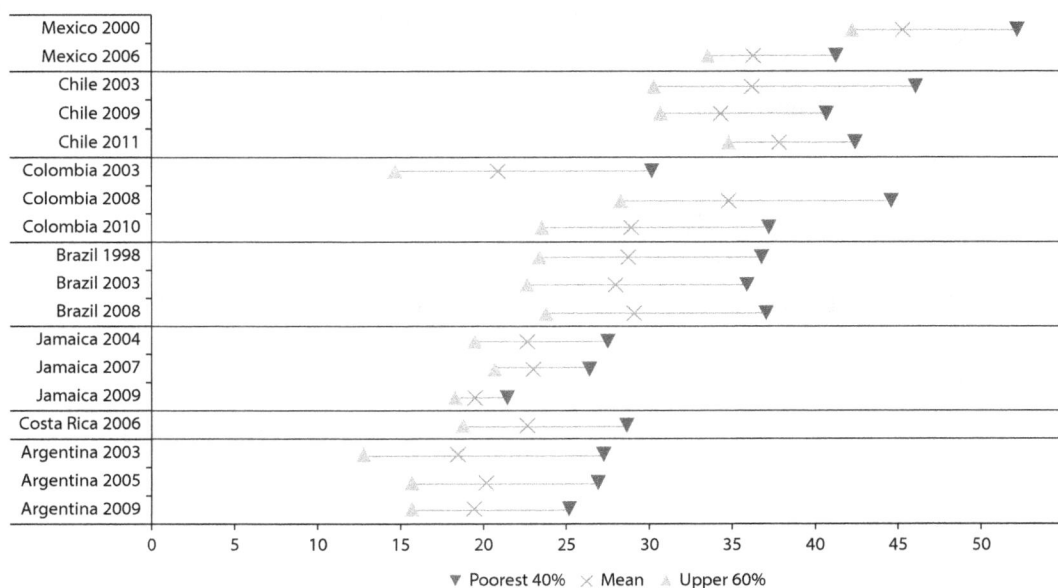

▼ Poorest 40% ⨯ Mean ▲ Upper 60%

Sources: Study estimates based on Argentina—EUGSS 2003, ENFR 2005 and 2009; Brazil—PNAD 1998, 2003, and 2008; Chile—CASEN 2003, 2009, and 2011; Colombia—ECV 2003, 2008, and 2010; Costa Rica—ENSA 2006; Jamaica—JSLC 2004, 2007, and 2009; Mexico—ENSA 2000, ENSANUT 2006.

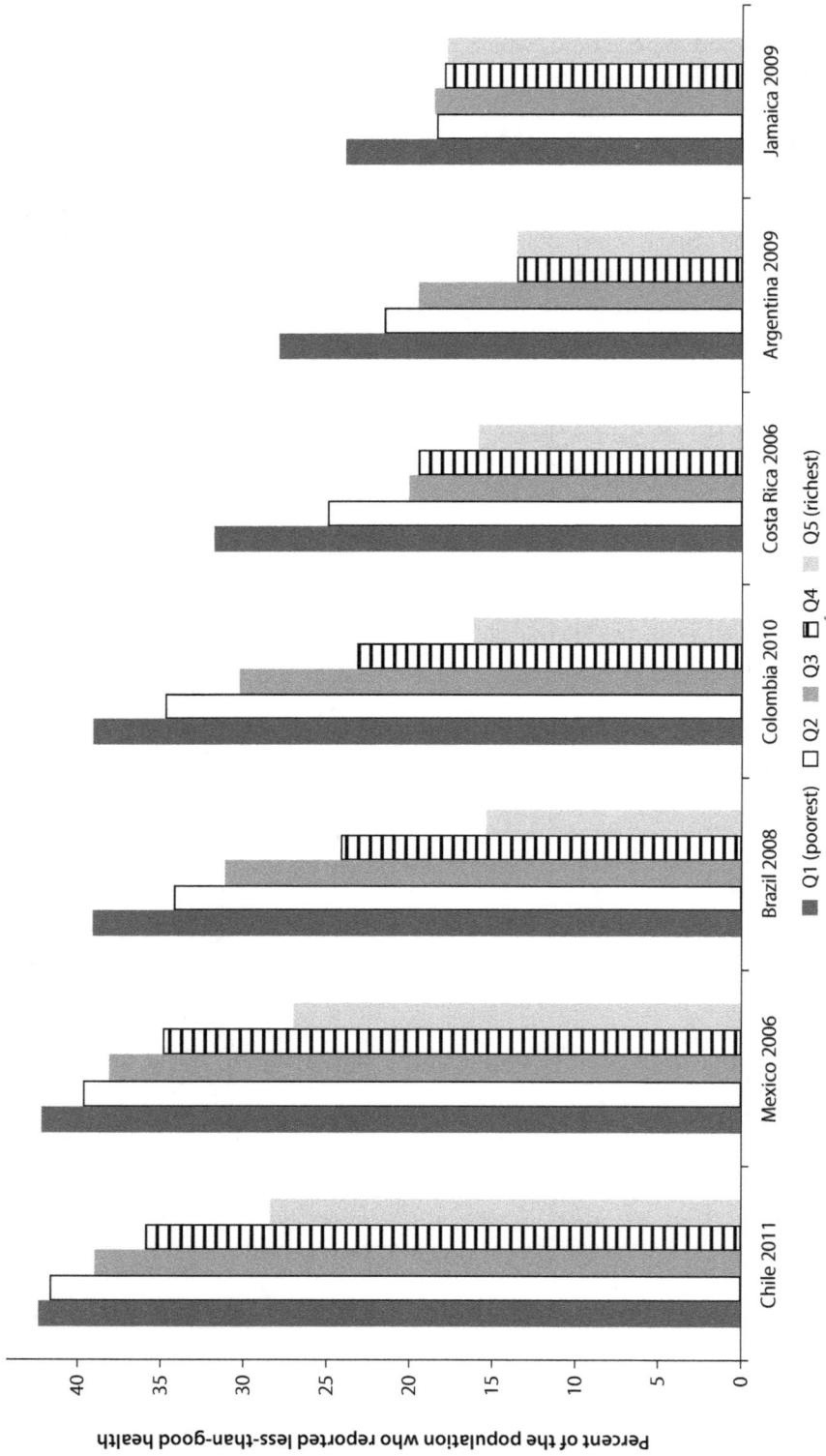

Figure 4.17 Gradient in Less-Than-Good Self-Assessed Health Status, 2010 (or Nearest Year)

Percent of the population who reported less-than-good health

Q1 (poorest)   Q2   Q3   Q4   Q5 (richest)

Chile 2011   Mexico 2006   Brazil 2008   Colombia 2010   Costa Rica 2006   Argentina 2009   Jamaica 2009

Sources: Study estimates based on Argentina—ENFR 2009; Brazil—PNAD 2008; Chile—CASEN 2011; Colombia—ENDS 2010; Costa Rica—ENSA 2006; Guatemala—ENSMI 1998 and 2008-09; Jamaica—JSLC 2009; Mexico—ENSANUT 2006.

In terms of SAH inequalities across the entire distribution, this variable is disproportionately distributed among the poor for all countries, with more poor people reporting worse health status than the rich (concentration indices, or CIs, are presented in appendix C). Over time, this variable is becoming more pro-poor and more inequitable in Argentina and Brazil, but less pro-poor or closing the gap in Chile, Colombia, and Jamaica. Mexico shows no change in this variable over time. The results are the same whether we measure the number or share of SAH responses, although the absolute measure shows less inequality for all countries. All results are statistically significant.

Chronic Conditions

Considerable progress has occurred in terms of mortality and morbidity in Latin America since the beginning of the century, when communicable diseases were among the leading causes of death. Today, approximately 48 percent of the population in the Americas die of 10 leading causes: ischemic heart diseases (9.21 percent), cerebrovascular diseases (7.70 percent), diabetes mellitus (6.54 percent), influenza and pneumonia (4.54 percent), cardiac insufficiency (3.56 percent), hypertensive diseases (3.45 percent), assaults resulting in homicide (3.45 percent), chronic diseases of the lower respiratory tract (3.30 percent), cirrhosis and other diseases of the liver (3.06 percent), and motor vehicle accidents (3.02 percent). Seven of the 10 leading causes of death belong to the group of chronic diseases. Data on morbidity combined with mortality and their causes provide critical information to decision makers on where to target health services and how to make health systems more effective and increase the odds of reducing unnecessary deaths (PAHO 2012).

In this study, the distribution of chronic conditions has been evaluated for reported medical diagnoses of asthma, depression, diabetes, and heart disease. In the information analyzed, we capture what we refer to as a "pseudo-prevalence" of NCDs. The survey questions (which are usually formulated, "Have you ever been diagnosed [by a physician or health professional] with one of these conditions?") do not ask about treatment. These survey questions do not capture those who have the condition but who either had no access to, or were not diagnosed by, a health professional. Effective health-promotion campaigns and better health care services for chronic conditions would be expected to reduce the prevalence rate for all conditions reported. Nevertheless, averages for all five chronic conditions have increased over time in most countries. These results have important implications for health services in terms of preventive actions and access to health care for diagnosis and treatment. An important target for health systems is to leverage health promotion and initiatives to prevent chronic disease, which are essential features of UHC. Ideally, surveys with biomarkers for major chronic conditions would be available, allowing for changes in actual prevalence to be distinguished from changes in access to diagnosis.

Countries for which data on the four NCDs have been analyzed include Argentina, Brazil, Chile, Costa Rica, Jamaica, and Mexico. In contrast to less-than-good SAH status discussed above, NCDs in the surveys show no clear socioeconomic gradient across countries (figure 4.18). These results are similar to findings for Colombia, in which socioeconomic differences, measured by education, in diabetes and hypertension treatment and risk-factor measures for NCDs (systolic blood pressure, fasting plasma glucose, body mass index (BMI), and total cholesterol) show no clear socioeconomic gradient for most measures (Di Cesare and others 2013). It is interesting that the few exceptions in figure 4.18 where a consistent gradient does exist—namely, Chile and Costa Rica, which are considered high performers (Jamison and others 2013)— pseudo-prevalence is pro-poor; one plausible explanation is be that, once barriers to access are lifted, disparities in the true prevalence of NCDs are revealed.

Asthma. According to the evidence, the prevalence of asthma in Latin America is as high as in developing countries on average (despite the region's higher income). Asthma has also been increasing over time (Pearce and others 2007) and is highly associated with low income and poor living conditions (Cooper and others 2009; Costa and others 2013). In addition, asthma diagnosis and control are still lacking for many patients in the region, and current levels of care fall short of international guidelines (Neffen and others 2005). Current trends in asthma prevalence pose a challenge to health systems by contributing to high levels of preventable hospitalizations. This presents an opportunity for public policy to address unequal access to health care services and social determinants of health, which greatly contribute to risk factors. Chile has the highest average rate of diagnosed asthma among the six countries reporting. Average asthma levels have been increasing over time in Argentina and Jamaica, while Brazil and Mexico report slight reductions.

Depression. Depression is the leading cause of disability and the most common mental disorder in the world (Marcus and others 2012). It affects 5 percent of the adult population in LAC and is more prevalent among women than men. Despite the potential for a good prognosis, about 60 to 65 percent of those with depression receive no health care, placing them at a higher risk for suicide. Approximately 63,000 people in the Americas take their own lives every year because of depression. Barriers to accessing care include the lack of trained health professionals and the absence of early diagnosis and treatment services, social stigma associated with mental disorders, and inappropriate financing for mental health services. In LAC, mental health gets less than 2 percent of the health budget (PAHO 2012). Depression can devastate the individual and adversely affect family and community alike; it is therefore important to provide service coverage for the early diagnosis and treatment of depression and other mental disorders. The elimination of barriers to accessing mental health services is an important target for health policies and system improvements. Our data show Chile with the highest levels of diagnosed depression among the four countries reporting on this disorder, with rates twice that of Mexico and three times that of Brazil. Over time, Brazil has

Figure 4.18 Diagnosed Asthma, Depression, Diabetes, and Heart Disease: Averages and Quintile Distribution, 2000–12 (or Nearest Year)

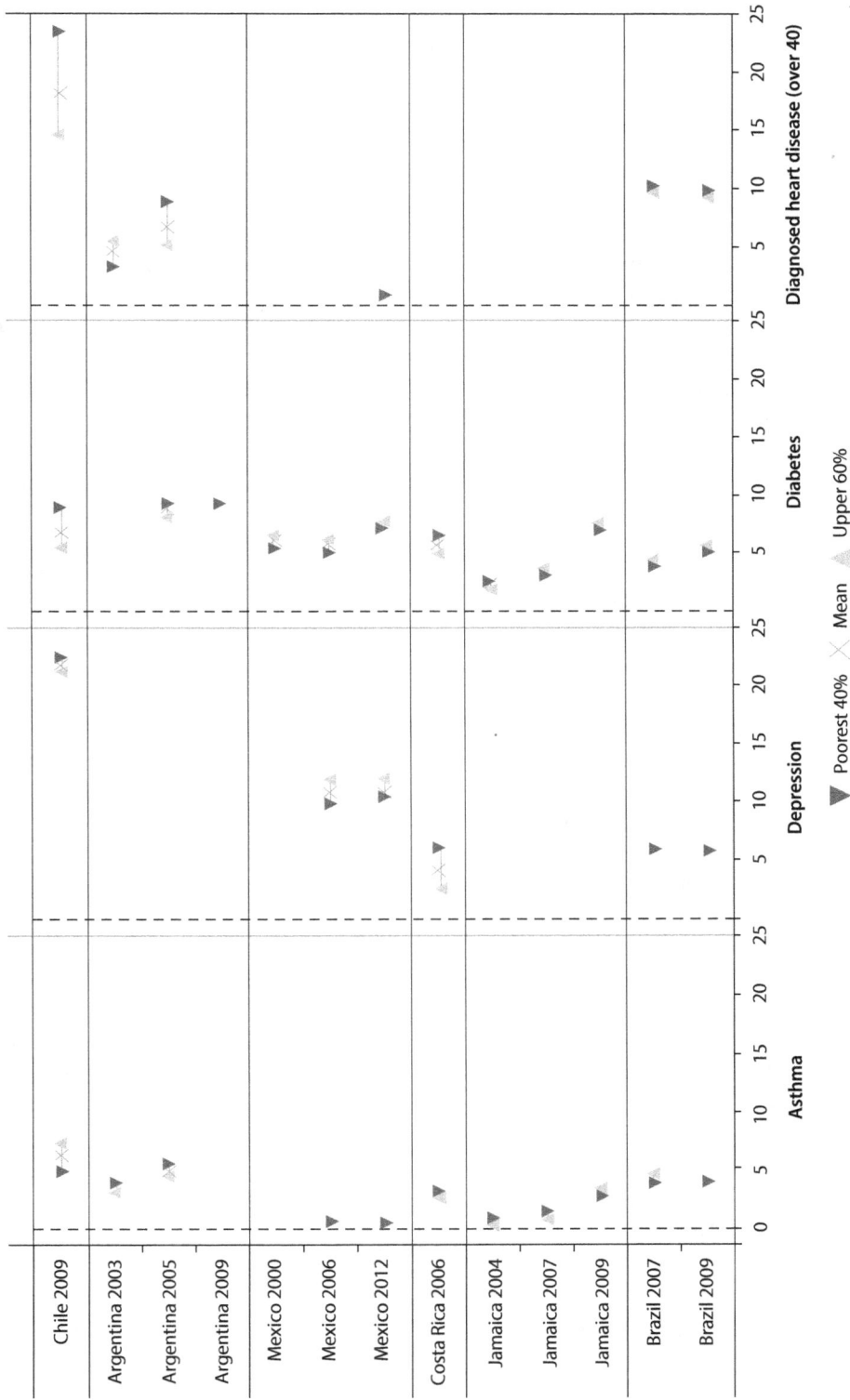

Sources: Study estimates are based on Argentina—EUGSS 2003, ENFR 2005 and 2009; Brazil—PNAD 2003 and 2008; Chile—2009; Costa Rica—ENSA 2006; Jamaica—JSLC 2004, 2007, and 2009; Mexico—ENSA 2000, ENSANUT 2006 and 2012.

113

shown a slight decrease, and Mexico a slight increase, in the average rates of diagnosed depression in the population. There is no gap between the rich and the poor in Brazil. In Mexico, the rich report more depression than the poor, while elsewhere the opposite is noted.

Diabetes. Diabetes is a leading cause of disability and the third leading cause of death in the Americas, accounting for 6.54 percent of all deaths. In 2011, the number of people in Latin America and the Caribbean with diabetes was estimated at 25 million, contributing to one of the highest rates of diabetes in the world. Approximately 44 percent of people with diabetes do not know they have it, contributing to higher levels of chronic complications and premature mortality (PAHO 2012). Available data on diagnosed diabetes show Argentina with the highest rate (9.6 percent), followed by Mexico (9.0 percent), Jamaica (7.2 percent), Chile (6.8 percent), Costa Rica (5.5 percent), and Brazil (5.0 percent). All countries with data for two or more years show an increase in the average levels of diabetes over time, especially Jamaica with a 4 percentage-point increase in five years. As with other chronic conditions, the quintile distribution for diagnosed diabetes has no well-defined socioeconomic gradient. These results should be interpreted with caution because the CIs are for the most part not statistically significant (see appendix C).

Ischemic Heart Disease. Ischemic heart disease is the number-one killer in the LAC region for both men and women—responsible for 9.21 percent of deaths. Unnecessary deaths from cardiac conditions, especially for ischemic heart disease, can be avoided through preventive actions (PAHO 2012). Figure 4.18 shows that approximately 6.5 percent of the population in Argentina has been diagnosed with a heart disease, compared with 7.5 percent in Mexico, 9.5 percent in Brazil, and 18 percent in Chile. Over time, average levels of diagnosed heart disease have been constant in Brazil, increased by 1 percentage point in Mexico, and by 2 in Argentina. Quintile distributions of diagnosed heart disease show no clear socio-economic gradient except in Argentina and Chile. Inequality patterns for heart disease in the four countries studied are uneven. Brazil and Mexico data show little change over time, and concentration indices are very close to zero, indicating little inequity in the distribution for heart disease in the population. Argentina had a highly pro-rich concentration index in 2003, but the direction of inequality was reversed in 2005, though this is not statistically significant.

There is strong evidence in the literature, mostly from developed countries, suggesting that the poor and those with little formal education or in marginalized and disadvantaged groups have a higher risk of dying due to NCDs when compared with other groups (Di Cesare and others 2013). Evidence from Chile and Mexico corroborates these findings (figure 4.19). Nevertheless, the results for the four NCDs studied here suggest that those in poorer socioeconomic groups have similar rates of NCDs as those in higher socioeconomic groups, although they report worse health status and have higher mortality for these conditions. As is discussed in the next session, poor access to health care services for diagnosis and

Figure 4.19 Mortality Rates for Leading Causes of Mortality, by Educational Attainment, Chile and Mexico, 2010 (or Nearest Year)

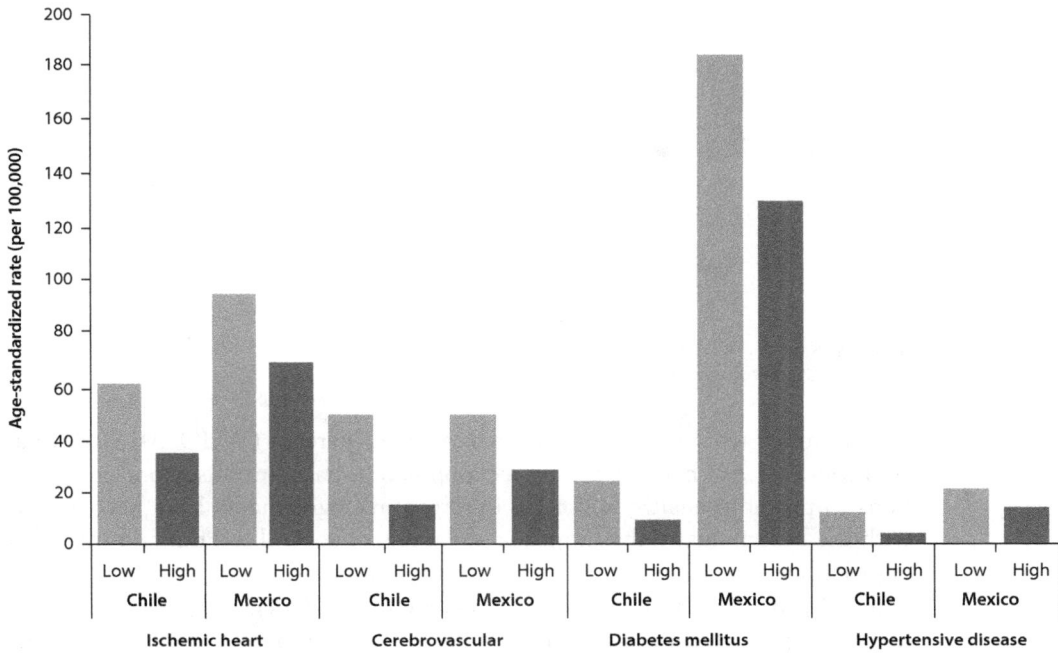

Source: Analysis by T. Dmytraczenko, F. Marinho, L. Alencar, and G. Almeida from Registration of Vital Statistics. Chile—2009; Mexico—2010.
Note: Educational attainment: Mexico—low = no schooling, high = primary and above; Chile—low = secondary and below, high = tertiary and above.

treatment of NCDs among the poor may contribute to the differences in reported prevalence. Understanding the barriers the poor encounter for the early diagnosis and treatment of NCDs will allow decision makers to design policies and health services to improve access for this group.

Risk Factors

Most NCDs are associated with preventable behaviors such as tobacco use, physical inactivity, unhealthy diet, and the harmful use of alcohol, which lead to risk factors such as raised blood pressure, overweight/obesity, hyperglycemia, and hyperlipidemia. According to World Health Organization (WHO) the leading NCD risk factor is raised blood pressure or hypertension (to which 13 percent of global deaths are attributed), followed by tobacco use (9 percent), high blood glucose (6 percent), physical inactivity (6 percent), and overweight and obesity (5 percent). Heart disease, ischemic stroke, and type 2 diabetes mellitus are associated with obesity, and so is mortality due to these conditions.

Obesity. As per figure 4.20, the highest level of obesity among adults is found in the Americas (26 percent) compared with all other WHO regions. This rate is

Figure 4.20 Age-Standardized Prevalence of Obesity in Adults Ages 20+ Years, by WHO Region and World Bank Income Group, Comparable Estimates, 2008

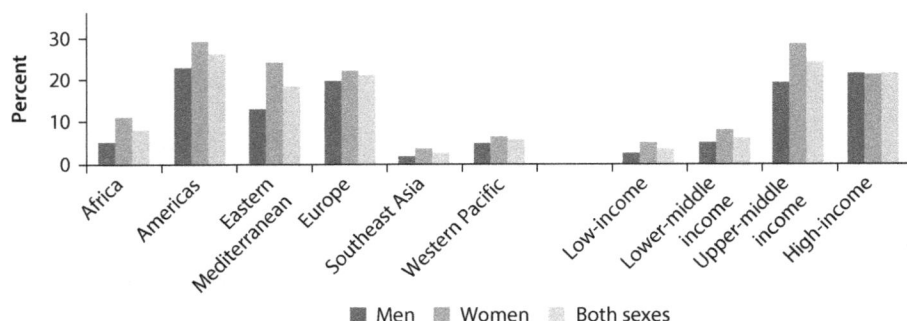

■ Men   ■ Women   ▨ Both sexes

Source: WHO 2011.
Note: Obesity is defined as body mass index ≥30 kg/m^2.

higher among women, 29 percent, than men, 23 percent (WHO 2011). Several countries in LAC have implemented population-based multisectoral interventions to promote healthy lifestyles. In Argentina, agreements have been signed with the food industry that impose regulations to control sodium and trans fats in processed foods, while the city of Bogota has built outdoor gyms and bicycle paths to promote physical activity (Bonilla-Chacín 2014). Programs that target the entire population are known to be effective (Torres and others 2013). But age-specific programs may be needed to address lifelong consequences of conditions such as obesity. For instance, evidence suggests that children who are overweight by the age of five years are most susceptible to becoming obese later in life, pointing to the importance of public health interventions for young children (Cunningham, Kramer, and Narayan 2014).

Figure 4.21 shows that average obesity rates are similar for men and women in Argentina and Colombia; in Chile it is substantially higher for women than men. Chile reports high obesity rates among both men and women, while Haiti reports the lowest obesity rates for the LAC region. An interesting and troublesome pattern is that, for all countries with historical data, the average rate of obesity for both men and women has increased over time. Brazil has the highest obesity-rate increase among women, from 10 percent in 1996 to 21 percent in 2006. Except for Argentina, Chile, and Colombia in 2010, women in the bottom 40 percent are less likely to be obese than those in the other groups. Most countries report less inequality over time. Disparities between the poor and the rich, men and women alike, are falling in all countries in relative and absolute terms. Exceptions: absolute inequality for obesity remained constant among men in Argentina and Colombia (see appendix C). The data should be viewed with the caveat that most of the surveys analyzed collect information on self-reported obesity without collecting BMI data.

Hypertension. Hypertension is the sixth-leading cause of death in the Americas, accounting for 3.45 percent of all deaths in the region. Approximately one in

Figure 4.21 Diagnosed Hypertension and Obesity: Averages and Quintile Distribution, 1995–2012 (or Nearest Year)

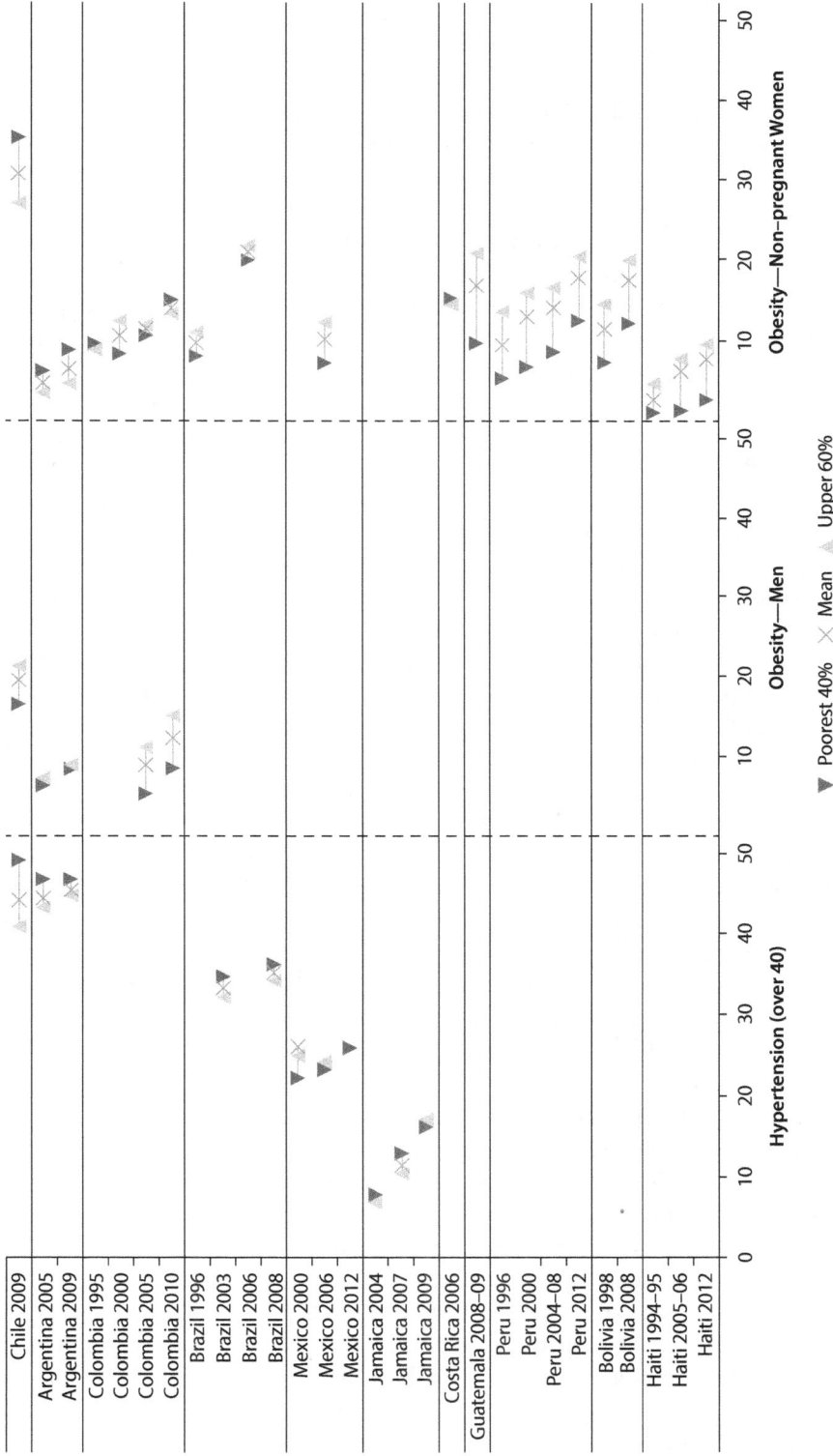

Legend: ▶ Poorest 40%   ✕ Mean   ▲ Upper 60%

Obesity—Men | Obesity—Non-pregnant Women | Hypertension (over 40)

Categories (y-axis): Chile 2009, Argentina 2005, Argentina 2009, Colombia 1995, Colombia 2000, Colombia 2005, Colombia 2010, Brazil 1996, Brazil 2003, Brazil 2006, Brazil 2008, Mexico 2000, Mexico 2006, Mexico 2012, Jamaica 2004, Jamaica 2007, Jamaica 2009, Costa Rica 2006, Guatemala 2008–09, Peru 1996, Peru 2000, Peru 2004–08, Peru 2012, Bolivia 1998, Bolivia 2008, Haiti 1994–95, Haiti 2005–06, Haiti 2012

Sources: DHS—Equity Datasheet, except for study estimates based on Argentina—ENFR 2005 and 2009; Brazil—PNDS 2006, PNAD 2003 and 2008; Chile—ENS 2009; Costa Rica—ENSA 2006; Guatemala—ENSMI 1998 and 2008–09; Jamaica—JSLC 2004, 2007, and 2009; Mexico—ENSA 2000, ENSANUT 2006 and 2012.

117

three adults in the Americas has hypertension, which increases risk of heart attack, stroke, and kidney disease (PAHO 2012). Hypertension was analyzed for Argentina, Brazil Chile, Jamaica, and Mexico. Survey questions for all countries ask about medical diagnosis of hypertension, except for Jamaica, where respondents are not asked whether the condition was diagnosed by a health professional. Average levels of hypertension for the last year reported are lower in Jamaica (15 percent), followed by Mexico (16 percent), Brazil (20 percent), Chile (29 percent), and Argentina (32 percent). Quintile distribution shows no clear gradient, except for Chile. In Argentina, Brazil, and Chile, the richest 20 percent report less hypertension than all other income groups. But, generally, concentration indices for hypertension in all countries, except for Chile and Jamaica in 2009, are either not statistically significant or close to zero, indicating no socioeconomic inequality. Inequality reversed direction in Jamaica: 2004 and 2007 data show the richest 20 percent reporting the lowest levels of hypertension, and in 2009 this group reported the highest levels for this condition, owing, perhaps, to a change in the survey question, which no longer required the respondent to report hypertension diagnosed by a health professional, as was the case in earlier surveys. Hypertension in Jamaica had the largest increase, rising from less than 5 percent in 2004 to 15 percent in 2009. This anomaly highlights the need to formulate survey questions according to best practices.

The results described above show a clear trend: the region is reporting an overwhelming increase in diabetes and heart disease and their associated risk factors, obesity and hypertension, in all income groups. Although little to no inequality is evident in the rates of arthritis, depression, diabetes, and hypertension, our findings show a clear pro-rich inequality in obesity among men and women, albeit the gap between the rich and the poor is diminishing in most countries. The latter is related to a sharper increase of obesity among the poorest quintile groups when compared with the increase in the richest-quintile groups. The importance of public health interventions and health promotion campaigns to address these critical results cannot be undermined. Health authorities have the opportunity to reduce deaths and disease by introducing public policies and providing universal coverage to services that promote healthy lifestyles, prevent disease, and provide timely treatment.

Service Utilization by Adults

To achieve effective service coverage, health systems that are universal should ensure all people receive needed quality health care without financial hardship. Assessment of needed health services requires the conceptualization and measurement of 'need', a difficult and often controversial exercise. A literature review in search for a common ground on defining need revealed at least four approaches. Need can be determined with (1) the use of objective and/or subjective measures for individual need, such as SAH status and morbidity versus clinical assessment ascribed by a health professional; (2) use of area characteristics as the basis for need versus individual health needs; (3) defining need of population groups based on age (life-course approach), gender, race/ethnicity, etc.; and (4) defining need as the individual capacity to benefit from health care (Dixon and others 2003).[6] Our rationale was to measure health care utilization in terms of purpose (curative and preventive services), type (specialized), and site (outpatient and hospital setting) based on an individual's need measured by health status and existing morbidities. Data on services coverage are still scarce in many Latin American and Caribbean countries, but some information is available for some key interventions and services, including breast cancer screening and outpatient, hospitalization, preventive, curative, and specialized services.

Breast cancer screening is directly linked to reduced morbidity and mortality among women, particularly after age 50. According to current best practice, mammography is a cost-effective preventive measure, though controversial evidence has recently questioned its benefit for early diagnosis and reduction in breast cancer–specific mortality for women in certain age groups (Miller and others 2014; Mukhtar, Yeates, and Goldacre 2013; Tabár and others 2011). These studies have revived the debate over suitable government guidelines and recommendations for screening. Still, breast cancer is responsible for more than 37,000 deaths in the region annually. Analysis of breast cancer mortality over time, calculated with the average annual percent change of age-standardized mortality rates, shows an increase in the average levels of breast cancer mortality in Colombia, Costa Rica, and Mexico during a period of approximately 10 years (2000 to circa 2010) and a decrease in Argentina, Brazil, Chile, and Peru during the same period. In 2010, Argentina had highest mortality rate of 20.3, but over time the country was able to reduce its mortality due to breast cancer, registering an annual percentage change from 2000 to 2010 of 1.27. With a rate of 9.92, Mexico has the lowest mortality rate attributable to breast cancer, although percentage changes during the 2000–10 period show an annual increase in deaths of 0.51 (PAHO 2013).

Guidelines for breast cancer screening are available for all countries studied, except Guatemala and Jamaica, although they vary on when and how often women should have mammograms. Our expectation was that countries would have higher coverage levels of mammography over time as well as a fairer distribution among income groups. Results indeed show average levels of mammography increasing in Argentina, Brazil, Colombia, and Mexico (figure 4.22). Highest levels of mammography for a three-year recall period are found in Mexico (81 percent) and Colombia (80 percent), followed by Argentina (71 percent), Brazil (59 percent), Chile (57 percent), and Costa Rica (33 percent). Figure 4.22 also shows that the better off have greater coverage than those in the bottom 40 percent of the income distribution, except in Mexico, and all countries have improved equity in utilization (see CIs in appendix C). Most notably, Mexico has made tremendous gains in improving access to breast cancer screening for the poor through its *Seguro Popular* program (Knaul and others 2012). It achieved a considerable increase in overall coverage for this targeted intervention, as well as a shift from a pro-rich distribution in 2006 to a pro-poor one in 2012. Elsewhere, a clear social gradient exists for mammography, showing

Figure 4.22 Breast Cancer Screening: Averages and Quintile Distribution, 2000–12 (or Nearest Year)

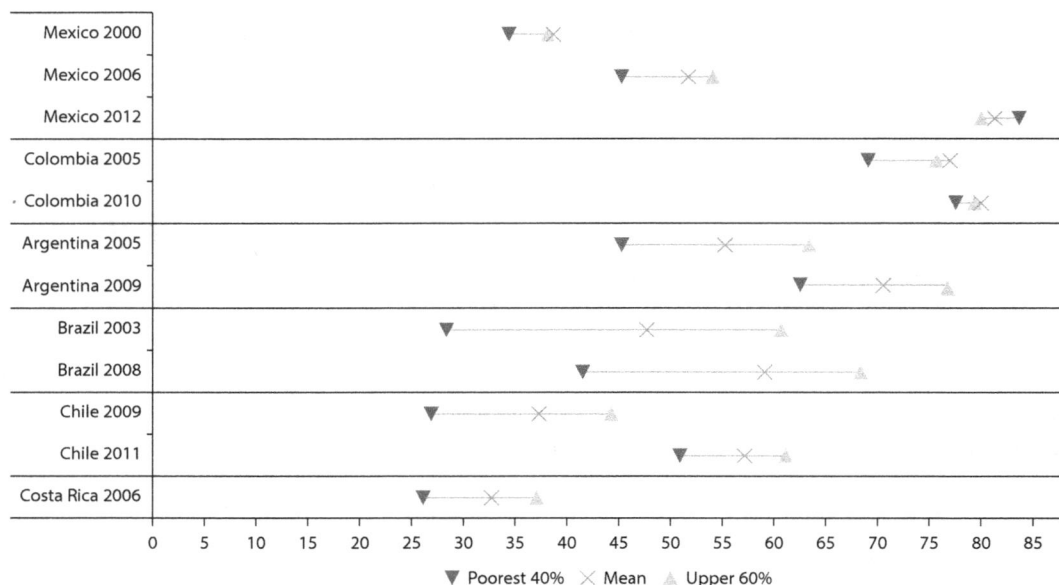

Sources: Study estimates based on Argentina—ENFR 2005 and 2009; Brazil—PNAD 2003 and 2008; Chile—ENS 2009; Colombia—ENDS 2005 and 2010; Costa Rica—ENSA 2006; Mexico—ENSA 2000, ENSANUT 2006 and 2012.
Note: Proportion of women ages 40–69 years who had a mammogram in the past three years, except for Colombia (ages 40–49 years). Mexico results were adjusted because the survey recall period was one year only.

greater use at higher income levels (figure 4.23). However, the Colombia and Mexico results must be interpreted with caution for the reasons noted in the section on cervical cancer screening.

Preventive Visits. The use of preventive health care services is essential for disease prevention, early diagnosis of diseases, screening for risk factors, and guidance on healthy lifestyles. So it is reasonable to expect that all adults should have at least one preventive-care visit annually. Five countries reported preventive visits for a recall period of a month (figure 4.24). Except for Argentina (77 percent), levels across the region are quite low: 21 percent in Chile, 20 percent in Brazil, 17 percent in Colombia, and 15 percent in Peru. Pronounced inequalities are evident in countries with a pro-rich distribution; Brazil and Colombia have concentration indices of 0.10 and 0.15, respectively (see appendix C). In Colombia, the distribution is becoming less skewed over time, whereas in Brazil the degree of inequality is unchanged. Overall trends show increased utilization of preventive health care services and less inequality among population groups in the majority of countries studied.

Quintile distributions show a socioeconomic gradient for Chile and Peru that is the inverse of that for all other countries (figure 4.25). In both countries, use

Figure 4.23 Gradient in Breast Cancer Screening, 2010 (or Nearest Year)

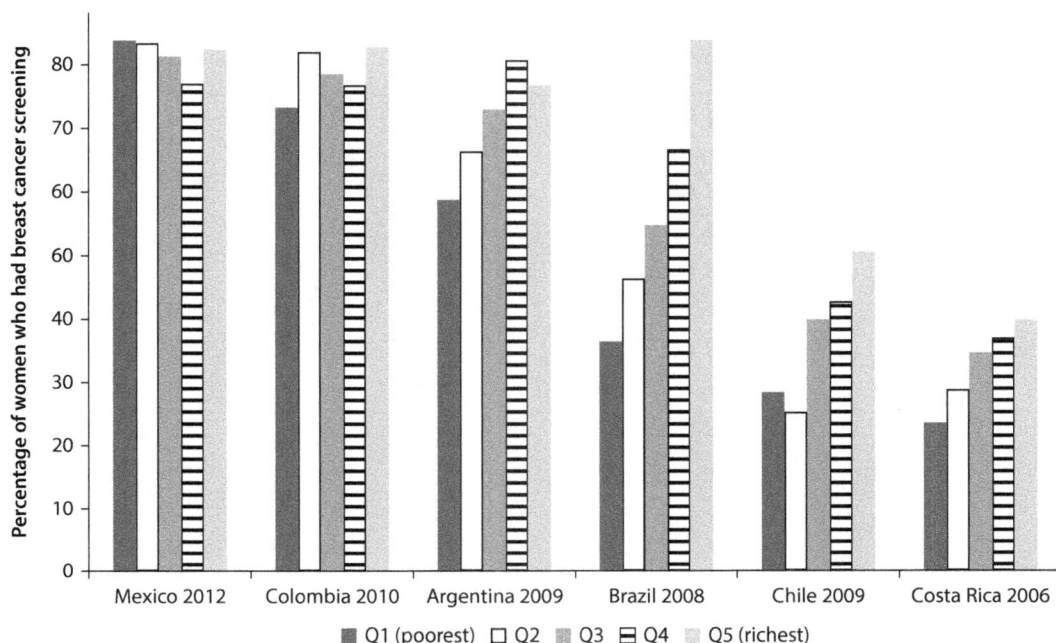

Sources: Study estimates based on Argentina—ENFR 2009; Brazil—PNAD 2008; Chile—ENS 2009; Colombia—ENDS 2010; Costa Rica—ENSA 2006; Mexico—ENSANUT 2012.
Note: Survey data have been normalized for a three-year recall period.

of preventive services declines as income increases, though the distribution is almost balanced in Peru. In Brazil and Colombia the relationship between utilization and income is uniformly positive, and, as noted above, the degree of inequality is greater. In Argentina average levels of preventive services are similar among the socioeconomic extremes (quintile 1 and 5), but higher for all other groups.

Curative Visits. In contrast to preventive visits—which are for maintaining health and preventing disease in the absence of symptoms—curative care treats and diagnoses injuries or illnesses either in outpatient or hospital settings. Survey questions for curative care are preceded by questions about the existence of an injury or illness requiring health care; therefore, answers on service utilization are restricted to those who reported a specific health problem or injury. Highest levels of curative visits in a month are reported for Mexico (86 percent), Jamaica (78 percent) and Colombia (78 percent), followed by Argentina (53 percent), Brazil (21 percent), Peru (19 percent), Guatemala (15 percent), and Chile (9 percent). Given the same needs, the rich are more likely to use curative care services in all countries studied, although the gap between the rich and the poor

Figure 4.24 Utilization of Outpatient, Inpatient, Preventive, and Curative Health Services: Averages and Quintile Distribution, 2000–12 (or Nearest Year)

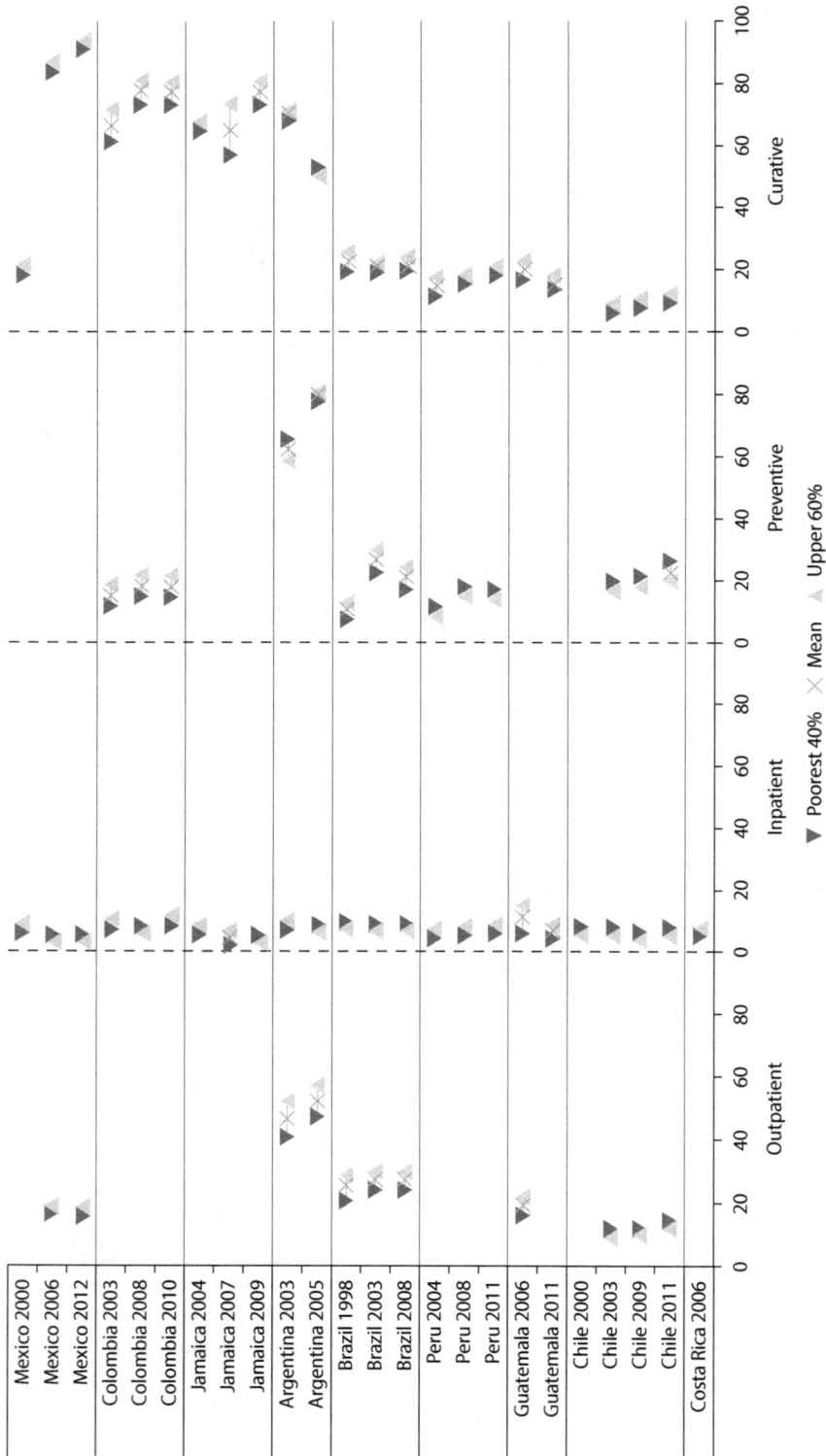

▼ Poorest 40% ✕ Mean ▲ Upper 60%

Sources: Study estimates based on Argentina—EUGSS 2003 and 2005; Brazil—PNAD 1998, 2003, and 2008; Chile—CASEN 2000, 2003, 2009, and 2011; Colombia—ECV 2003, 2008, and 2010; Costa Rica—ENSA 2006; Jamaica—JSLC 2004, 2007, and 2009; Guatemala—ENCOVI 2006 and 2011; Mexico—ENSA 2000, ENSANUT 2006 and 2012; Peru—ENAHO 2004, 2008, and 2011.
Note: For Chile, physician visits were used as a proxy for outpatient visits.

Figure 4.25 Gradient in Preventive Visits, 2010 (or Nearest Year)

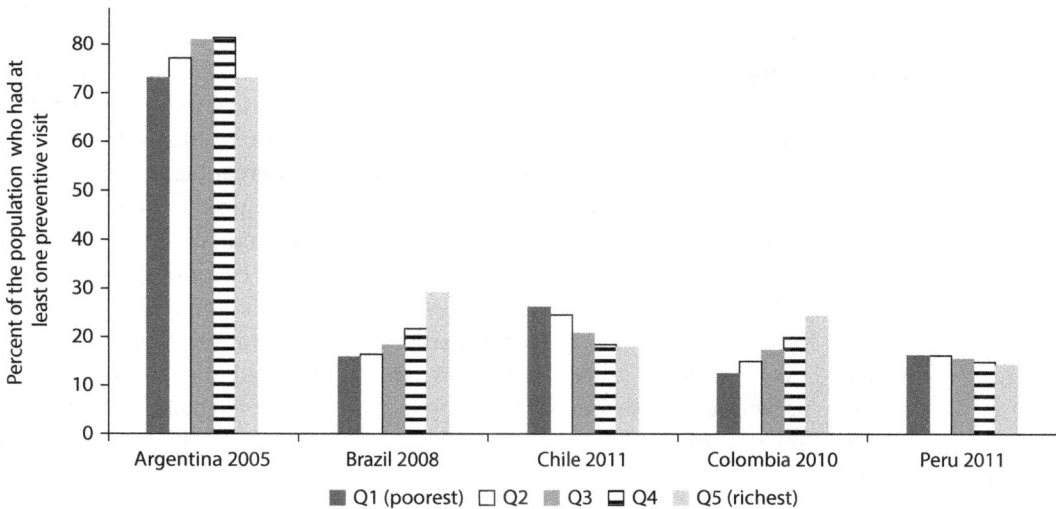

Sources: Study estimates based on Argentina—EUGSS 2005; Brazil—PNAD 2008; Chile—CASEN 2011; Colombia—ECV 2010; Peru—ENAHO 2011.
Note: Survey data have been normalized for a 3-month recall period.

is narrowing. The only exception is Colombia, where inequality indices remained fairly constant over time.

Although it may be fair to expect that all ill or injured individuals will receive care (100 percent coverage for needed services), it is problematic to assume that more curative care is better, particularly when we are unable to discriminate between care delivered in an outpatient versus hospital setting. Available survey data are not granular enough to let us distinguish improvements in access to inpatient services for those who needed it from care received in a hospital setting that could otherwise have been managed at the primary-care level, avoiding unnecessary hospitalization. Without further information to discern the reason for increases or decreases in this variable, interpretation is limited. These limitations are further discussed in the next chapter.

Outpatient and Inpatient Services. Outpatient and hospital services refer to the site/place where services were received and level of service within the health-service delivery network. Outpatient or ambulatory services may include curative, preventive, specialized, or primary health services, among others. These services may be delivered by physicians or other health care professionals. Hospital services are those that provide inpatient care requiring at least one night of hospitalization. In general, the proportion of population using outpatient health services is low: 51 percent in Argentina, 27 percent in Brazil, 16 percent in Mexico, 15 percent in Guatemala, and 14 percent in Chile. Although these proportions have increased by 7 percentage points in Argentina, 3 in Chile, and 2 in Brazil, they have decreased by 4 percentage points in

Guatemala and 1 in Mexico. Like curative and preventive services, outpatient services are pro-rich for all countries, although inequalities have decreased over time. Compared with outpatient services, the proportion of the population receiving inpatient services in all countries is much smaller, varying from 4 percent in Jamaica to 8 percent in Argentina, Brazil, and Colombia. Over time, levels of hospitalization have remained stable in Argentina, Brazil, Chile, and Colombia; they decreased in Jamaica and Mexico by 2 percentage points and in Guatemala by 4. In Peru they increased by 2 percentage points. Most hospital services are equally distributed among the rich and the poor, or show a slightly pro-rich inequality. Guatemala and Jamaica are the only exceptions, with pro-rich inequality higher than most countries. As with curative services, it is problematic to assume that more/fewer outpatient and hospital services are better/ worse. Fewer avoidable hospitalizations and more outpatient services for primary prevention and needed health services are desirable goals; but available survey data do not lend themselves to this type of analysis. These issues are discussed in further detail in the next chapter.

Financial Protection across Income Groups

Most countries in the region saw a statistically significant decline in catastrophic expenditures. There are wide variations in this measure, and the association with income or coverage is weak. Without exception, medicines are a heavier burden on the poor than the wealthy, though the gap is narrowing. In relative terms few households are falling into poverty due to health expenditures, but this still means that millions of people are not being protected from financial hardship.

Populations that pay heavily out of pocket for health services at the point of service delivery are at greater risk of incurring large expenditures and suffering financial shocks due to illness than those whose health services are financed through prepaid pooled resources. A common metric used to assess vulnerability to health shocks is the share of households incurring catastrophic health spending, which is defined as out-of-pocket payments that exceed a certain threshold of household consumption (Wagstaff and van Doorslaer 2003; Xu and others 2003).

Figure 4.26 presents results of the analysis using 25 percent of nonfood consumption as the threshold above which out-of-pocket payments are considered catastrophic. Catastrophic health expenditures vary widely in the countries studied, ranging from 1 percent in Costa Rica to more than 21 percent in Chile. As one might expect, wealthier countries (Brazil and Mexico) have low levels of catastrophic spending (below 5 percent), mid-income countries such as Colombia and Peru fall in the middle range (5–10 percent), and lower-income Guatemala in the high range (above 10 percent). The association with income, however, is weak. Perhaps more surprisingly, catastrophic spending does not correlate strongly with coverage. Catastrophic spending is

Figure 4.26 Incidence of Catastrophic Health Expenditures, 2004–10 (or Nearest Year)

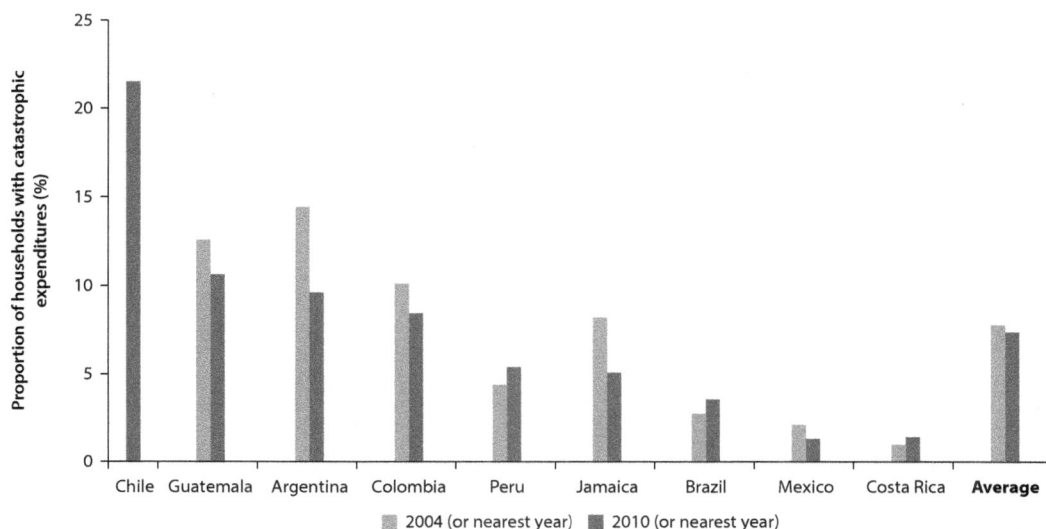

Sources: Study estimates based on Argentina—ENGH 1997 and 2005; Brazil—POF 2002–03 and 2009–09; Chile—ESGS 2006; Colombia—ECV 2008 and 2010; Costa Rica—ENIG 2004 and 2013; Guatemala—ENCOVI 2006 and 2011; Jamaica—JSLC 2007 and 2009; Mexico—ENIGH 2000 and 2010; Peru—ENAHO 2004 and 2008.
Note: Differences in mean between time periods significant at 1 percent, except in Colombia (not significant). Catastrophic health expenditures defined at the 25 percent threshold of nonfood consumption.

lower in Peru than one might expect given its lower income and coverage compared with other countries. It is extremely high in Chile, a country with nearly universal population coverage and the highest income per capita in Latin America. In the first decade of the millennium, most countries in the region saw a statistically significant decline in catastrophic expenditures; Brazil and Peru were the exception, but the increase was marginal (one percentage point or less).

Xu and others (2003), in a 59-country study of catastrophic health expenditures at the 40 percent capacity-to-pay threshold,[7] found an overall positive correlation between the proportion of households incurring catastrophic spending and the share of total health expenditures financed out of pocket. They also found substantial variability between countries at each level. In the mid- to late 1990s, Latin American countries (for example, Argentina, Brazil, Colombia, Paraguay, and Peru) were shown to have relatively high rates of catastrophic expenditures (figure 4.27). In the decades since, rates have declined substantially, most notably in Brazil, Mexico, and Peru; in other countries, changes in catastrophic expenditures were marginal. Though the trend is toward fewer households incurring catastrophic spending, these figures mask some variation within the period. In Jamaica, for example, the share rose above the 4 percent mark in 2004 before dipping down to 2.5 percent in 2009. In Brazil, rates were slightly

Figure 4.27 Proportion of Households with Catastrophic Expenditures versus Share of Out-of-Pocket Payment in Total Health Expenditures

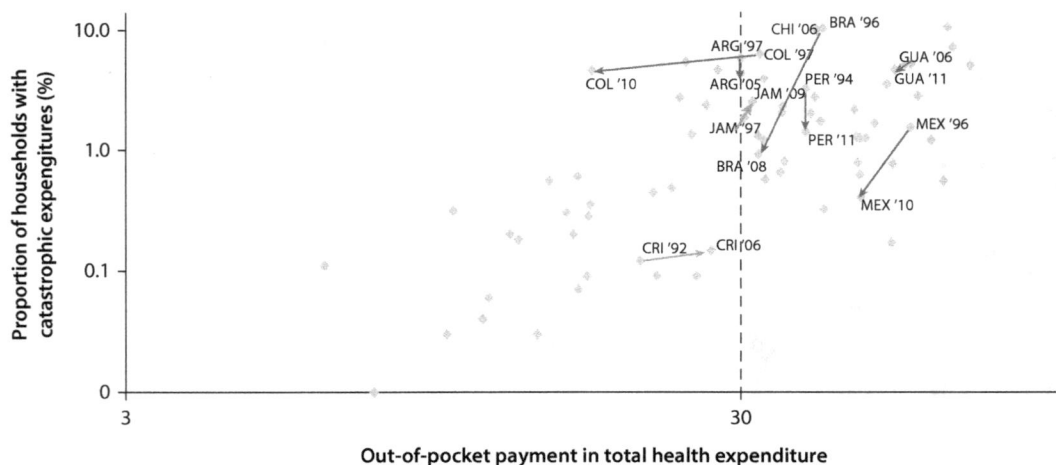

Source: Knaul and others 2012; Xu and others 2003.
Note: Catastrophic health expenditures defined at the 40 percent threshold of household capacity-to-pay.

higher in 2008 (0.9 percent) than in 2003 (0.6 percent); both these changes were statistically significant.

In line with Xu and others' earlier findings, catastrophic expenditures correlate positively with the share of out-of-pocket payments in total health spending. Colombia is an outlier. Its catastrophic spending is relatively high (4.6 percent) given the portion of total expenditure financed through out-of-pocket payments (17 percent, which is among the lowest in a region where out-of-pocket payments accounted for 32 percent of total financing for health on average in 2012). Though out-of-pocket payments have increased in absolute terms in the countries studied (see chapter 1), as a share of total financing, they have either declined or remained unchanged in all but Costa Rica, which saw a 1 percentage-point increase in the out-of-pocket share of total financing.

Comparable data on the composition of out-of-pocket payments was available for five of the nine countries studied. In all cases other than Colombia, medicines represent the largest expenditure item, absorbing 45 percent of out-of-pocket outlays on average and as much as three-quarters of household spending in Brazil, up 10 percentage points from the previous survey year. In contrast, a change of similar magnitude, but in the opposite direction, was seen in Peru. There was no change in Colombia or Mexico. Without exception, medicines are a heavier burden on the poor than the rich because they consume a larger share of the health budget of poor households; the gap is narrowing, however, in all countries. Jamaica was not included in this group because data do not allow for a comparison.

Nonetheless, it is interesting to look at the Jamaica case more closely given that the government has been implementing two medicine subsidy programs since 2003: the National Health Fund and the Jamaica Drugs for the Elderly Program. Although there was little movement (a 1.7 percentage-point decline) in the overall share of out-of-pocket spending on medicines, there were important distributional changes. The burden of expenditures for medicines has been reduced primarily in the bottom three quintiles, though more so for the middle and lower-middle classes (quintiles two and three) than the poorest.

Outpatient services are the second-highest expenditure item but, in contrast to medicines, represent a larger share of wealthier households' spending—though the gap is narrowing (except in Mexico and Peru, which have showed little change). Inpatient services tend to absorb a more modest share of out-of-pocket payments (less than 10 percent), except in Colombia and Mexico, where their share is 30–37 and 18–23 percent respectively. In the case of Mexico, the distribution across income groups is fairly even; in Colombia it is pro-rich. The share or distribution of household spending on lab and diagnostic services has shown little change. This last finding is surprising in light of the rising burden of NCDs; diagnostic tests are important in the detection and management of these conditions.

This illustrates some of the shortcomings of expenditure analysis. It relies on reporting of actual expenditures and, hence, tells us nothing about items that households spent no money on. The poor may in fact be forgoing necessary diagnostic services because they cannot afford them. Indeed, we know from the previous section that the poor lag behind the rich in utilization of key diagnostic services such as cervical and breast cancer screening. The data on out-of-pocket payments cannot capture this because no purchase is made and, so, it does not appear as a household expenditure. Likewise, little can be gleaned about the nature of the health goods and services procured. Were they elective or necessary or, for that matter, known to be effective? Further, a reduction in financial barriers, often a feature of programs to advance UHC, may result in more purchases of health-related services owing to latent demand. For these reasons, it is difficult to interpret data on the incidence of catastrophic payments across the income distribution. Ideally, we would have more granular information about the nature of these expenditures, particularly whether they are elective or not.

Figure 4.28 shows the concentration index for catastrophic payments, as well as changes over time, where available. In most countries, catastrophic expenditures are pro-rich, but that is not the case across the board. In Brazil, Colombia, Guatemala, and Jamaica, these payments are concentrated among the poor, though to a lesser extent in Colombia, where disparities are narrowing. Disparities, when measured across the entire population distribution, are widening in several countries irrespective of whether catastrophic expenditures are pro-rich or pro-poor; in all cases the differences are statistically significant.

Figure 4.28 Concentration Index for Catastrophic Health Expenditures, 2004–10 (or Nearest Year)

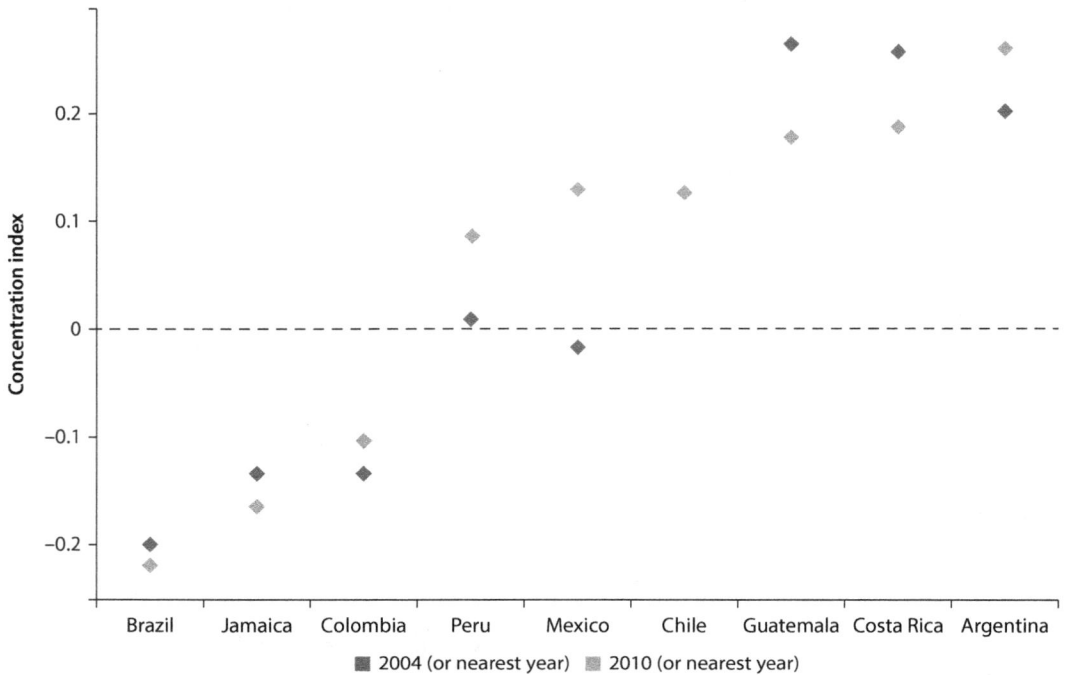

Sources: Study estimates based on Argentina—ENGH 1997 and 2005; Brazil—POF 2002–03 and 2009–09; Chile—ESGS 2006; Colombia—ECV 2008 and 2010; Costa Rica—ENIG 2004 and 2013; Guatemala—ENCOVI 2006 and 2011; Jamaica—JSLC 2007 and 2009; Mexico—ENIGH 2000 and 2010; Peru—ENAHO 2004 and 2008.
Note: The concentration index is pro-poor when it is below zero and pro-rich when it is above zero. Catastrophic health expenditures defined at the 25 percent threshold of nonfood consumption.

Policy makers may be particularly interested in whether the poor are being disproportionately burdened with expenditures on health. Figures 4.29 and 4.30 show, respectively, the incidence of catastrophic health expenditures among the poorest 40 percent of the population compared with the incidence in the richest 60 percent of the population and the scale of impoverishment due to health payments. Impoverishment is measured as the difference between what the poverty headcount would have been if households did not make health payments compared with the actual poverty headcount. In all countries catastrophic expenditures for the bottom 40 percent and the overall population have moved in tandem, mostly declining over time, with the exception of Brazil and Peru where, as noted above, there has been a slight increase. The poverty headcount attributable to health payments is lowest in Costa Rica, Argentina and Mexico, where it has also declined, and largest in Peru and Jamaica. The gap has been narrowing in Colombia and Guatemala, but increasing in Brazil and Peru.

Figure 4.29 Incidence of Catastrophic Health Expenditures among the Poorest 40 Percent of the Population, 2000–10 (or Nearest Year)

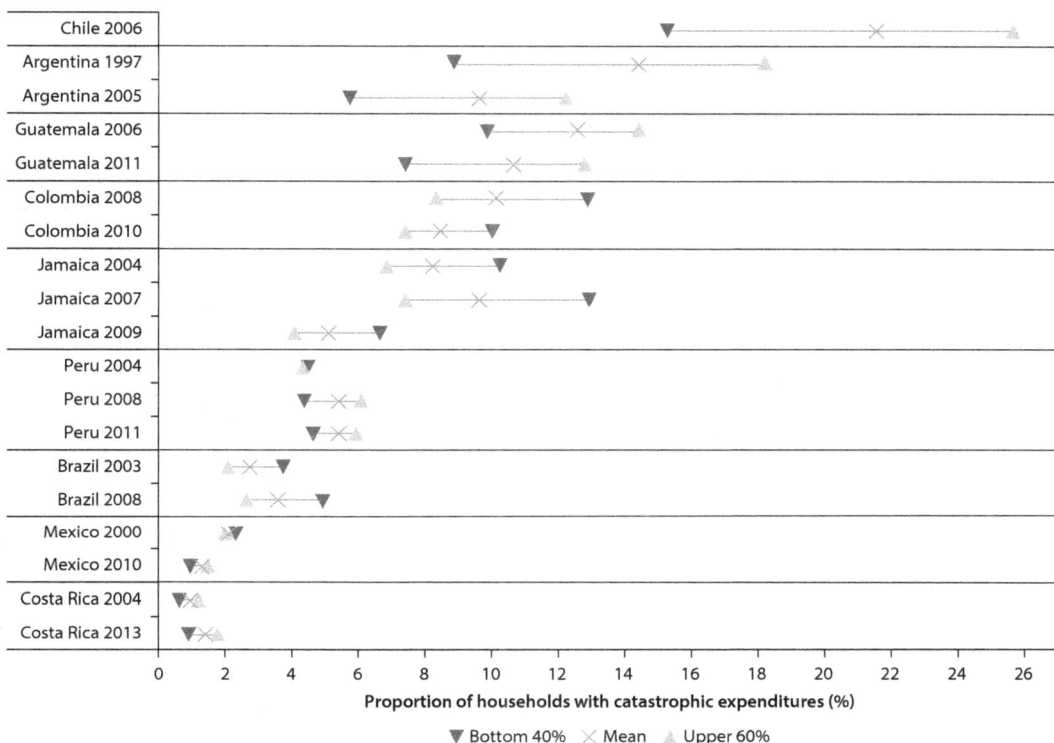

Proportion of households with catastrophic expenditures (%)

▼ Bottom 40% ✕ Mean ▲ Upper 60%

Sources: Study estimates based on Argentina—ENGH 1997 and 2005; Brazil—POF 2002–03 and 2009–09; Chile—ESGS 2006; Colombia—ECV 2008 and 2010; Costa Rica—ENIG 2004 and 2013; Guatemala—ENCOVI 2006 and 2011; Jamaica—JSLC 2007 and 2009; Mexico—ENIGH 2000 and 2010; Peru—ENAHO 2004 and 2008.
Note: Catastrophic health expenditures defined at the 25 percent threshold of nonfood consumption.

Tracking Progress through Summary Measures

The data presented in the previous section does not directly answer the question about whether there is a causal link between the programs implemented and the changes that occurred in health outcomes, service utilization, or financial protection. A number of comprehensive evaluations have been carried out in the region that do establish that health reforms have had a positive impact (Dow and Schmeer 2003; Frenz and others 2013; Gertler, Martinez, and Celhay 2011; Macinko and others 2006; Rasella, Aquino, and Barreto 2010). Giedion, Alfonso, and Díaz (2013) conducted a review of the literature on impact of universal coverage schemes in developing countries and conclude that the strength of the evidence varies depending on the result measured. Evidence is strongest of the positive impact on access to health care. Further, the studies indicate that this

Figure 4.30 Impoverishment Attributable to Out-of-Pocket Payments for Health Care, 2000–10 (or Nearest Year)

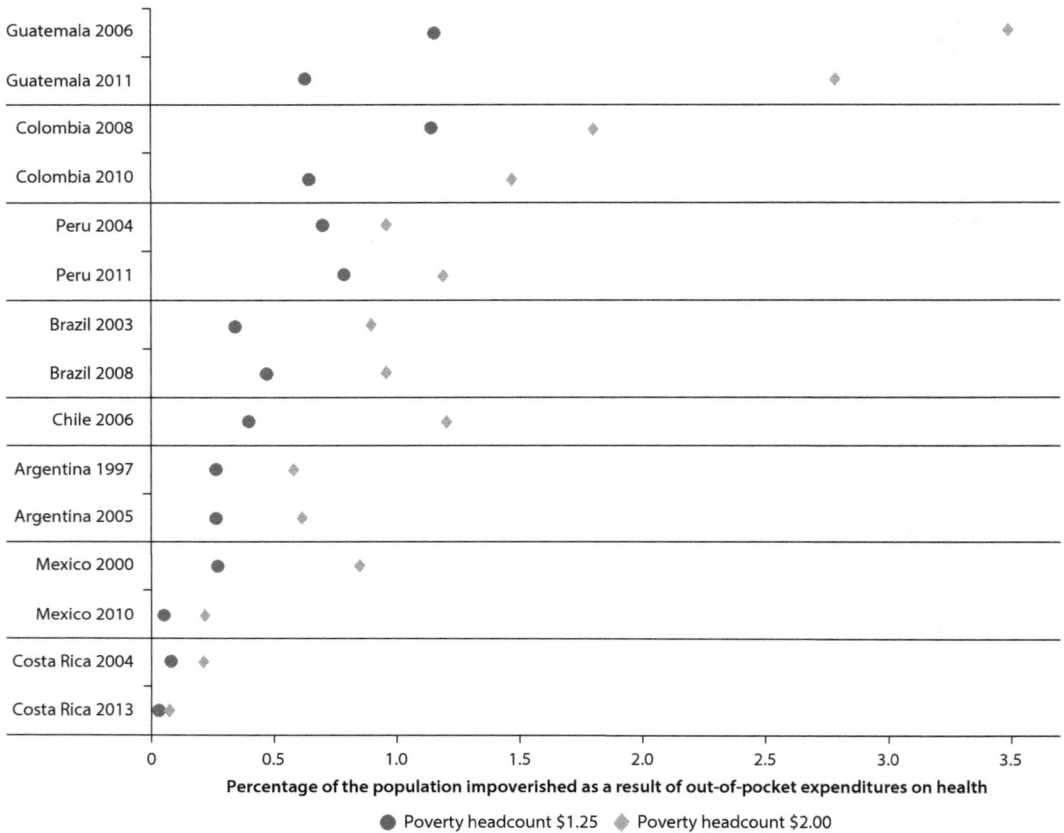

Percentage of the population impoverished as a result of out-of-pocket expenditures on health

● Poverty headcount $1.25   ◆ Poverty headcount $2.00

Sources: Study estimates based on Argentina—ENGH 1997 and 2005; Brazil—POF 2002–03 and 2009–09; Chile—ESGS 2006; Colombia—ECV 2008 and 2010; Costa Rica—ENIG 2004 and 2013; Guatemala—ENCOVI 2006 and 2011; Jamaica—JSLC 2007 and 2009; Mexico—ENIGH 2000 and 2010; Peru—ENAHO 2004 and 2008.

impact is heterogeneous, with benefits accruing mostly to the worse-off socio-economic groups. This suggests that monitoring equity in utilization of health services may be a good proxy measure of progress toward universal health care coverage across countries.

The service utilization data analyzed in detail in the previous sections have been compiled below in a way that allows for countries to assess their progress in increasing the level and distribution of service coverage over time and relative to other countries in the region. The quadrant marked in green delineates the range in which both the level of service utilization is above the regional average and relative inequality across income groups is less than the regional median. Services have been grouped into two broad categories. The first includes repro-ductive, maternal, newborn, and child health services that are proven to be cost-effective in preventing maternal and child deaths (Jamison and others 2006,

2013); these are MDG-related services. The second groups services for the general population and some NCD interventions. All selected service delivery indicators have the characteristic that more of the service is preferable to less, they are bounded to be between zero and 100 percent and the desirable coverage target is 100 percent.

The region has generally high levels of MDG-related interventions, particularly maternal health services for which service coverage approaches 100 percent (figure 4.31). Furthermore, with few exceptions, countries are moving in the right direction, with coverage levels increasing and utilization becoming less pro-rich over time. Coverage is particularly equitable for public health programs such as family planning and immunization; many countries have reached near complete equality in contraceptive prevalence. It should be noted that immunization rates obtained from population-based surveys are invariably lower than results reported using administrative data, which yields coverage figures for the region as a whole in the 93–96 percent range depending on the vaccine (PAHO 2013).

Figure 4.31 Tracking Progress in Level and Distribution of MDG-Related Services, 1995–2010 (or Nearest Year)

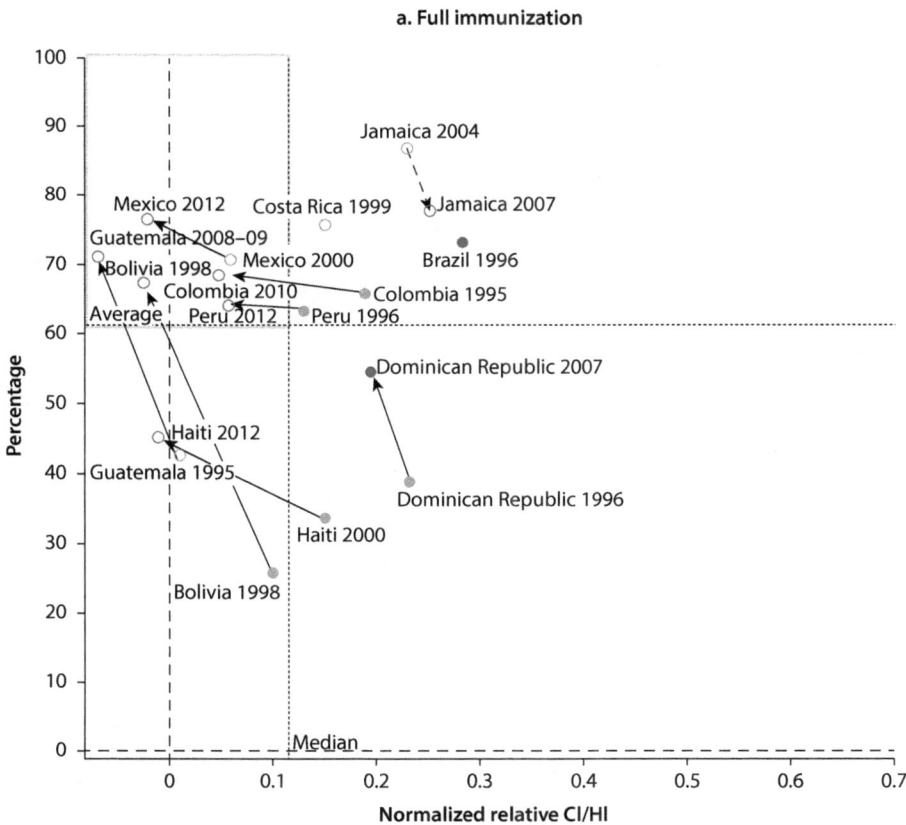

a. Full immunization

figure continues next page

Toward Universal Health Coverage and Equity in Latin America and the Caribbean
http://dx.doi.org/10.1596/978-1-4648-0454-0

Figure 4.31   Tracking Progress in Level and Distribution of MDG-Related Services, 1995–2010 (or Nearest Year) *(continued)*

b. Medical treatment of acute respiratory infection

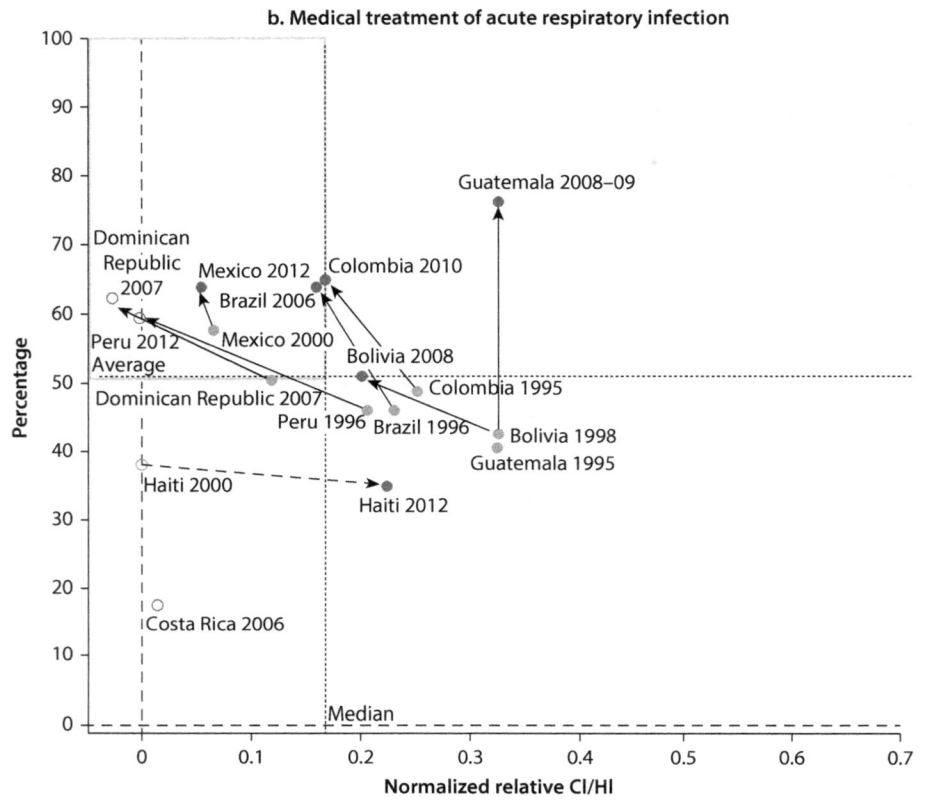

Figure 4.31 Tracking Progress in Level and Distribution of MDG-Related Services, 1995–2010 (or Nearest Year) (continued)

c. Contraceptive prevalence

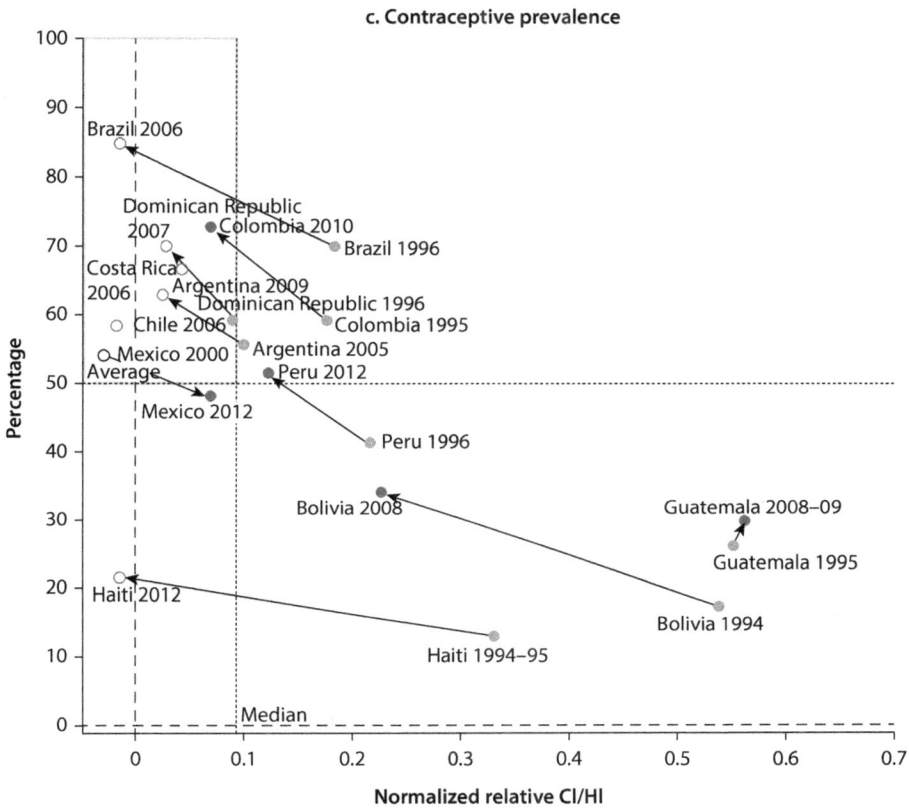

figure continues next page

Figure 4.31 Tracking Progress in Level and Distribution of MDG-Related Services, 1995–2010 (or Nearest Year) *(continued)*

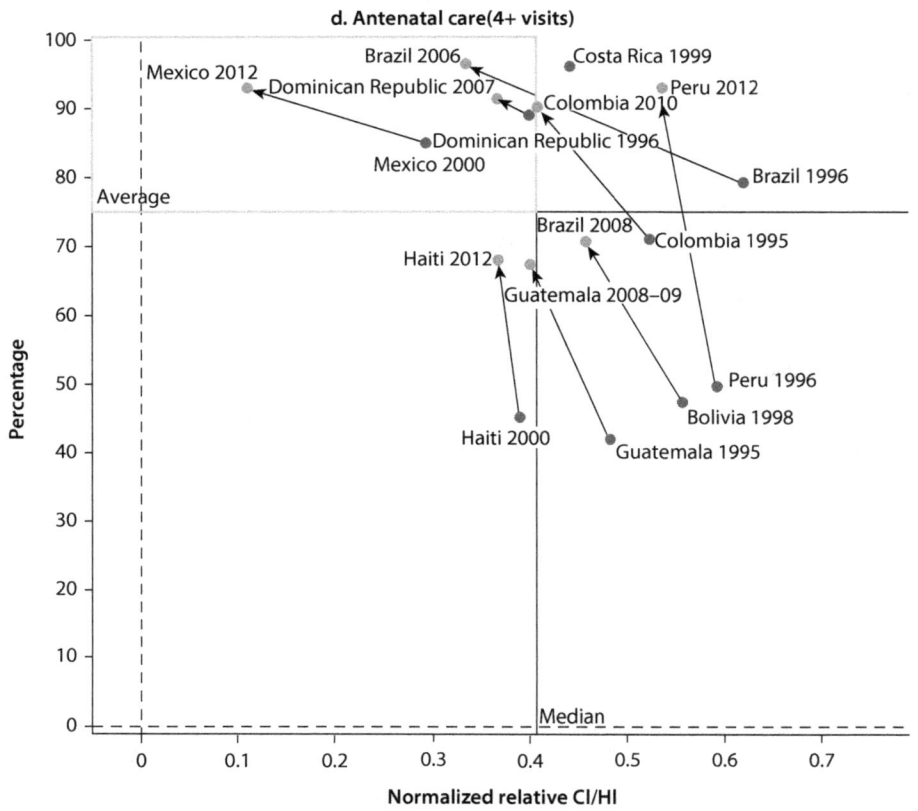

d. Antenatal care(4+ visits)

Toward Universal Health Coverage and Equity in Latin America and the Caribbean
http://dx.doi.org/10.1596/978-1-4648-0454-0

Figure 4.31 Tracking Progress in Level and Distribution of MDG-Related Services, 1995–2010 (or Nearest Year) *(continued)*

e. Skilled birth attendance

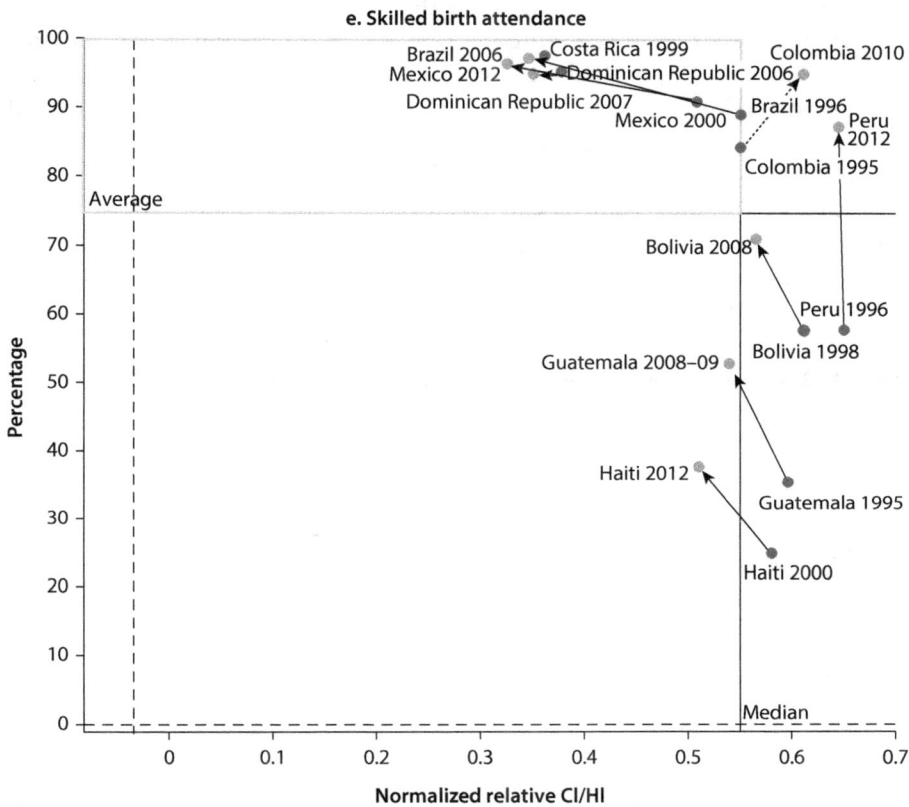

Note: The northwest quadrant refers to high average, low inequality; the northeast quadrant refers to high average, high inequality; the southwest quadrant refers low average, low inequality; and the the southeast quadrant refers to low average, high inequality. Dots represent CI/HI statistically significant at 5 percent. Circles represent CI/HI not statistically significant at this level. Blue represents the oldest survey year, while orange represents the most recent or a single survey year. CI/HI = concentration index/horizontal inequity index.

The relative position of countries, however, is generally maintained. Peru is an exception both in that the 2004–08 figures place it below the average and that they show decline in immunization coverage. Primary care services, such as medical treatment of acute respiratory infections and antenatal care, are more pro-rich than public health programs but less so than skilled deliveries, which are mostly provided in a hospital setting in the region. Brazil, the Dominican Republic, and Mexico fare well in the level and distribution of coverage across these primary-care services. It would have been interesting to compare their performance to that of the LAC countries that were used by the Lancet Commission—which revised the case for investments in health on the occasion of the 20th anniversary of the 1993 World Development Report—as a reference because they achieve high levels of health status in 2011 despite having been

Toward Universal Health Coverage and Equity in Latin America and the Caribbean
http://dx.doi.org/10.1596/978-1-4648-0454-0

classified as lower-middle income countries two decades earlier (Jamison and others 2013). Surprisingly, however, neither Chile nor Costa Rica has trend data from surveys for maternal and child health variables. Demographic health surveys are generally the source for this information, and developing countries often received financial support and technical assistance for implementation from the U.S. Agency for International Development. Chile and Costa Rica did not benefit from this support, perhaps precisely because of their high level of achievement in health and human development more generally.

Without exception, countries in the region are progressing toward greater coverage of preventive visits and screening for cervical and breast cancers (figure 4.32). But coverage for NCD interventions is considerably lower than for

Figure 4.32 Tracking Progress in Level and Distribution of NCD Services, 1995–2010 (or Nearest Year)

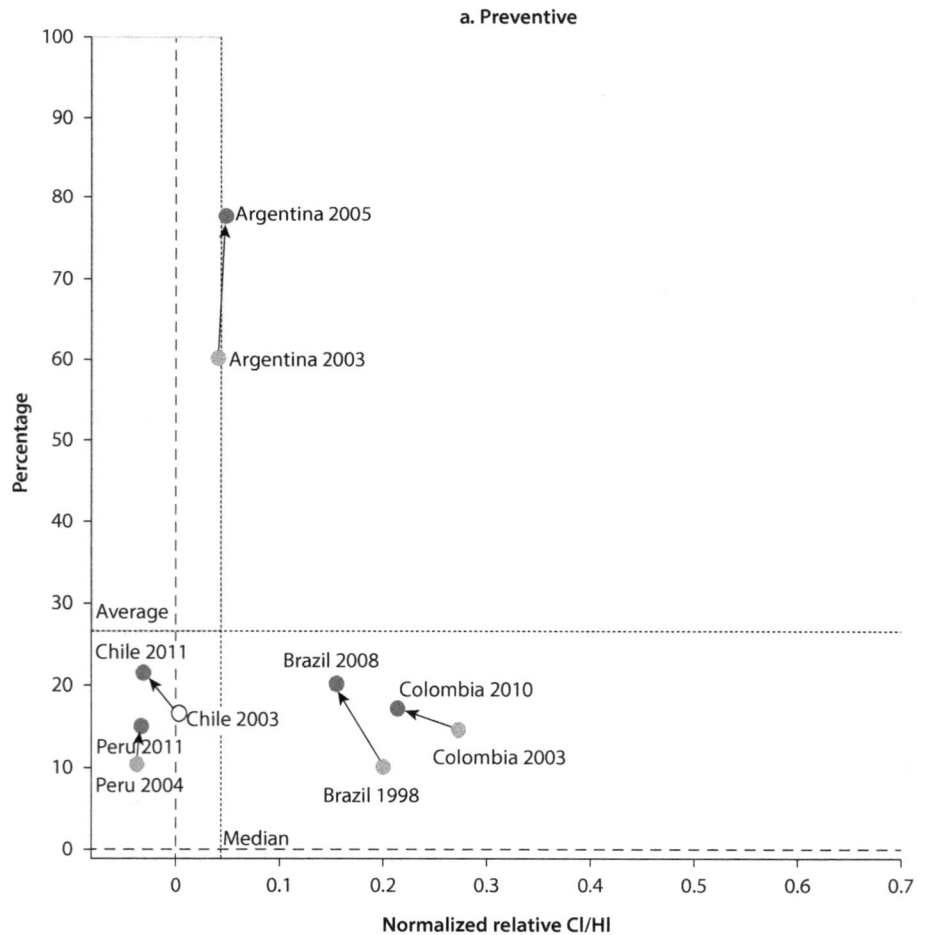

a. Preventive

Figure 4.32 Tracking Progress in Level and Distribution of NCD Services, 1995–2010 (or Nearest Year) *(continued)*

b. Cervical cancer screening

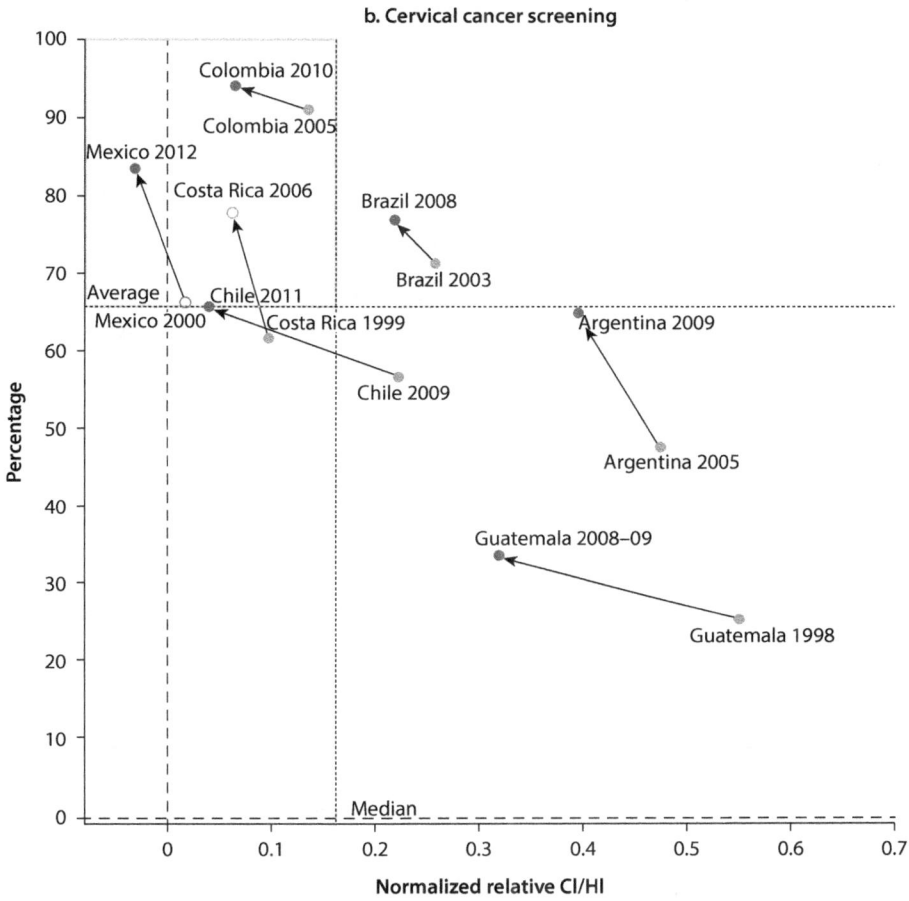

figure continues next page

Toward Universal Health Coverage and Equity in Latin America and the Caribbean
http://dx.doi.org/10.1596/978-1-4648-0454-0

Figure 4.32 Tracking Progress in Level and Distribution of NCD Services, 1995–2010 (or Nearest Year) *(continued)*

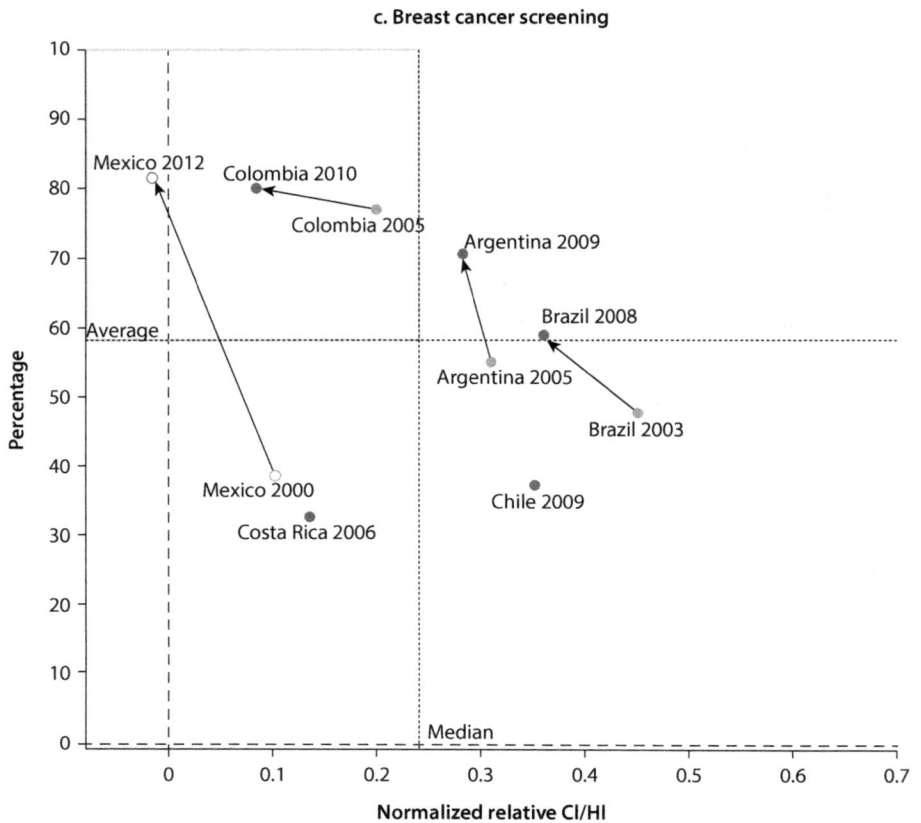

c. Breast cancer screening

Note: The northwest quadrant refers to high average, low inequality; the northeast quadrant refers to high average, high inequality; the southwest quadrant refers low average, low inequality; and the the southeast quadrant refers to low average, high inequality. Dots represent CI/HI statistically significant at 5 percent. Circles represent CI/HI not statistically significant at this level. Blue represents the oldest survey year, while orange represents the most recent or a single survey year. CI/HI = concentration index/horizontal inequity index.

reproductive, maternal, and child health services. Coverage of preventive visits is especially low. With few exceptions, these services are utilized more by the rich than the poor, though disparities are narrowing. Services delivered in a primary care setting, such as general preventive visits and cervical cancer screening, are less skewed toward the better off than mammography, which requires special-ized care and imaging equipment. In contrast, Pap smear cytology is a low-cost intervention, making the low coverage in some countries the more surprising.

The summary indicators presented here are heavily skewed toward preventive interventions, confirming other indicator review findings that revealed that there is a paucity of good treatment and coverage indicators for developing countries (WHO and World Bank 2014). This is particularly apparent for services related to the treatment and management of noncommunicable diseases, which is a major shortcoming in light of the growing burden associated with this category of diseases. The complexity of the essential package of best buys for clinical intervention of noncommunicable disease control puts into question whether population surveys are the appropriate instrument with which to track progress in delivering these services. For instance, it is fairly simple to determine through a household interview whether a pregnant woman had a delivery assisted by a skilled attendant or a child received a full course of vaccination (though as discussed earlier the results may still deviate from administrative data). In contrast, the interventions in the WHO essential package for ischemic heart disease, for example, include counseling and multidrug therapy for people who have had a heart attack or are at high risk (≥30 percent) of a cardiovascular event in the next 10 years, and treatment of heart attacks with aspirin (Jamison and others 2013). While medicines for cardiovascular risk reduction can be packaged into polypills, there are a variety of drug combinations that are prescribed depending on individual patient characteristics. This complexity makes it challenging to isolate a service delivery indicator that would have a target population identifiable thorough a household interview and for whom the coverage target would be 100 percent.

Administrative records provide more granular data for monitoring treatment and management of noncommunicable and chronic diseases, particularly if we are to consider quality, discussed in the next chapter. Nevertheless, assessing the equity dimension (which we argue is essential to monitoring progress toward UHC), requires analysis of administrative data stratified by measures of socioeconomic status or other relevant social determinants. Because health information systems tend not to record the income of the patient, some studies have used place of residence as a proxy variable for stratification by socioeconomic status. The analysis is more robust when geographic areas are homogeneous, which generally requires information on neighborhood of residence. For the most part, this would entail refining the health information systems being used in developing countries. Analyses of NCDs will likely include a combination of survey and administrative data.

In their comprehensive review of evaluations of universal coverage schemes, Giedion, Alfonso, and Díaz (2013) find evidence of their positive impact on financial protection; it is less convincing, however, than the evidence of their impact on service utilization. There are fewer studies on the effect on financial protection, and the evidence is stronger that the programs result in declines in out-of-pocket spending more so than in catastrophic health expenditures. This may be due to the limitations of this type of measure, which were discussed in the previous section. Though only four studies in the review assessed impact on impoverishment, three found a positive effect. This suggests that impoverishment may be a better measure than catastrophic health expenditures for monitoring progress across the financial protection dimension of UHC.

The picture is less clear when we look at our results on progress regarding financial protection. Mexico is the only country moving in the right direction, with declining catastrophic expenditures, a reduction in impoverishment due to health spending, and a shrinking share of out-of-pocket payments in total health expenditures. Colombia has on the one hand seen a decline in catastrophic expenditures and impoverishment, but on the other a rise in out-of-pocket share of total health spending; the opposite is true in Brazil. Peru saw all three indicators worsen. Impoverishment caused by health expenditures is lowest in Costa Rica and Mexico, despite the high out-of-pocket expenditures in the latter. Chile is an outlier, with highest level of catastrophic health expenditures among study countries. It is unfortunate and surprising that for both Chile and Costa Rica the periodicity of the data is sparse for the financial protection indicators. Likewise, Brazil's next survey gathering this information is scheduled for 2015, broadening the current five-year gap by at least two years.

Giedion, Alfonso, and Díaz (2013) also reviewed the impact of universal coverage schemes on health status and find that most studies are inconclusive, though a few did demonstrate a positive impact. Macinko and others (2006) find that the Family Health Program contributed to the decline in child mortality and other outcomes in Brazil; in a midterm evaluation of Plan Nacer in Argentina, Gertler, Martinez, and Celhay (2011) found that very low birth weights and early neonatal deaths declined in two provinces; Dow and Schmeer (2003) concluded that expanded health insurance in Costa Rica caused infant and child mortality to decline, although it explained only a small part of the declines when they controlled for confounding factors. Although improved health status may be the ultimate goal of programs to advance UHC, other social determinants are at play, several of them outside the purview of the health sector. Countries must monitor health-outcome indicators, of course, but alone, these are insufficient for thorough assessments of programs to advance UHC.

Improvements in utilization and financial protection are more immediate objectives of these programs. This clear relationship, supported by impact-evaluation studies, suggests that they are good measures to monitor progress toward UHC. Although useful for countries to benchmark their evolution both over time and relative to other countries, monitoring these summary measures should in no way substitute for in-depth evaluations of the impact of individual programs. The studies analyzed by Giedion, Alfonso, and Díaz (2013) reveal that the impact of universal coverage schemes on utilization and financial protection varies depending on program design and implementation. The complexities of individual programs detailed in the previous chapter cannot be fully captured through simple measures.

Finally, we note that variations in access and utilization of health services stem from availability and quality of care, transportation, affordability, waiting time, service hours, cultural and language barriers, discrimination, and information about and understanding of risk factors, among others. These dynamics contribute to inequalities in health outcomes, including premature mortality and higher disease prevalence among the poor and disadvantaged (WHO 2005). An individual's socioeconomic position does not exist in isolation and can produce a cycle of disadvantages, including limited access to health care, education, information, and other goods and services (UNDP 2005), all of which can impact health behavior. The reduction of gaps between the rich and the poor in utilization of needed health care requires the elimination of barriers to access so this cycle of disadvantage can be interrupted. Monitoring and evaluating service coverage and financial protection at local and national levels becomes essential to ensure that corrective actions and programs can be implemented so everyone can access the services they need.

Notes

1. Uruguay was not included because we lacked access to survey data for the period under study.
2. See table 3.1 for a categorization of countries according to the level of segmentation of their health systems.
3. Coverage of vaccines against seasonal influenza and haemophilus influenza has increased, which partly explains the reduction in respiratory infections.
4. It should be noted these immunization rates, obtained from population-based surveys, are significantly below those reported in the annual PAHO publication *Immunization in the Americas*, which relies on administrative data.
5. This can be seen more clearly in the disaggregated data in appendix C.
6. Need as "capacity to benefit" is said to be the ability of an individual to benefit from health care. According to Dixon and others (2011), capacity to benefit implies that those with worse health status have a greater need for health care.
7. Capacity to pay is defined as income after basic subsistence is met, where subsistence is average food consumption of households in the 45th to 55th percentile range.

References

Almeida, Gisele, and Flávia Mori Sarti. 2013. "Measuring Evolution of Income-Related Inequalities in Health and Health Care Utilization in Selected Latin American and Caribbean Countries." *Revista Panamericana de Salud Pública* 33 (2): 83–89.

Bitrán, Ricardo, Rodrigo Muñoz, and Lorena Prieto. 2010. "Health Insurance and Access to Health Services, Health Services Use and Health Status in Peru." In *The Impact of Health Insurance in Low and Middle Income Countries*, edited by Maria-Luisa Escobar, Charles C. Griffin, and R. Paul Shaw. Washington, DC: Brookings Institution Press.

Bonilla-Chacín, Maria Eugenia, ed. 2014. *Promoting Healthy Living in Latin America and the Caribbean: Governance of Multisectoral Activities to Prevent Risk Factors for Noncommunicable Diseases*. Washington, DC: World Bank.

Bott, S., A. Guedes, M. Goodwin, and J. A. Mendoza. 2012. *Violence against Women in Latin America and the Caribbean: A Comparative Analysis of Population-Based Data from 12 Countries*. Washington, DC: Pan American Health Organization.

Breslau, Naomi, and Edward Peterson. 1996. "Smoking Cessation in Young Adults: Age and Initiation of Cigarette Smoking and Other Suspected Influences." *American Journal of Public Health* 86 (2): 214–20.

Cercone, James, Etoile Pinder, Jose Pacheco Jimenez, and Rodrigo Briceno. 2010. "Impact of Health Insurance on Access, Use, and Health Status in Costa Rica." In *The Impact of Health Insurance in Low and Middle Income Countries*, edited by Maria-Luisa Escobar, Charles C. Griffin, and R. Paul Shaw. Washington, DC: Brookings Institution Press.

CONAPO (Consejo Nacional de Población). 2011. "Índice de marginación por entidad federativa y municipio 2010." Mexico City. http://www.conapo.gob.mx.

Cooper, P. J., L. C. Rodrigues, A. A. Cruz, and M. L. Barreto. 2009. "Asthma in Latin America: A Public Heath Challenge and Research Opportunity." *Allergy* 64 (1): 5–17.

Costa, Eduardo, Mauricio Bregman, Denizar V. Araujo, Claudia H. Costa, and Rogerio Rufino. 2013. "Asthma and the Socio-Economic Reality in Brazil." *World Allergy Organization Journal* 6 (1): 20.

Council on Scientific Affairs. 1986. "Alcohol and the Driver." *JAMA* 255 (4): 522–27.

Couttolenc, Bernard, and Tania Dmytraczenko. 2013. "Brazil's Primary Care Strategy." UNICO Study Series 2, World Bank, Washington, DC.

CSDH (Commission on Social Determinants of Health). 2008. *Closing the Gap in a Generation: Health Equity through Action on the Social Determinants of Health.* Geneva: WHO.

Cunningham, S. A., M. R. Kramer, and K. M. V. Narayan. 2014. "Incidence of Childhood Obesity in the United States." *New England Journal of Medicine* 370: 403–11.

Di Cesare, Mariachiara, Young-Ho Khang, Perviz Asaria, Tony Blakely, Melanie J. Cowan, Farshad Farzadfar, Ramiro Guerrero, Nayu Ikeda, Catherine Kyobutungi, Kelias P. Msyamboza, Sophal Oum, John W. Lynch, Michael G. Marmot, and Majid Ezzati, on behalf of The Lancet NCD Action Group. 2013. "Inequalities in Non-Communicable Diseases and Effective Responses." *The Lancet* 381 (9866): 585–97.

Dixon, Anna, Julian Le Grand, John Henderson, Richard Murray, and Emmi Poteliakhoff. 2003. "Is the NHS Equitable? A Review of Evidence." LSE Health and Social Care Discussion Paper 11, London School of Economics, London.

———. 2011. "Is the NHS Equitable?: A Review of Evidence." LSE Health and Social Care, London School of Economics and Political Science, London.

Dow, William H., and Kammi K. Schmeer. 2003. "Health Insurance and Child Mortality in Costa Rica." *Social Science & Medicine* 57: 975–86.

Fink, Günther, Isabel Günther, and Kenneth Hill. 2011. "The Effect of Water and Sanitation on Child Health: Evidence from the Demographic and Health Surveys 1986–2007." *International Journal of Epidemiology* 40: 1196–204.

Fiszbein, Ariel, Norbert Rudiger Schady, and Francisco H. G. Ferreira. 2009. *Conditional Cash Transfers: Reducing Present and Future Poverty.* Washington, DC: World Bank.

Forouzanfar, Mohammad H., Kyle J. Foreman, Allyne M. Delossantos, Rafael Lozano, Alan D. Lopez, Christopher J. L. Murray, and Mohsen Naghavi. 2011. "Breast and Cervical Cancer in 187 Countries between 1980 and 2010: A Systematic Analysis." *The Lancet* 378 (9801): 1461–84.

Frenz, Patricia, Iris Delgado, Jay S. Kaufman, and Sam Harper. 2013. "Achieving Effective Universal Health Coverage with Equity: Evidence from Chile." *Health Policy and Planning* 29 (6): 717–31.

Gakidou, Emmanuela, Krycia Cowling, Rafael Lozano, and Christopher J. L. Murray. 2010. "Increased Educational Attainment and Its Effect on Child Mortality in 175 Countries between 1970 and 2009: A Systematic Analysis." *The Lancet* 376 (9745): 959–74.

Gertler, Paul, Sebastian Martinez, and Pablo Celhay. 2011. "Impact of Plan Nacer on the Use of Services and Health Outcomes: Intermediate Results Using Administrative Data from Misiones and Tucuman Provinces." World Bank, Washington, DC.

Giedion, Ursula, Eduardo Andrés Alfonso, and Yadira Díaz. 2013. "The Impact of Universal Coverage Schemes in the Developing World: A Review of the Existing Evidence." UNICO Studies Series 25, World Bank, Washington, DC.

Giedion, Ursula, and Manuela Villar Uribe. 2009. "Colombia's Universal Health Insurance Scheme." *Health Affairs* 28 (3): 853–63.

Gonzalez, Rogelio, Jennifer Harris Requejo, Jyh Kae Nien, Mario Merialdi, Flávia Bustreo, and Ana Pilar Betran. 2009. "Tackling Health Inequities in Chile: Maternal, Newborn, Infant, and Child Mortality between 1990 and 2004." *American Journal of Public Health* 99 (7): 1220–26.

Gragnolati, Michele, Magnus Lindelow, and Bernard Couttolenc. 2013. *Twenty Years of Health System Reform in Brazil: An Assessment of the Sistema Único de Saúde.* Washington, DC: World Bank.

HHS (United States Department of Health and Human Services). 2014. *The Health Consequences of Smoking—50 Years of Progress: A Report of the Surgeon General.* Centers for Disease Control and Prevention, Coordinating Center for Health Promotion, National Center for Chronic Disease Prevention and Health Promotion, Office on Smoking and Health. Atlanta, GA: HHS.

Ider, E. L., and Y. Benyamini. 1997. "Self-Rated Health and Mortality: A Review of Twenty Seven Community Studies." *Journal of Health and Social Behavior* 38: 21–37.

IHME (Institute of Health Metrics and Evaluation). 2010. "Global Burden of Disease Compare, Latin America and Caribbean, DALYs, Both Sexes, under 5 Years." University of Washington, Seattle. http://viz.healthmetricsandevaluation.org /gbd-compare.

IHME (Institute of Health Metrics and Evaluation) and World Bank. 2013. *The Global Burden of Disease: Generating Evidence, Guiding Policy: Latin America and Caribbean Regional Edition.* Seattle, WA: Institute of Health Metrics and Evaluation.

Jamison, Dean T., Joel G. Breman, Anthony R. Measham, George Alleyne, Mariam Claeson, David B. Evans, Prabhat Jha, Anne Mills, and Philip Musgrove, eds. 2006. *Priorities in Health.* Washington, DC: World Bank.

Jamison, Dean T., Lawrence H. Summers, George Alleyne, Kenneth J. Arrow, Seth Berkley, Agnes Binagwaho, Flávia Bustreo, David Evans, Richard G. A. Feachem, Julio Frenk, Gargee Ghosh, Sue J. Goldie, Yan Guo, Sanjeev Gupta, Richard Horton, Margaret E. Kruk, Adel Mahmoud, Linah K. Mohohlo, Mthuli Ncube, Ariel Pablos-Mendez, K. Srinath Reddy, Helen Saxenian, Agnes Soucat, Karen H. Ulltveit-Moe, and Gavin Yamey. 2013. "Global Health 2035: A World Converging within a Generation." *The Lancet* 382 (9908): 1898–955.

Jimenez, Jorge, and Maria Ines Romero. 2007. "Reducing Infant Mortality in Chile: Success in Two Phases." *Health Affairs* 26 (2): 458–65.

Knaul, Felicia Marie, Eduardo González-Pier, Octavio Gómez-Dantés, David García-Junco, Héctor Arreola-Ornelas, Mariana Barraza-Lloréns, Rosa Sandoval, Francisco

Caballero, Mauricio Hernández-Avila, Mercedes Juan, David Kershenobich, Gustavo Nigenda, Enrique Ruelas, Jaime Sepúlveda, Roberto Tapia, Guillermo Soberón, Salomón Chertorivski, and Julio Frenk. 2012. "The Quest for Universal Health Coverage: Achieving Social Protection for all in Mexico." *The Lancet* 380 (9849): 1259–79.

Laxminarayan, Ramanan, and Lori Ashford. 2008. "Using Evidence about 'Best Buys' to Advance Global Health." Disease Control Priorities Project.

Liu, Li, Hope L. Johnson, Simon Cousens, Jamie Perin, Susana Scott, Joy E. Lawn, Igor Rudan, Harry Campbell, Richard Cibulskis, Mengying Li, Colin Mathers, and Robert E. Black, for the Child Health Epidemiology Reference Group of WHO and UNICEF. 2012. "Global, Regional, and National Causes of Child Mortality: An Updated Systematic Analysis for 2010 with Time Trends Since 2000." *The Lancet* 379 (9832): 2151–61.

Lora, Eduardo. 2012. "Health Perceptions in Latin America." *Health Policy and Planning* 27 (7): 555–69.

Macinko, James, Frederico C. Guanais, Maria de Fatima, and Marinho de Souza. 2006. "Evaluation of the Impact of the Family Health Program on Infant Mortality in Brazil, 1990–2002." *Journal of Epidemiology and Community Health* 60 (1): 13–19.

Marcus, M., M. T. Yasamy, M. Van Ommeren, D. Chisholm, and S. Saxena. 2012. "Depression: A Global Public Health Concern." World Federation of Mental Health, World Health Organization, Perth, Australia.

Mayhew, D. R., A. C. Donelson, D. J. Beirness, and H. M. Simpson. 1986. "Youth, Alcohol and Relative Risk of Crash Involvement." *Accident, Analysis & Prevention* 18 (4): 273–87.

Miller, Anthony B., Claus Wall, Cornelia J. Baines, Ping Sun, Teresa To, and Steven A. Narod. 2014. "Twenty Five Year Follow-Up for Breast Cancer Incidence and Mortality of the Canadian National Breast Screening Study: Randomised Screening Trial." *British Medical Journal* 348:1–10.

Mossey, Jana M., and Evelyn Shapiro. 1982. "Self-Rated Health: A Predictor of Mortality among the Elderly." *American Journal of Public Health* 72 (8): 800–8.

Mukhtar, Toqir K., David R. G. Yeates, and Michael J. Goldacre. 2013. "Breast Cancer Mortality Trends in England and the Assessment of the Effectiveness of Mammography Screening: Population-Based Study." *Journal of the Royal Society of Medicine* 106 (6): 234–42.

Neffen, Hugo, Carlos Fritscher, Francisco Cuevas Schacht, Gur Levy, Pascual Chiarella, Joan B. Soriano, and Daniel Mechali. 2005. "Asthma Control in Latin America: The Asthma Insights and Reality in Latin America (AIRLA) Survey." *Revista Panamericana de Salud Pública* 17 (3): 191–97.

O'Donnell, Owen A., and Adam Wagstaff. 2008. *Analyzing Health Equity Using Household Survey Data: A Guide to Techniques and Their Implementation.* Washington, DC: World Bank.

OECD (Organisation for Economic Co-operation and Development). 2004. *Towards High-Performing Health Systems.* Paris: OECD.

———. 2011. *Health at a Glance 2011: OECD Indicators.* Paris: OECD. doi: 10.1787/health_glance-2011-en.

Omer, Saad B., Daniel A. Salmon, Walter A. Orenstein, M. Patricia de Hart, and Neal Halsey. 2009. "Vaccine Refusal, Mandatory Immunization, and the Risks for Vaccine-Preventable Diseases." *New England Journal of Medicine* 360 (19): 1981–88.

PAHO (Pan American Health Organization). 2012. "Health in the Americas: Regional Outlook and Country Profiles." PAHO, Washington, DC.

———. 2013. *Cancer in the Americas: Country Profiles 2013*. Washington, DC: PAHO.

———. 2014. "Strategy for Universal Access to Health and Universal Health Coverage." Document CD53/5, Rev 2, 53rd Directing Council, PAHO, Washington, DC.

Pearce, Neil, Nadia Ait-Khaled, Richard Beasley, Javier Mallol, Ulrich Keil, Ed Mitchell, and Colin Robertson. 2007. "Worldwide Trends in the Prevalence of Asthma Symptoms: Phase III of the International Study of Asthma and Allergies in Childhood (ISAAC)." *Thorax* 62 (9): 758–66.

Rasella, Davide, Rosana Aquino, and Mauricio L. Barreto. 2010. "Reducing Childhood Mortality from Diarrhea and Lower Respiratory Tract Infections in Brazil." *Pediatrics* 126 (3): e534–40.

Richardson, Vesta, Joselito Hernandez-Pichardo, Manjari Quintanar-Solares, Marcelino Esparza-Aguilar, Brian Johnson, Cesar Misael Gomez-Altamirano, Umesh Parashar, and Manish Patel. 2010. "Effect of Rotavirus Vaccination on Death from Childhood Diarrhea in Mexico." *New England Journal of Medicine* 362 (4): 299–305.

Rudan, Igor, Cynthia Boschi-Pinto, Zrinka Biloglav, Kim Mulholland, and Harry Campbell. 2008. "Epidemiology and Etiology of Childhood Pneumonia." *Bulletin of the World Health Organization* 86 (5): 408–16.

Seguridad, Justicia y Paz. 2013. "Metodología del ranking (2013) de las 50 ciudades más violentas del mundo." http://www.seguridadjusticiaypaz.org.mx/biblioteca/summary/5-prensa/177-por-tercer-ano-consecutivo-san-pedro-sula-es-la-ciudad-mas-violenta-del-mundo.

Shengelia, Bakhuti, Ajay Tandon, Orvill B. Adams, and Christopher J. L. Murray. 2005. "Access, Utilization, Quality, and Effective Coverage: An Integrated Conceptual Framework and Measurement Strategy." *Social Science and Medicine* 61 (1): 97–109.

Tabár, Laszlo, Bedrich Vitak, Tony Hsiu-His Chen, Amy Ming-Fang Yen, Anders Cohen, Tibor Tot, Sherry Yueh-Hsia Chiu, Sam Li-Sheng Chen, Jean Ching-Yuan Fann, Johan Rosell, Helena Fohlin, Robert A. Smith, and Stephen W. Duffy. 2011. "Swedish Two-County Trial: Impact of Mammographic Screening on Breast Cancer Mortality during 3 Decades." *Radiology-Radiological Society of North America* 260 (3): 658.

Torres, A., O. L. Sarmiento, C. Stauber, and R. Zarama. 2013. "The Ciclovia and Cicloruta Programs: Promising Interventions to Promote Physical Security and Social Capital in Bogotá, Colombia." *American Journal of Public Health* 103 (2): e23–30.

UNDP (United Nations Development Program). 2005. *Inequality in Health and Human Development*. New York: UNDP.

UNICEF (United Nations Children's Fund), World Health Organization, World Bank, and United Nations. 2013. *Levels and Trends in Child Mortality Report 2013: Estimates Developed by the UN Inter-Agency Group for Child Mortality Estimation*. New York: UNICEF.

USPSTF (U.S. Preventive Services Task Force). 2012. "Screening for Cervical Cancer—Clinical Summary of U.S. Preventive Services Task Force Recommendation." Agency for Healthcare Research and Quality, U.S. Department of Health and Human Services, Washington, DC. http://www.uspreventiveservicestaskforce.org/uspstf/uspscerv.htm.

van Doorslaer, E., and C. Masseria. 2004. *Income-Related Inequalities in the Use of Medical Care in 21 OECD Countries*. Paris: OECD.

Victora, Cesar G., Estela M. L. Aquino, Maria do Carmo Leal, Carlos Augusto Monteiro, Fernando C. Barros, and Celia L. Szwarcwald. 2011. "Maternal and Child Health in Brazil: Progress and Challenges." *The Lancet* 377 (9780): 1863–76.

Wagstaff, Adam. 2011. "The Concentration Index of a Binary Outcome Revisited." *Health Economics* 20 (10): 1155–60.

Wagstaff, Adam, Marcel Bilger, Zurba Sajaia, and Michael Lokshin. 2011. *Health Equity and Financial Protection*. Washington, DC: World Bank.

Wagstaff, Adam, and Eddy van Doorslaer. 2000. "Measuring and Testing for Inequity in the Delivery of Health Care." *Journal of Human Resources* 35 (4): 716–33.

———. 2003. "Catastrophe and Impoverishment in Paying for Health Care: With Applications to Vietnam 1993–1998." *Health Economics* 12 (11): 921–33.

WHO (World Health Organization). 2005. "Action on the Social Determinants of Health: Learning from Previous Experiences." Commission on Social Determinants of Health. World Health Organization, Geneva.

———. 2008. *The World Health Report 2008: Primary Health Care—Now More Than Ever*. Geneva: WHO.

———. 2010. *The World Health Report—Health Systems Financing: The Path to Universal Coverage*. Geneva: WHO.

———. 2011. *Global Status Report on Alcohol and Health*. Geneva: WHO. http://www .who.int/substance_abuse/publications/global_alcohol_report/en.

WHO and World Bank. 2014. "Monitoring Progress toward Universal Health Coverage at Country and Global Levels: A Framework." Joint WHO/World Bank Group Discussion Paper, WHO and World Bank, Washington, DC.

World Bank. 2012. "Datasheet for Bolivia, Brazil, Colombia, Dominican Republic, Guatemala, Haiti and Peru." http://web.worldbank.org/WBSITE/EXTERNAL /TOPICS/EXTHEALTHNUTRITIONANDPOPULATION/EXTPAH/0,,contentM DK:23159049~menuPK:400482~pagePK:148956~piPK:216618~theSit ePK:400476,00.html.

Xu, Ke, David B. Evans, Kei Kawabata, Riadh Zeramdini, Jan Klavus, and Christopher J. L. Murray. 2003. "Household Catastrophic Health Expenditure: A Multicountry Analysis." *The Lancet* 362 (9378): 111–17.

CHAPTER 5

Assessing Progress toward Universal Health Coverage: Beyond Utilization and Financial Protection

Magnus Lindelow, Saskia Nahrgang, Tania Dmytraczenko, Fatima Marinho, and Lane Alencar

Abstract

Assessments of the movement toward universal health coverage tend to focus on the utilization of health services, formal entitlement or eligibility to access services, and measures of financial protection. However, if our concern is to assess to what extent all persons can obtain the health care they need without financial hardship, indicators in these areas have important limitations. Indeed, expansion of health care coverage, in the sense of making health services available and more affordable, does not automatically translate into improved health outcomes. With this issue in mind, chapter 5 complements analyses of patterns of utilization, coverage, and financial protection in Latin America and the Caribbean (LAC) with a review of what is known about the links between utilization and health outcomes. In doing so, it looks at questions of unmet need for health care, timeliness of care, and quality of health services. These are areas in which measurement tends to be harder than in the case of utilization and financial protection. Nonetheless, although there are limited routine data that are comparable across countries, studies and monitoring data from selected countries provide enough of a picture to highlight the importance of these issues and hopefully to spur efforts to develop more systematic approaches for collecting and reporting on timeliness and quality of care in the region.

Introduction

Although often not explicitly stated in the definition of universal health coverage (UHC)—"to ensure that everyone who needs health services is able to get them, without undue financial hardship" (WHO and World Bank 2014, 1)—the concept hinges on the notion that people are able to access *quality* services that are effective in dealing with the conditions that afflict them. However, assessments of progress toward UHC tend to focus on formal entitlements and eligibility to access services (for example, insurance coverage), utilization of health services (for example, number of consultations or percentage of a target population receiving a particular intervention), and measures of financial protection (for example, share of population falling below the poverty line because of health expenditures). These are clearly critical issues. But if the concern is to assess the extent to which all persons can get the health care they need without financial hardship, the traditional indicators have important limitations (see, for example, Savedoff 2009).

Consider the case of heart disease, which now accounts for a large share of mortality and the burden of disease in LAC. For patients with increased risk of heart disease, or experiencing complications associated with this condition, their health care needs are complex. UHC would mean the broad implementation of proven primary prevention programs. It would also mean early diagnosis and, once diagnosed, effective management through regular monitoring of blood pressure and cholesterol, support to change health-related behaviors such as smoking and diet, and prescription of appropriate medication. And it would mean timely and effective emergency care in the event of a heart attack or stroke. This example highlights the complexity of the concept of *need* for health services, which is central to the definition of UHC. It also emphasizes the importance of *quality* and *timeliness* in ensuring that health care needs are met.

The limitations of simple indicators of utilization and financial protection are also apparent in the case of antenatal care (ANC). A typical coverage indicator focuses on the percentage of pregnant women that attend a defined number of ANC consultations. But for these visits to improve pregnancy outcomes, the care needs to be effective. The nurse or doctor needs to communicate effectively with the pregnant woman, correctly perform appropriate tests and exams, ensure that test results are communicated and acted on in a timely manner, identify risks, take appropriate actions, etc.

These examples make it clear that expanded benefits coverage, in the sense of making health services available and more affordable, will not automatically translate into improved health outcomes; such gains depend equally on improving the quality of care. Indeed, even among high-income countries with a long history of universal population coverage, there are large disparities in health outcomes. These disparities are in part due to broader economic, social, and environmental factors. However, these differences across countries persist even when focusing on indicators that closely track the performance of the health system, such as amenable mortality, survival from cancer or heart attack, or the rate of complications from chronic conditions such as diabetes. In addition, significant variation in timeliness and quality *within* countries also persist. Those who are poor face greater problems not only in accessing care but also in receiving adequate care from providers. Putting aside for a moment the diverse interpretations of the timeliness and quality of health care, and how these should be measured, let us acknowledge that they (1) are key dimensions of health-system performance and (2) can drive a significant wedge between utilization and outcomes.

The aim of this chapter is to complement analyses of patterns of population coverage, service utilization, and financial protection in LAC by selectively reviewing the links between utilization and health outcomes. Specifically, it will look at questions of unmet need, timeliness of care, and quality of health services. These issues are central to UHC—health care needs cannot be effectively met without a clear sense of what people need, and unless the care provided is timely and of adequate quality. In keeping with the earlier chapters, this chapter also considers distributional issues in relation to timely access and quality. Although limited, it suggests that disadvantages in access and financial protection faced by the poor and other vulnerable groups are compounded by disparities in the quality of health services available to them.

The chapter is intended to stimulate a greater appreciation of why it is important to systematically monitor and analyze timeliness and quality of health care and connect such efforts to policy analysis and public debate on UHC. The focus of the chapter is intentionally selective. It does not review all policies and programs in LAC with an eye toward improving quality and timeliness of access, as such an effort would warrant a report in its own right. It also does not purport to be a comprehensive analysis of health-system performance. Indeed, many important dimensions of health-system performance are left out of this chapter, either because they are covered elsewhere in this report, or because they are only indirectly related to achievement of UHC (for example, efficiency).[1] Finally, the chapter is also selective in the countries analyzed and in the extent of comparative analysis. For many countries in the region, data are limited regarding unmet need, timeliness, and quality. The data we have also lack standardization and so do not lend themselves to comparability. Notwithstanding these limitations, studies and monitoring data from selected countries provide enough of a picture to highlight the importance of these issues and hopefully to stimulate efforts to develop more systematic approaches for collecting and reporting on timeliness and quality of care in the region.

The chapter is organized into five sections. The first section provides a framework for looking at UHC beyond basic indicators of utilization and financial protection. Building on this framework, the second section provides an overview of the challenges that arise in assessing progress toward UHC when the target population for a particular intervention, or the need for health services, is not apparent. Section three highlights the importance of timeliness in access to care, and the growing concern with waiting lists and waiting times in the region. The fourth section provides an overview of the importance of the technical quality of health care in determining whether improvements in access and utilization of health services translate into improved health outcomes. The final section discusses how quality and the effectiveness of the health system can be assessed based on research and indicators focused on actual health outcomes.

Toward Universal Health Coverage and Equity in Latin America and the Caribbean
http://dx.doi.org/10.1596/978-1-4648-0454-0

Beyond Utilization of Health Services: Framing the Issues

For some types of health interventions, coverage is comparatively easy to assess. For instance, in the case of basic interventions with a clearly defined target group, such as childhood vaccinations, simple measures of coverage provide a relatively accurate picture of the extent to which needs have been met.[2] For some interventions, however, it is much harder to assess whether a patient has received the right services, at the right time, delivered appropriately, and with adequate follow-up. Three issues, in fact, arise. First, if the target population for an intervention is based on diagnosis rather than specific demographic criteria (for example, hypertension or diabetes), coverage is difficult to determine. Second, for many types of care, timeliness of access is important, and this tends not to be captured by most utilization data. Third, the care provided needs to be appropriate (i.e., consistent with recommended clinical practice) given a particular (and correct) diagnosis.

These concerns resonate with a long-standing and established literature on quality of health care, which has highlighted how, through combinations of underuse, overuse, and inappropriate use of medicines and procedures, many health systems underperform on outcomes and efficiency. One commonly used definition of "quality of health care" is "the degree to which health care services for individuals and populations increase the likelihood of desired outcomes and are consistent with current professional knowledge" (Institute of Medicine of the National Academies 2001; Lohr 1990; WHO 2006). With medical technology and practice becoming increasingly complex, the rise in chronic diseases requiring coordination and continuity of care, and growing concern about escalating costs, the question of health care quality has gained prominence. The monitoring and improvement of quality is now central to many national frameworks for health-system performance.

Although there is broad agreement on a general definition of quality, details concerning the elements of quality and approaches to measurement vary across frameworks and studies. In some cases, health care quality is defined narrowly, focusing on effectiveness, safety, and patient-centeredness or responsiveness of care (Arah and others 2006; Kelley and Hurst 2006). The delivery of health care consistent with good clinical practice, however, is inherently intertwined with access. Many quality frameworks therefore expand the definition of quality to include timeliness, equity, and efficiency (Arah and others 2006; Campbell, Roland, and Buetow 2000; WHO 2006). Moreover, the measurement of health care quality typically covers dimensions of structure, process, and outcome, with "structure" referring to characteristics of health care facilities and providers, "process" to the interactions between providers and patients, and "outcomes" to evidence on changes in patient's health status (Donabedian 1980).

The concept of *effective coverage* is one approach that has been introduced to link coverage with quality by quantifying the gap between actual and potential benefits from health services (Shengelia, Murray, and Adams 2003). Effective coverage is defined as the expected health gain from a particular intervention relative to the potential health gain possible with the optimal performance of providers in a given health system. A number of factors can drive a wedge between the potential and expected health gain, including lack of infrastructure, equipment, and providers (resource availability gap); limited physical access to providers for some groups (physical availability gap); cost barriers (affordability gap); conflicts with religious beliefs or cultural practices (cultural acceptability gap); the services provided may be inappropriate or of poor quality, limiting their effectiveness (strategic choice and provider-related quality gaps); and a failure of patients to adhere to suggested treatment (adherence gap). This resonates with the concept of "effectiveness" in the health care quality literature, which refers to the degree of achieving desirable outcomes given the correct provision of evidence-based health care services to all who could benefit but not to those who would not benefit (Arah and others 2006).[3]

This chapter adopts a narrower approach, which seeks to address key gaps relative to earlier chapters and much of the existing literature on UHC within the constraints of available data and evidence. Specifically, it focuses on what is known about unmet need, timeliness, and quality of care (in the narrow sense of consistency with good clinical practice) in LAC, and how problems in these areas are related to one of the key goals of all health systems—namely, to improve the level and distribution of health outcomes in the population. To frame these issues, it is helpful to consider a simplified care pathway, starting with timely detection and diagnosis, passing through timely access to care, technical quality of health services and patient compliance, and ending with health outcomes (figure 5.1). Basic indicators of access can shed some light on the first two links in this chain, but only very partially, and they have nothing to say about technical quality or whether access translates into health outcomes. To address these gaps, the proposed framework draws on the quality literature and existing quality frameworks to identify complementary indicators. The remainder of the chapter goes through each of the areas to review data and evidence from the LAC region on the links between access and outcomes.

The proposed framework clearly leaves many important issues outside the purview of the analysis. The issues of availability, access, and affordability are covered in detail in chapter 4 and are also the mainstay of international and national efforts to monitor UHC. The chapter also adopts a limited perspective on quality, excluding issues of satisfaction (and related issues such as responsiveness, patient-centeredness, and cultural acceptability) as well as patient safety on the grounds that less directly relate to UHC (the chain between need, utilization, and outcome) and because the region has little comparable data. Finally, the chapter includes only a limited discussion of measures of structural quality, including human resources, medical technology, and pharmaceuticals. Chapter 4 includes some discussion of the level and distribution of health-system resources or inputs, and the focus of this chapter is rather on the capacity and organizational issues that stand in the way of improved quality and outcomes.

Toward Universal Health Coverage and Equity in Latin America and the Caribbean
http://dx.doi.org/10.1596/978-1-4648-0454-0

Figure 5.1 A Simple Framework of Indicators for Assessing UHC

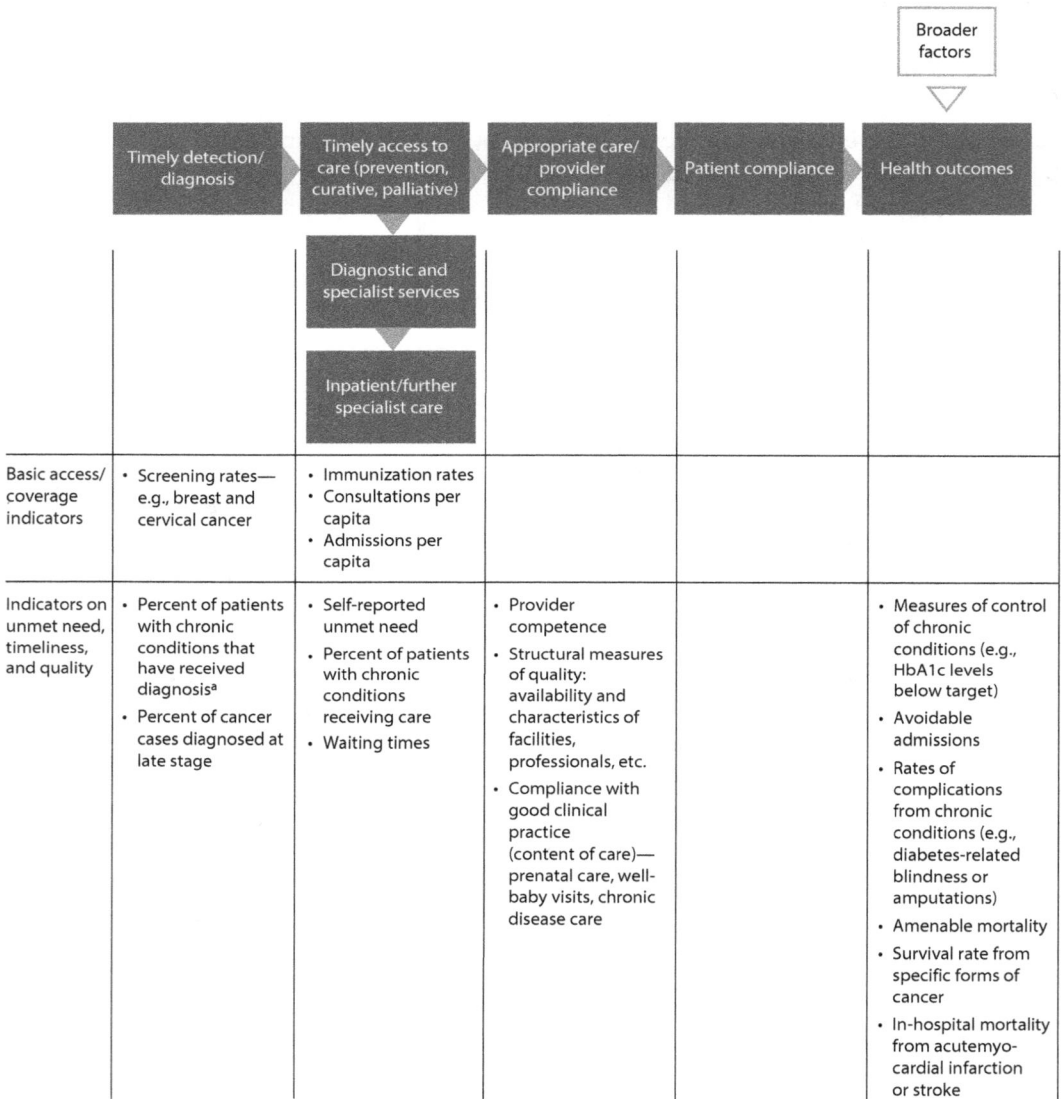

Broader factors

| Timely detection/ diagnosis | → | Timely access to care (prevention, curative, palliative) | → | Appropriate care/ provider compliance | → | Patient compliance | → | Health outcomes |

Diagnostic and specialist services

Inpatient/further specialist care

	Timely detection/ diagnosis	Timely access to care (prevention, curative, palliative)	Appropriate care/ provider compliance	Patient compliance	Health outcomes
Basic access/ coverage indicators	• Screening rates— e.g., breast and cervical cancer	• Immunization rates • Consultations per capita • Admissions per capita			
Indicators on unmet need, timeliness, and quality	• Percent of patients with chronic conditions that have received diagnosis[a] • Percent of cancer cases diagnosed at late stage	• Self-reported unmet need • Percent of patients with chronic conditions receiving care • Waiting times	• Provider competence • Structural measures of quality: availability and characteristics of facilities, professionals, etc. • Compliance with good clinical practice (content of care)— prenatal care, well-baby visits, chronic disease care		• Measures of control of chronic conditions (e.g., HbA1c levels below target) • Avoidable admissions • Rates of complications from chronic conditions (e.g., diabetes-related blindness or amputations) • Amenable mortality • Survival rate from specific forms of cancer • In-hospital mortality from acutemyo-cardial infarction or stroke

Note: a. Number of patients with chronic conditions based on estimated prevalence or biomarkers in surveys.

UHC, Unmet Need, and the Diagnosis of Disease

A central premise of the concept of UHC is that health care needs are effectively met. Although the need for health care is often clear in the case of acute conditions, effective care for most chronic conditions depends on diagnosis and treatment even before symptoms are apparent. Yet, in many countries, a significant proportion of hypertensive and diabetic patients have not been diagnosed. Similarly, cancer is often detected and diagnosed at late stages. These examples highlight the need for detailed information from specialized surveys and administrative data to monitor progress toward UHC.

The first step in ensuring that health care needs are effectively attended to is to ensure that patients and providers recognize needs in a timely manner. As noted earlier, some needs are easy to establish. For instance, most countries have clear schedules for ANC and childhood immunizations that apply to a defined target population (all pregnant women and children within a defined age range, respectively). With services of this nature, there is a readily available basis for determining the extent to which health care needs are being met. Another approach to assess unmet need is to simply ask households whether there was a time in the last six or 12 months when they felt they needed care but did not receive it. Such data are often collected in household surveys, and can shed light not only on unmet need but also on the reasons why perceived needs were not met (box 5.1).

With conditions such as hypertension, diabetes, and cancer, the capacity of individuals to self-diagnose and assess their health care needs is limited, either because of the complexity of the condition or because it may be asymptomatic. Diabetes and hypertension are both major independent risk factors for cardiovascular diseases (CVDs), and the main causes of death in LAC for the past two

---

Box 5.1 Illustrations of Data on Unmet Need from the OECD and Brazil

The OECD reports routinely on unmet need for health care (see, for example, OECD 2011). Data for indicators on unmet need come from national and cross-national health-interview surveys, including the European Union Statistics on Income and Living Conditions survey (EU-SILC) and the international health policy surveys conducted by the Commonwealth Fund. Respondents are typically asked if there was a time in the last 12 months when they felt they needed health care services but did not receive them, with follow-up questions on why the need for care was unmet.

In many OECD countries, unmet need is very low (less than 3 percent across all income groups). Some countries have higher unmet need, however, particularly among low-income households. For instance, more than 10 percent of households in the bottom quintile report unmet need for health care in the last year in Greece, Italy, and Poland.

Some LAC countries also have data on unmet need. For example, several rounds of Brazil's national household survey, the *Pesquisa Nacional por Amostra de Domicílios*, have asked about nonuse of health care services when there is a perceived need. In the case of Brazil, no clear trend is evident over the past decade in nonuse of services for individuals who report an illness episode. It reports an important shift, though, in the relative importance of reasons for not seeking care (Gragnolati, Lindelow, and Couttolenc 2013). In particular, the share of households reporting lack of money (for services or transport) as a reason for not using needed services has declined over the past two decades, particularly for those at the lower end of the income distribution. Similarly, there is evidence that the expansion of infrastructure and staffing has made services more available, with fewer households reporting access or transport as reasons for not seeking care. Meanwhile, facility-related reasons (lack of or unfriendly staff, inadequate scheduling, waiting time) have increased, becoming the chief motive for not seeking care.

---

decades.[4] These costs are at least in part avoidable. Simply by controlling blood glucose levels, the risk of a CVD event can be reduced by 42 percent and the risk of heart attack, stroke, or death from CVD by 57 percent (DCCT/EDIC Study Research Group 2005). Moreover, complications associated with prolonged hyperglycemia can be avoided, and a number of clinical trials have shown that a reduction in blood pressure can lower the risk of myocardial infarction by 20–25 percent, stroke by 35–40 percent, and heart failure by 50 percent (Staessen, Wang, and Thijs 2001).

For conditions like hypertension and diabetes, timely diagnosis and treatment depend on access to effective primary care, appropriate referrals to diagnostic services and specialist care, and quality follow-up care. So, how should progress toward UHC be assessed in these cases? Indicators on access to and use of primary care and coverage of screening programs provide some insight. But a more meaningful assessment of progress toward UHC would also focus on whether patients with particular conditions have been diagnosed in a timely manner and are receiving care consistent with good practice. These assessments are more complicated. Still, a number of studies have shed light on the timeliness of diagnosis or detection, illustrating the broader health-system challenges of trying to achieve UHC goals.

Most estimates of the prevalence of diabetes and hypertension are based on self-reporting in household or phone surveys, in which respondents are asked whether they have been diagnosed with a particular chronic condition by a medical professional. Depending on the context, however, many individuals with chronic conditions have not had a diagnosis, and self-reported prevalence rates therefore tend to underestimate actual prevalence, with underreporting likely to vary systematically with geographic location and socioeconomic status. More reliable estimates of the prevalence of chronic diseases come from comprehensive disease registries or national health examination surveys that include measurement of vital signs. For instance, Gakidou and others (2011) use health-examination surveys from several countries, including Colombia and Mexico, to assess how significant this underreporting is. They find that around half of individuals with diabetes or hypertension in Colombia and Mexico have never had their condition diagnosed, thus precluding effective management, compared with between 10 and 30 percent of diabetic and hypertensive individuals in the United States and the United Kingdom (figure 5.2). Similarly, the Colombian survey reports that 12 percent of diagnosed women received no treatment. Moreover, for patients with diabetes, complications like retinopathy and diabetic foot syndrome are also systematically underdiagnosed and undertreated.

These findings have profound implications for how we think about coverage. If we focus only on individuals who have been diagnosed with diabetes or hypertension (or both), and who would be likely to identify themselves as having diabetes or hypertension in a household survey or phone surveillance interview, only a relatively small percentage (2–20 percent depending on sex and condition) are not receiving treatment. But if we take into account that many diabetic and hypertensive individuals have not been diagnosed, then less than half of

Figure 5.2 Diagnosis and Treatment of Diabetes and Hypertension

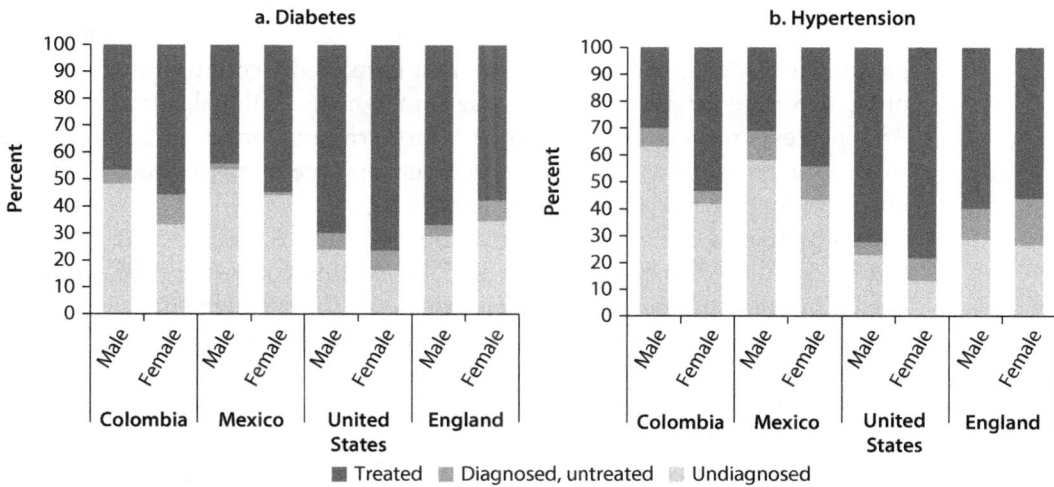

Source: Gakidou and others 2011.

those in need of treatment are receiving it.[5] Studies of this nature highlight significant coverage gaps in diagnosis and treatment. Of course, surveys that capture measurement of vital signs tend to be rare and cannot provide the basis for routine monitoring of UHC. Still, by providing reliable estimates of coverage gaps, they can help identify the scale of the problem in a particular context and more reliable estimates of the target population that can be used to estimate coverage based on administrative data.

Timely detection and diagnosis are equally important with regard to cancer. An estimated 1.7 million cases of cancer will be diagnosed in the LAC region in 2030, with more than 1 million cancer deaths annually. Although the overall incidence of cancer is lower in Latin America (age-standardized rate of 163 per 100,000) than in Europe (264 per 100,000) or the United States (300 per 100,000), the mortality burden is greater (Ferlay and others 2008).[6] In part, this is due to presentation at more advanced stages (clinical stage three and four), but problems in accessing effective cancer care are also a factor. Indeed, for some types of cancer, including breast cancer, cervical cancer, and colorectal cancer, chances of cure and survival increase substantially if they are detected and treated at an early stage.[7]

Comprehensive and comparable regional data on the timeliness of diagnosis of cancer are difficult to come by. Evidence from a few countries illustrates the problem. For instance, a study of cancer care by the Brazilian Federal Audit Tribunal (TCU 2011) found that weaknesses in primary care coupled with lack of access to both diagnostic procedures and specialist care meant that 60 percent of cancer patients were diagnosed at a late stage, reducing the prospects of effective treatment and survival.[8] The problem of late diagnosis was also highlighted by the AMAZONE study, which focused on breast cancer in Brazil (Simon and others 2009). This study also documented disparities between the public and private sectors (almost 37 percent of patients in public institutions were diagnosed at a late stage versus 16.2 percent from private institutions) and between different parts of the country (46.2 percent of women were diagnosed at a late stage in the north of Brazil, compared with 25.1 percent in the wealthier south).[9] Furthermore, doctors in Brazil report that a staggering 80 percent of breast cancer cases are brought directly to their attention by patients (Cazap and others 2010).

Similar findings have been reported from Mexico. A study by the National Cancer Institute reported that out of 744 patients covered by the Mexican Health Insurance (*Seguro Popular*) and with newly diagnosed breast cancer, more than 80 percent presented with locally advanced or metastatic disease (Mohar and others 2009). In comparison, 60 percent of newly diagnosed women in the United States have breast cancer detected at an early stage, with the help of mammography (Chávarri-Guerra and others 2012; National Cancer Institute 2011). This is consistent with information from a cross-sectional study and reports from Mexico finding that 90 percent of breast cancers were diagnosed through a self-detected breast lump (Lopez-Carillo and others 2001).

A number of factors contribute to late detection and diagnosis of cancer. Low screening rates are an important factor. Lee and others (2012) estimate that the screening rate for breast cancer in the public system in Brazil is well below both the WHO recommendation to screen more than 70 percent of the target population and the national goal to screen 60 percent of women aged 50–69 years (Anderson and others 2010).[10] Low screening rates, in turn, are related to local beliefs and sociocultural factors, but also poor availability and quality of services (Marinho and others 2008). For example, a Mexican study showed that it is far less likely for a woman to have a Pap smear and a mammogram if she resides in a marginalized rural community (Sosa-Rubí, Walker, and Serván 2009). Similarly, a study on perceived barriers and benefits to cervical cancer screening among low-income women in five countries in Latin America (Ecuador, El Salvador, Mexico, Peru, and República Bolivariana de Venezuela) found that the main barriers identified by all participants are accessibility and availability of quality services (Agurto and others 2004).

Delays in diagnosis can also be related to other health-system factors, in particular challenges in accessing procedures to confirm the diagnosis. This is illustrated in a study from Mexico based on a prospective review of 166 new breast cancer cases at a major public hospital in Mexico City. It found that for a subset of patients with confirmed stage I–IIIC breast cancer, the average time interval from symptom onset to the first primary-care consultation was 1.8 months. An additional 6.6 months then passed between the first primary-care consultation and the confirmation of diagnosis, and 0.6 months until initiation of treatment (Bright and others 2011). Another study from Mexico on factors associated with variable outcomes of acute lymphoblastic leukemia, a cancer of the white blood cells, which can be curable if detected early, reconstructed the prediagnostic symptomatic period for both survivors and nonsurvivors (Lora and others 2011). The study found long lags between the onset of symptoms and diagnostic confirmation (43.5 ± 22.5 days). These are both relatively small-scale studies from better-served parts of the country; it is very possible that delays are even greater in other parts of the country.

Hypertension, diabetes, and cancers account for a very large share of the burden of disease and mortality in the region. For all these conditions, timely diagnosis is critical for the disease to be effectively managed and treated, and is perhaps the most important aspect to consider in the monitoring of UHC. Yet, as we have seen, even with available and affordable primary health care services and screening programs, significant unmet need may remain. Although by no means straightforward, it is possible to establish systems for routine monitoring of the share of the diabetic and hypertensive patients that have been diagnosed and are under managed care, and of the stage of diagnosis for different forms of cancers. Indicators of this nature would go a long way toward addressing important information gaps in relation to UHC coverage.

Timeliness in Access to Care

Waiting to access needed health care is a feature of most health systems. However, unless waiting lists are limited and well- managed, delays in treatment may have a detrimental impact on patient outcomes. This fact has led many OECD countries to establish systems for systematic monitoring of waiting times. Such efforts are also under way in some LAC countries, but data are still limited.

Once a diagnosis or need for health care has been established, the next step in the chain between the availability of services and health outcomes is for the patient to be able to actually access the needed services. In some cases, this may be a matter of a first contact or consultation with a primary health care provider. But in many cases, the care pathway is more complex, with patients needing one or more diagnostic procedures, a consultation with a specialist, and perhaps follow-up care.

One prerequisite of UHC is that health services be available and affordable. Even if these prerequisites are met, however, demand for services is likely to outstrip supply. In systems where health services are not rationed on the basis of ability to pay, waiting becomes the default means of allocating scarce health-system resources. Indeed, even in high-performing health systems, access is rarely immediate, and the journey along the care pathway can involve repeated delays and other access problems.

Limited waiting times for nonurgent procedures—whether an outpatient consultation, diagnostic procedures, or elective surgery—are not necessarily an important concern. Waiting lists ensure that capacity is fully utilized and avoid inefficiency. In a well-functioning system, waiting lists allow health professionals to effectively prioritize access based on a hierarchy of need to avoid adverse outcomes associated with waiting (Siciliani, Borowitz, and Moran 2013). But in many instances, excessive waiting times and ineffective prioritization can put patients at risk. In addition, even if long-term health outcomes are not compromised, waiting can produce significant pain and anxiety for the patient.[11]

Waiting time has long been a health-sector policy concern in OECD countries, and is gaining prominence in the LAC region as well. Significant challenges include access to specialist care, diagnostic procedures, and inpatient services. Improvements in access to and quality of primary care have revealed significant suppressed demand for medium- and high-complexity care.

In general, waiting lists and waiting times depend on both demand- and supply-side factors, but the relationship is not straightforward. Demand for particular health services from the public system (and inflow to a waiting list) depends on health status (which, in turn, depends on demographics, lifestyles, and other factors), technology, coverage, effectiveness of primary care, patient preferences, and the cost and availability of outside options. These outside options in particular include services provided by the private sector and financed through out-of-pocket payment or private health insurance (Siciliani, Borowitz, and Moran 2013). In turn, the outflow from waiting lists depends primarily on service-delivery capacity (beds, health professionals, equipment, etc.) and productivity. A simple story of what is happening in countries that are expanding health care coverage is hence that improvements in access to primary care, combined with demographic and epidemiological changes, are generating rapidly growing demands for diagnostic and specialist services, and that investment in these services has not been meeting the growing demand. At the same time, weaknesses in referral and counter-referral systems make prioritization difficult, contribute to inequities in access, and hamper the productivity of specialist and hospital services (for example, by high level of no-shows to appointments).

Although the concepts of waiting lists (number of people waiting for a particular service) and waiting times (time period between identification of need and access to service) are easy to understand, measurement is by no means straightforward (Siciliani, Borowitz, and Moran 2013). Insofar as countries routinely measure and report on waiting times—many do not—measurement tends to focus on particular categories of services such as primary-care consultations, specific procedures (for example, cataract surgery, coronary bypass, hip replacement), specialist consultations (for example, ophthalmology, orthopedics), or urgent care (for example, cancer treatment). But measurement may start and end at different points in the patient journey, making cross-country comparisons difficult. For instance, measurement of waiting time could start with a GP referral to a specialist, with confirmation of diagnosis and decision to treat by a specialist, or admission to a waiting list for treatment. Increasingly, OECD countries are moving to measurement approaches that try to capture the full patient journey.

One approach to get comparable data is to interview patients. The Commonwealth Fund International Health Policy Survey took this approach, which provides data on waiting times for selected OECD countries (figure 5.3).

Data on waiting lists and waiting times in Latin America and the Caribbean are more limited. One way to gauge the level of concern with waiting times in the region is through opinion polls or public perception surveys.[12] Deloitte recently

Figure 5.3 Waiting Times in Selected OECD Countries

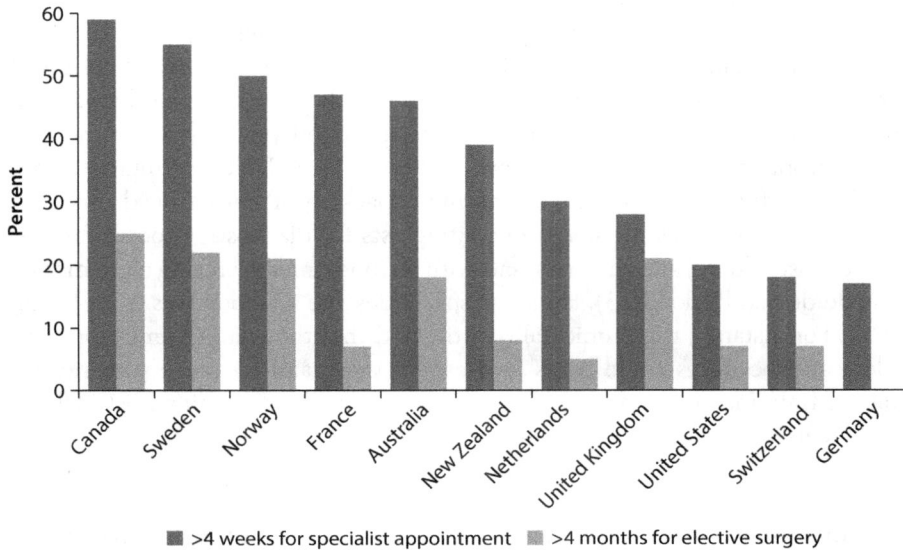

>4 weeks for specialist appointment   >4 months for elective surgery

Source: OECD 2012 based on 2010 data from Commonwealth Fund International Health Policy Surveys.
Note: Waiting times for specialist and elective surgery were the time between the patient being advised they needed care and the appointment. Only those respondents who had specialist consultations or elective surgery in the last year or two were asked to specify waiting times.

undertook perception surveys of adults in Brazil and Mexico (Deloitte 2011a, 2011b). In these surveys, waiting times were reported as an important reason for not seeking care (the second most important reason in Brazil [38 percent]; the third most important reason in Mexico).[13] Moreover, waiting time was the most poorly rated aspect of the health system performance defined by the study in both countries (81 percent giving an unfavorable or very unfavorable rating in Brazil; 74 percent in Mexico). In Colombia, the Ministry of Health (MoH) conducts a periodic survey of patient perceptions as part of a broader performance management system. In contrast to information from Brazil and Mexico, the Colombia survey presents a relatively positive picture, with most patients being able to access general and specialist consultations within 10 days (85 and 55 percent respectively) and more than 80 percent being confident that they will receive the care they need in the event of a serious condition (MinSalud 2012).

In contrast, a recent opinion poll in Brazil (CNI 2012) found very high levels of dissatisfaction with the health system, especially with delays in access to consultations or exams and a lack of doctors, although dissatisfaction was significantly lower among those who actually had direct experience using the health system.[14] The Mais Médicos Program, which seeks to address medical staff shortages in primary care in underserved areas, was established in 2013 as a response to this problem. In another recent survey, respondents also highlighted as key concerns the lack of doctors and long waiting times in hospitals and for referral services (IPEA 2011). Reflecting these concerns, these surveys also highlight the importance of private health plans for respondents as a means to ensure more rapid access to health care (IESS 2011; IPEA 2011).[15]

Data from opinion polls can be powerful, but are often based on relatively small samples, and answers tend to be very sensitive to how questions are asked. Harder data on waiting lists and waiting times in the region are harder to come by, but evidence from a few countries in the region provides a sense of the scale of the problem. For example, a recent analysis by the Health Secretariat of the São Paulo Municipality found an enormous backlog of unmet need, finding a total of 800,244 cases registered in waiting lists for diagnostic procedures, specialist consultations, and surgeries, and with waiting times averaging eight months (Estado de São Paulo 2013). For some specialties, the situation was considerably worse. For instance, the municipality estimated that the waiting times for gynecological procedures could be as long as five years, and for some surgeries the waiting time may be as much as nine years. Inevitably, the waiting list includes individuals who may have opted to seek care in the private system, who no longer need care, or who have died. The number of patients actually waiting will be lower than the total number on the list.

In the case of Colombia, data on judicial processes also offer insights into the problem of waiting lists. In 2007, the largest number of legal actions filed before the Constitutional Court of Colombia was in connection with claims for medical care (25 percent), followed by requests related to medication (19.6 percent), and in third place are those relating to waiting lists (16.7 percent) (Vargas López 2010).

Similarly, waiting lists are increasingly subject to routine monitoring in Chile, where the problem has long been recognized and led to the development of Plan AUGE in 2005 (table 5.1), with waiting list monitoring and guaranteed waiting times for a growing range of conditions. The conditions covered under AUGE have been gradually expanded and the list now includes 80 conditions. In 2010, FONASA had a waiting list of more than 183,000 patients (equivalent to nearly 2 percent of all consultations for the conditions covered by the waiting list) (Paraje and Vásquez 2012). This situation, which was associated with widespread public dissatisfaction as well as avoidable admissions and mortality, has since improved, although the extent of this improvement is the subject of debate.

Data on waiting *lists* provide clear indications of where there are bottlenecks in the health system but do not necessarily shed much light on waiting *times*. Data on cancer care from some countries in the region make it clear, however, that waiting times can in some cases be very long. In the case of Brazil, the challenge of late diagnosis referred to earlier in the chapter is compounded by delays in accessing treatment. Using administrative data on payments for radiation and chemotherapy from 2010, a study by the Federal Audit Authority (TCU 2011) shows that the median waiting time for chemotherapy in 2010 was 76.3 days (from the point of confirmed diagnosis), with only 35.6 percent of patients receiving treatment within 30 days. In addition, many patients face considerable delays in accessing diagnostic procedures or specialist care to confirm a diagnosis. In the case of radiation therapy, the corresponding figures were 113.4 days and

Table 5.1 The Experience of Waiting-Time Guarantees in Selected Countries

Country	Description
Brazil	Legislation guaranteeing access to treatment for cancer patients within 60 days from confirmed diagnosis was introduced in 2013. The systems for monitoring and enforcing the guarantee are still being developed, but enforcement is expected to be based on administrative sanctions and patients resorting to litigation of the right to health.
Chile	The *Plan AUGE* was introduced in 2005. The Regime of Explicit Guarantees in Health (Law 19,966) defines a package of medical benefits consisting of a prioritized list of diagnoses and treatments with Explicit Guarantees (initially 25, expanded to 40 in 2006, 66 in 2010, and 80 in 2014). Guarantees are defined in terms of access, timeliness, quality, and financial protection, and with associated clinical protocols. For example, the guarantee for colorectal cancer involves: • Within 45 days after diagnosis entitlement for biopsy and preoperative tests • Within 30 days from indication access to treatment (surgery, chemotherapy, and associated tests) • Within 90 days from the medical indication a follow-up exam There is also a maximum of copayments related to the monthly price paid by each individual. To ensure that the guarantee is met, the scheme involves vouchers/public subsidy for beneficiaries of the public scheme (FONASA) to use the services in the private sector if the guarantee cannot be met in the public sector. After almost a decade of implementing AUGE there have been notable improvements in outcomes, including for arterial hypertension, diabetes mellitus type I and II, depression, childhood epilepsy, and HIV/AIDS. The proportion of cases that receive treatment (calculated over a potential demand) has increased noticeably and the mortality rates of these conditions declined. For hypertension, diabetes mellitus type I, and HIV/AIDS, hospitalization rates declined (likely as a consequence of improved outpatient treatments), while others have increased (type II diabetes mellitus, childhood epilepsy, depression). But the financial sustainability of the guarantee is a growing challenge (Bitrán and others 2010). There is also some evidence that improvements in quality (linked to protocols) may have contributed to a reduction in hospital mortality for acute myocardial infarction (Nazzal and others 2008) and increase in prenatal detection of congenital heart disease (Concha and others 2008).
Uruguay	Maximum waiting times for accessing different specialties have been introduced: • 24 hours for general medicine, pediatrics, and gynecology. • 48 hours for general surgery. • 30 days for medical and surgical specialties. • 180 days from their indication for nonurgent surgical procedures. Enforcement of the guarantee is based on threat of withholding public subsidies (per capita payments).

15.9 percent. As a point of comparison, nearly all patients receive treatment within 30 days in the United Kingdom and Canada, and median waiting times range from 5 to 25 days depending on the type of treatment.

Although data about waiting times in the region are scant, concern about the health consequences of excessive delays in access to care have combined with judicial processes and political pressure to prompt many countries in the region to take action to reduce waiting times. Table 5.1 shows a brief summary of actions taken by some countries in the region to tackle the waiting time issue.

Quality of Care

This chapter has argued for the importance of complementing basic UHC indicators on utilization and financial protection with data and research on unmet need, timeliness of access, and quality. However, it is also possible to assess more directly whether the health system is contributing to improved outcomes. This section illustrates this possibility by looking at treatment outcomes for hypertension and diabetes, cancer survival and amenable mortality.

Toward Universal Health Coverage and Equity in Latin America and the Caribbean
http://dx.doi.org/10.1596/978-1-4648-0454-0

It is important to consider both the perceived and the technical quality of care. For lack of data to elucidate issues of perceived quality of care in the region, this section discusses only elements of technical quality. Timely detection and diagnosis is a prerequisite for effective care, and the timeliness of care can have important implications for outcomes. Another important factor that determines the effectiveness of care is the appropriateness, or technical quality, of health care services. In a narrow sense, this means that care is delivered in compliance with defined technical standards—i.e., does the nurse or physician ask the right questions, perform the appropriate tests and exams, reach the correct diagnosis, communicate effectively with the patient, and prescribe appropriate treatment?

There is an extensive literature from OECD countries that seeks to assess the technical quality of care for different types of health services. For instance, a review of the literature on quality of care in the U.S. covers a broad range of areas, including antibiotic use, respiratory illness, prenatal care, asthma, diabetes, hypertension and heart disease, mental health, and cancer (Schuster, McGlynn, and Brook 2005). There are also numerous efforts to define indicators for routine monitoring of health care quality, both in the context of country-specific health system performance framework and across countries in the OECD (see, for example, AHRQ 2013; Arah and others 2006; Kelley and Hurst 2006). Many of these indicators focus on outcome measures of quality, but also include efforts to monitor process dimensions of quality (Marshall, Leatherman, and Mattke 2004). Many OECD countries have also adopted mechanisms to promote quality improvement, including through use of financial incentives, development and dissemination of clinical guidelines, accreditation mechanisms, etc.

The literature on technical quality of health care in the LAC region is scant, and although most countries have quality-improvement initiatives of some sort, there are few examples of routine monitoring of technical quality. For instance, according to a PAHO review, only six out of 25 countries surveyed in 2000 had formal procedures for accreditation of health services and facilities (Ross, Zeballos, and Infante 2000). In part, this is because systematic analysis and monitoring of health care quality typically depends on detailed patient-record data, ideally in electronic form, or in-depth surveys. This is therefore an area of research and health system monitoring that is likely to evolve rapidly as countries in the region upgrade their health information systems. For now, however, evidence on health care quality can be gleaned from a few focused studies on prenatal care and cancer care.

Overall, coverage of maternal and child health care services, in particular, prenatal care, has improved significantly in the LAC region in recent decades, and nearly 90 percent of pregnant women in the region now receive at least four antenatal-care visits. But, as discussed in the first section of this chapter, the extent to which expanded coverage translates into improved outcomes depends in large part on the quality of care provided—i.e., the extent to which health care professionals manage to identify key risks, take appropriate action, and communicate effectively with the patient.

A number of studies from Brazil illustrate significant quality issues in prenatal care. A recent study from Rio de Janeiro interviewed 2,353 pregnant women, asking about date of initiation of prenatal care, the number of visits, and type of diagnostic exams performed (Domingues and others 2012). Based on criteria from the PHPN index,[16] only 38.5 percent of respondents had received adequate care. Moreover, almost a third of hypertensive women reported not to have obtained antihypertensive medication. The most important shortcomings were related to the timely completion of the first and second laboratory routine exams. Among women aged 28–33, only 41 percent completed recommended exams; for women aged 34–37, not even 20 percent had completed the first routine exam by the time they were expected to have results from the second one. Most clinical exams, such as blood-pressure measurement, weight recording, and monitoring of fetal heart sounds, achieved high levels of completion (between 73 and 98 percent). But only between 23 and 55 percent of cases received recommended information (for example, advice about labor, referral to the maternity service, and breast-feeding counseling) (Domingues and others 2012). Along similar lines, a study from the city of Pelotas found very high coverage and number of prenatal visits, but only 77 percent of women underwent a vaginal examination and almost a third of nonimmunized women did not receive tetanus toxoid (Barros and others 2005). Finally, a study of four maternity hospitals in Aracaju, in Northeast Brazil, also confirms high level of ANC coverage, with more than six prenatal-care visits on average (Ribeiro and others 2009). Only 33.9 percent of women were classified, however, as having adequate prenatal care utilization,[17] and a large share of women did not have a breast exam and were not counseled on breast-feeding. Inadequate care was furthermore less likely to occur in women who sought private care (11 percent) as compared with those seeking public care (39 percent).

Beyond prenatal care, studies from Brazil have also documented quality issues in delivery care, but in this case the overuse of medicines and procedures is the primary problem. For example, there is evidence that excessive labor induction through medication and caesarean sections has contributed to a rise in preterm births in the city of Pelotas (from 6.3 percent in 1982 to 16.2 percent in 2004), with adverse implications for infant mortality and morbidity (Barros and others 2005). Overuse of caesarean sections is a broader problem in Brazil, with 43 percent of births by caesarean section in 2010 (Victora and others 2011).[18]

An assessment of the quality of deliveries in 14 hospitals in the Dominican Republic also helps explain how high rates of institutional deliveries can coexist with high maternal mortality ratios (Miller and others 2003).[19] The study showed that the major referral hospitals, where more than 40 percent of births in the country occur, were overcrowded and understaffed, with inexperienced residents overseeing care provided by medical students, interns, and nurses. Uncomplicated labor and deliveries were over medicalized, complicated deliveries were not managed appropriately, and emergencies were not dealt with in a timely fashion.

Low technical quality of maternal and child health services is likely to have many determinants, including the working environment, incentives, availability of equipment and material, and provider skills. Among these factors, skills and provider competence have recently received increased attention, and a number of studies done globally provide evidence on the level and distribution of skills based on tests or vignettes (Das and Hammer 2014). In line with this literature, a recent study from the Dominican Republic aimed to assess the competence of primary care doctors for providing care and treatment to pregnant women and children under one year of age according to national standards. A sample of 66 doctors had to complete a written exam and a clinical case simulation. Only 8 percent of the doctors achieved sufficiently high scores to qualify as adequate caregivers for pregnant women, and none of them was considered adequate to provide care to children below the age of one (Pérez-Then and others 2008).

Regarding cancer care, the best indicator of the quality is arguably the survival rate for confirmed cases, ideally analyzed by stage at diagnosis. Given the complexity of cancer care, structural quality measures, such as the availability and functionality of technologically advanced equipment, specialist physicians, and hospital bed capacity, are also relevant indicators of quality and important determinants of outcomes. As in other regions, oncology services in LAC tend to be concentrated in major cities, contributing to inequalities in access to services and outcomes. For example, in Peru, 10 of the country's 18 radiation therapy units are located in Lima or other larger cities, whereas 20 of the country's 25 regions lack radiotherapy centers. In Mexico, there are 20 linear accelerators for 32 states, and seven of these are located in Mexico City (Goss and others 2013).

But it is also possible to assess the technical quality of cancer care by focusing on the process of care. One of the critical points in this regard concerns diagnostic procedures and associated follow-up care. The challenges are apparent from a case control study (invasive cancer and healthy controls) in four Colombian states, which found that almost 50 percent of cervical cancer screenings (Pap smears) were false negatives, and only about 65 percent of cases had a follow-up exam after a positive cytology result (Murillo and others 2011). Furthermore, results for cervical cancer screening (Pap smears) from remote states were found to be suboptimum: when the same smears were evaluated at a national laboratory, up to 61 percent of normal or negative smears had abnormal findings. A similar study found persistently high levels of false negative cervical cytology results of up to 53 percent in Mexico (Lazcano-Ponce and others 2008).

Weaknesses in the quality of diagnostic procedures and laboratory testing in Mexico have also been found to be compounded by inappropriate use of invasive diagnostic procedures, in particular the use of colposcopy in combination with Pap screening (Madrigal de la Campa, Lazcano Ponce, and Infante Castaneda 2005). Follow-up care after abnormal cytology screening is often also weak. Indeed, a study found that only 25 percent of patients received appropriate follow-up care, which may explain the lack of impact of cervical cancer screening in the country (Gage and others 2003).

Problems in providing high-quality diagnostics have also been found in relation to breast cancer in Brazil. One study found low levels of concordance in diagnosis between different pathologists examining the same sample (60 percent concordance in a sample of 329 biopsies) (Salles and others 2008). A separate study found that a relatively high proportion (22 percent) of fine-needle-aspiration biopsy procedures obtained inadequate material for further cytopathological analysis, which could be related to provider incompetency or technical difficulty due to less advanced equipment or a combination of those (INCA 2010; Lee and others 2012).

Beyond diagnosis, quality of cancer care is also related to the appropriateness of treatment regimens, including chemotherapy, as well as palliative care. The adoption of updated regimens for chemotherapy has been slow in the region, particularly in remote areas. For instance, WHO reported that tamoxifen for breast cancer was not available in Bolivia, El Salvador, Nicaragua, Paraguay, and Saint Kitts and Nevis, despite being available in most countries for cost as low as US$0.10 per pill.

Similarly, when asked about the availability of modern treatments for cancer care in the public system in Brazil, responding oncologists confirmed that the uptake of more updated regimens is a problem (65 percent). Around 15 percent mentioned the limited availability of trastuzumabe, another medicine used for the treatment of breast and other types of cancer (TCU 2011). Project AMAZONE from Brazil, a study funded by GBECAM involving 4,912 women with breast cancer across 28 treatment centers, confirmed that observation. The study found that newer generations of chemotherapeutics and specific treatments for hormone-sensitive breast cancer, like adjuvant trastuzumabe, were used more frequently in patients treated in private health facilities (56 percent) than in patients treated in public (5.6 percent) or philanthropic (10 percent) health facilities. This is related to the fact that, despite their importance for appropriate treatment decisions, more sophisticated diagnostic methods, such as hormone receptor and growth factor determination, are not widely available in the public sector. These methods can have important implications for treatment choices. For instance, the Mexican Cancer Institute (INCAN) reported that physicians changed their treatment recommendations in 31 out of 96 cases on the basis of genetic profiling of tumors, with a decrease from 48 to 34 percent in chemotherapy recommendation (Bargallo-Rocha and others 2015), yet most treatment centers do not perform these tests.

Finally, availability of effective palliative care is very limited in most countries in the region (Goss and others 2013; Lee and others 2012; Torres and others 2007). In many Latin American countries, resources are mainly directed to curative rather than palliative treatment, reflected in the overall small number of palliative centers that are almost exclusively available in the public health system.[20] The insufficient offering of such services is accompanied by limited availability of potent analgesics (pain medication) and few specialists in the area of palliative care, and average consumption of opioids in the region remains well below world levels, which translates into inadequate pain management (Callaway and others 2007; WHO 2013).[21]

Overall, it is clear that the technical quality of health care service, whether in relation to maternal and child health, cancer, or other areas, is a critical aspect in determining whether health care needs have been met. High rates of coverage of prenatal care and institutional deliveries do not necessarily translate into good health outcomes. Similarly, expansion of cancer screening without commensurate improvements in the availability and quality of diagnostic procedures, and access to up-to-date treatment regimens, is unlikely to translate into significant improvements in cancer survival. This highlights the need to complement monitoring the availability and use of services with a greater focus on quality. With improved information systems, there are ways to routinely monitor important dimensions of quality, but surveys and other approaches to collect data will continue to be important tools as well. The evidence also highlights challenges in terms of lack of pathologists and related health professionals, low levels of training and continuing education, and weaknesses in accreditation and quality-control systems.

Health Outcomes: Why Timeliness and Quality Matter

This chapter has argued for the importance of complementing basic UHC indicators on utilization and financial protection with data and research on unmet need, timeliness of access, and quality. However, it is also possible to assess more directly whether the health system is contributing to improved outcomes. This section illustrates this possibility by looking at treatment outcomes for hypertension and diabetes, cancer survival and amenable mortality.

The true test of a health system is not only whether it ensures equitable access to health services based on need but also whether it produces good and equitable health outcomes. Timeliness and quality are very important, as they can drive a significant wedge between the potential and actual health gains from realized access to services. It is beyond the scope of this chapter to discuss each of these areas in detail, and a comprehensive discussion of trends and patterns in the region is in any event hampered by the lack systematic and comparable data. Nonetheless, existing studies and data highlight the value of some specific indicators in strengthening the monitoring and analysis of coverage and health system performance.

Specifically, this section covers four types of indicators. First, much of the chapter has focused on the diagnosis and management of hypertension and diabetes. In the case of these two conditions, there are studies that go beyond process measures of quality to assess to what extent treatment targets are actually being achieved. Second, indicators of complications related to diabetes and hypertension, and of avoidable hospital admissions, can be important for benchmarking and monitoring performance of the health systems, capturing both problems of access to and effectiveness of primary care. Third, an extension of the indicators of complications and admissions as measures of health-system performance is to assess "amenable mortality"—namely, the extent of mortality that could have been avoided through effective health care. Finally, in the case of cancer, registries could provide the basis for an analysis of survival rates, which in turn are powerful indicators of how successful the health system is in detecting, diagnosing, and treating cancer.

Achieving Treatment Targets in Chronic Disease Management

The risk of death and complications associated with diabetes and hypertension can be significantly reduced if the conditions are effectively managed to maintain blood sugar and blood pressure within a controlled range. The extent to which this is achieved, however, will depend both on patients being appropriately diagnosed and on the technical quality of health care offered to these patients. LAC results highlight many missed opportunities to reduce the burden of three major risk factors for CVD (diabetes, arterial hypertension, and hypercholesterolemia) and suggest that diabetes and related risk factors are not managed effectively.

A recent analysis of health examination surveys from seven countries, including Colombia and Mexico, found not only that a substantial proportion of individuals with diabetes remain undiagnosed and untreated, but also that the proportion of individuals reaching treatment targets was very low (Gakidou and others 2011). For instance, patients with diabetes reaching treatment targets for blood glucose, arterial blood pressure, and serum cholesterol was very low, ranging from 1 percent of male patients in Mexico to about 12 percent in the United States. More than 70 percent of individuals with diabetes in all countries were not reaching the blood glucose treatment targets set by the International Diabetes Federation.[22]

These findings are consistent with results from a systematic literature review on the quality of diabetes care in low- and middle-income countries in the LAC region—the proportion of patients reaching treatment targets varied widely for glycemic control (13.0–92.9 percent), hypertension (4.6–92.0 percent), and lipids (28.2–18.3 percent). Most of the literature analyzed for this review came from Brazil, Jamaica, and Mexico. The review also found that screening for non-CVD end organ dysfunction was the most commonly missed component of care regarding management of diabetes in the region. The authors acknowledge that the low reporting of only 1 percent of patients having been screened for such diabetes-related dysfunctions could be secondary to documentation weaknesses. But the consistent lack of data on this aspect points toward a neglected aspect of diabetes care.

Complications and Avoidable Admissions

The number of avoidable or "unnecessary" hospital admissions is another important measure of access to and quality of primary care. Estimates from the Inter-American Development Bank (Guanais, Gómez-Suárez, and Pinzón 2012) suggest that the LAC region had 8–10 million avoidable hospitalizations in 2009. A high impact of avoidable hospitalization by chronic diseases was found in Argentina, Colombia, Costa Rica, and Mexico; countries with lower income, such as Ecuador and Paraguay, showed a larger effect of preventable conditions.

Within the broad category of avoidable admissions, it is also possible to focus on complications or procedures associated with specific conditions. For instance, lack of or poor management of diabetes can lead to complications such as diabetic foot syndrome and amputations. One study from Brazil showed that 66.3 percent of amputations performed in general hospitals occur in patients with diabetes. Furthermore, 85 percent of amputations are preceded by ulcers that can be effectively treated in a primary health care setting (Gamba 1998). The economic impact of prolonged hospital admissions and amputations resulting from diabetic foot is significant. Data from the Brazilian state of Sergipe showed a 49 percent increase in the cost related to amputations from 2008 to 2010 (DATASUS). In the public system alone, 13 amputations were done per week in the state, 9 of which were attributed to diabetes. Similarly, a retrospective chart review of diabetic patients attending a screening program in the State of Pernambuco in Brazil found a pattern of urban-rural disparity, with 40 percent of patients from rural areas having diabetic retinopathy, compared with 25 percent of patients from urban areas (Escarião and others 2008).

Amenable Mortality

One approach to assessing both coverage and quality of the health system is to study the extent to which the system is contributing to improving health outcomes through an analysis of trends in amenable mortality—i.e., deaths that could have been avoided in the presence of timely and effective health care. This approach is based on data from national death registers, which record the cause of death based on standardized disease classification standards.[23] Mortality from specific conditions is then defined as amenable to timely and effective health care, and this permits an analysis of trends and patterns (for example, variation between countries or regions) of mortality that could have been avoided. The premise of this analysis is that improvements or spatial differences in the coverage and/or effectiveness of the health system over time will be reflected in data on amenable mortality.[24]

A number of studies have been undertaken to compare trends and levels of amenable mortality in OECD countries (McKee and McMichael 2008; Nolte and McKee 2003, 2004, 2012), but there is little systematic evidence from the LAC region. Some studies have been undertaken in Brazil, which have found significant declines in amenable mortality. For instance, Malta and others (2010) looked at trends in amenable mortality in infants (children under 1) during the period 1997–2006. They found a significant decline in both deaths amenable to health care (37 percent) and deaths from ill-defined causes (75 percent, indicating improved access to health care), while mortality from other causes remained stable (a reduction of 2.2 percent). This was likely to be driven at least in part by improvements in coverage and quality of the health system. For instance, mortality from pneumonia fell by 52.7 percent, with effective primary care likely to have played an important role. But other factors, in particular improvements in living conditions and public health interventions that affect the incidence of different health conditions, will also have played a role. Although the study presents a positive picture of the health system overall, it also reports an increase of 28 percent in mortality amenable to adequate prenatal care. This is hard to reconcile with improvements in coverage of prenatal care, but the authors speculate that poor quality of prenatal care may have played a role.

A more recent study focused on a cohort of children in Pelotas (Gorgot and others 2011; Santos and others 2011) found that most of the mortality in children was avoidable, with most of the mortality amenable to adequate maternal care during pregnancy (70 percent of deaths), and most deaths taking place in the first year of life (92 percent). This points to an increase in premature deaths and quality issues in prenatal care as key contributing factors. The study also documents a socioeconomic gradient, with children born to women in the lowest quintile having a three times higher probability of dying from amenable causes than those born to women in the highest quintile, in part due to the fact that preterm births are nearly twice as high in the lowest quintile. Effective smoking cessation and provision of progesterone to high-risk women could contribute to a reduction of mortality. The increase in mortality that could be avoided through effective prenatal care may also be partly due to an increase in maternal conditions that affect the fetus (for example, diabetes), and improved diagnosis and more accurate classification of deaths.

Along similar lines, Abreu, César, and França (2007) studied trends in amenable mortality for children and adults between 1983 and 2002 in 117 municipalities. Comparing the periods 1983–1992 and 1993–2002, they found a significant reduction in amenable mortality, while mortality from other causes remained stable. They also noted a significant difference between women and men in amenable mortality, with ischemic heart disease accounting for most of this difference (there was also a large sex difference in mortality from other causes, most likely due to different rates of deaths due to violence and accidents) (Abreu, César, and França 2009).

We analyzed data from the WHO mortality database for the period 1985–2010 to investigate trends in mortality rates due to amenable causes for two age groups—0–14 years old and 15–69 years old—in eight countries. The top amenable causes were selected from the list proposed by Nolte and McKee (2003); malnutrition and nutritional anemias were included as underlying causes of death because of their importance as a social determinant of health, even though they are amenable to broader social policies—not just health policies. [25] Some causes classified as amenable by Nolte and McKee were not included either due to low incidence in the region or because there were data gaps in defining the cause of death.

Figure 5.4 shows that, for the age group under 15 years of age, amenable mortality due to intestinal infectious diseases, malnutrition and nutritional anemias, and pneumonia and influenza accounted for 14–55 percent of total deaths

Figure 5.4 Proportional Mortality by Infectious Amenable Causes, 1985 and 2010—Age Group 0–14 Years

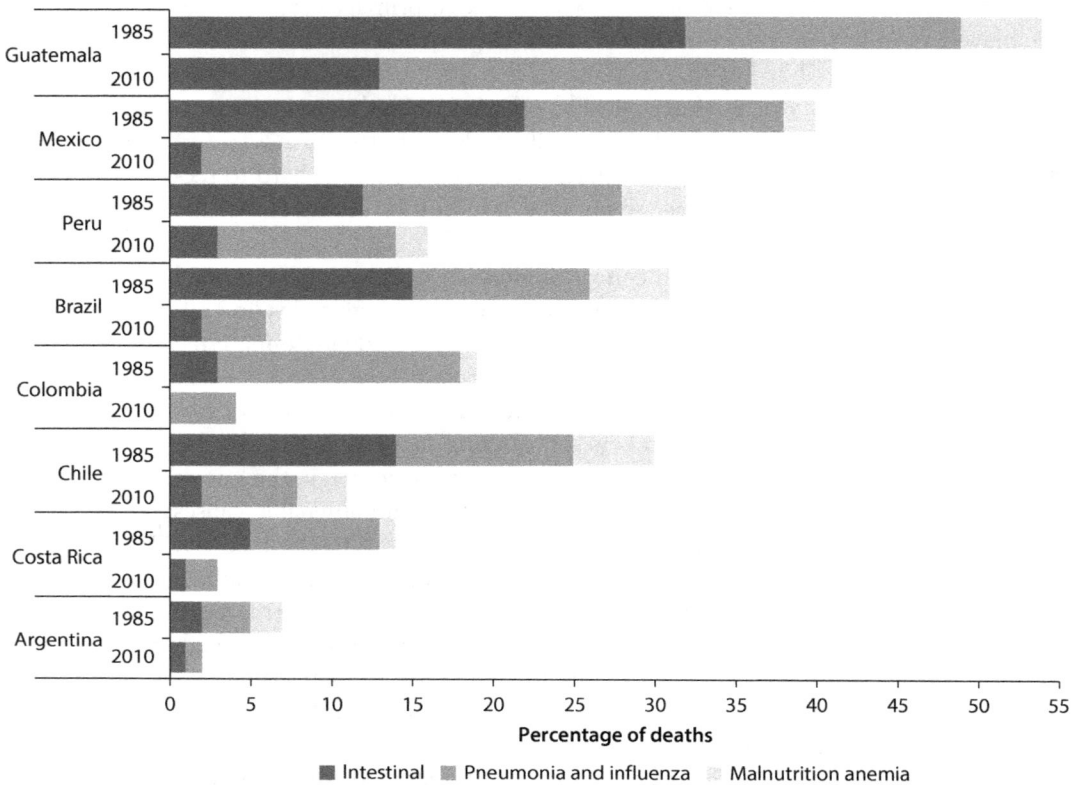

Legend: ■ Intestinal ■ Pneumonia and influenza ▨ Malnutrition anemia

x-axis: Percentage of deaths

Source: World Bank estimates with data from WHO Mortality Database, modified.
Note: Amenable causes include intestinal infectious disease (ICD9 001-009, ICD-10 E40-56, D50-53); malnutrition and nutritional anemias (ICD-9 260-68, ICD-10 A00-9); and pneumonia and influenza (ICD-9 480-86, 487; ICD-10 J10-18).

in the studied countries, with Chile and Costa Rica having the lowest proportion and Guatemala the highest. By 2010, all countries had seen a reduction in the share of amenable mortality, although improvements varied considerably, with the largest absolute drops occurring in Mexico and Brazil and the largest relative gains in Chile, Costa Rica, Mexico, and Brazil, where deaths due to these amenable causes have fallen below 10 percent of total deaths. In addition, in all countries except Guatemala there was a greater decline observed for amenable mortality than for any other causes considered amenable to health care and health policies (table 5.2). This confirms findings from earlier research in Brazil and suggests that, in all countries studied, the health policies and programs implemented over the period did make a noticeable contribution toward improving child health outcomes and explain in part the reduction of child mortality observed in the region.

The picture regarding amenable mortality in the age range of 15–69 years is more mixed. In 1985, amenable mortality due to the specified

Table 5.2 Standardized Death Rates by Selected Amenable and Other Causes of Death, 1985 and 2010—Age Group 0–14 Years

		Argentina	Brazil	Chile	Colombia	Costa Rica	Guatemala	Mexico	Peru
Intestinal infectious diseases	1985	10.1	50.0	6.2	36.2	10.1	344.4	70.1	48.1
	2010	1.4	2.3	0.2	2.1	1.0	20.3	2.9	1.8
	Percent	86	95	96	94	90	94	96	96
Malnutrition and nutritional anemias	1985	7.7	18.1	1.6	11.9	2.0	56.0	6.8	15.6
	2010	0.6	1.1	0.1	3.2	0.0	9.5	2.3	1.0
	Percent	92	94	94	73	98	83	66	93
Pneumonia and influenza	1985	12.7	39.3	27.8	28.5	15.2	174.0	49.2	68.5
	2010	3.4	5.0	3.1	5.6	0.9	34.8	5.6	9.9
	Percent	74	87	89	80	94	80	89	86
Amenable[a]	1985	30.5	107.5	35.6	76.7	27.3	573.9	126.1	132.0
	2010	5.4	8.4	3.6	10.8	1.8	64.4	10.8	12.4
	Percent	82	92	90	86	93	89	91	91
Other	1985	431.2	341.9	188.7	258.1	192.7	553.1	315.5	442.7
	2010	223.2	114.4	73.4	100.7	68.3	118.9	122.4	79.3
	Percent	48	67	61	61	65	92	61	82

Source: World Bank estimates with data from WHO Mortality Database, modified.
Note: The direct standardization method was applied using the 2000 WHO standard world population.
a. Amenable causes include intestinal infectious disease (ICD-9 001-009, ICD-10 E40-56, D50-53); malnutrition and nutritional anemias (ICD-9 260-68, ICD-10 A00-9); and pneumonia and influenza (ICD-9 480-86, 487; ICD-10 J10-18).

noncommunicable diseases in the age group accounted for 15–37 percent of deaths, depending on the country (figure 5.5). Most countries had a small to moderate reduction in the share of amenable mortality, with the range in 2010 narrowing to 12–29 percent. Brazil saw the largest absolute drop, and Brazil and Argentina the greatest decline in relative terms. Table 5.3 shows that levels of amenable causes of death among adults fell in all countries, but only in some— Argentina, Brazil, Chile, Colombia, and Costa Rica—did death rates for the specific amenable causes analyzed decrease more than death rates from other causes. In the last 25 years, trends for specific chronic diseases have varied considerably. Death by cerebrovascular disease decreased in all eight countries, while deaths by colon and rectum cancers increased across the board. These results must be interpreted with caution because improvements in the registration of cause of death, particularly due to noncommunicable diseases, confounds actual changes in mortality. Nonetheless, the findings corroborate evidence from other sources that the health care systems are not fully responding to the emerging needs for diagnosis, management, and treatment of chronic illnesses.

Cancer Survival

Data on cancer survival shed light on effectiveness of cancer care in terms of the prospect of survival.[26] In the OECD, there is now sufficient data based on registries to permit benchmarking countries on cancer survival, and such data have provided an important impetus for countries to develop plans and

Figure 5.5 Proportional Mortality by Specific Amenable Causes, 1985–2010—Age Group 15–69 Years

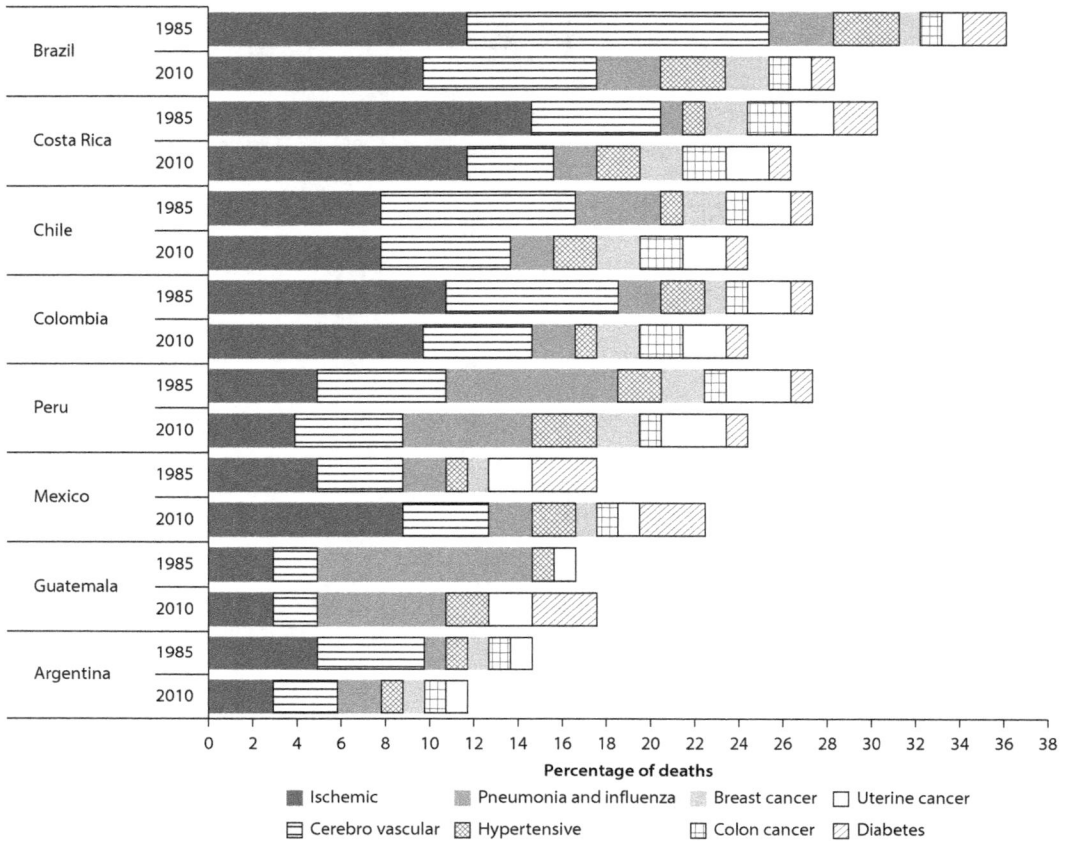

Source: World Bank estimates with data from WHO Mortality Database, modified.
Note: Amenable causes include hypertensive disease (ICD-9 401-5; ICD-10 I10-13, I15); cerebrovascular disease (ICD-9 430-38; ICD-60-69); ischemic heart disease (ICD-9 410-14; ICD-10 I20-25); malignant neoplasm of colon and rectum (ICD-9 53-54; ICD-10 C18-21); malignant neoplasm of breast and uterus (ICD-9 74, 179, 180, 182; ICD-10 C50, C53-55); and diabetes mellitus (ICD-9 250; ICD-10 E10-14).

strategies for improving the performance of cancer care (OECD 2013). In the case of breast cancer, survival differs widely across countries, from more than 80 percent in Norway and Switzerland to less than 60 percent in the cases of Poland or Brazil.

Cancer registries in the LAC region are significantly less developed, and there is little systematic data on survival. A study found mortality differences between patients with cervical cancer in urban and rural areas, which were attributed to less education, underemployment, and lack of social insurance coverage (Palacio-Mejia and others 2003). Similar findings have been reported for childhood cancers, with worse survival rates in regions with poorer socioeconomic conditions, more rural populations, and among those farther away from specialized cancer care centers (Perez-Cuevas and others 2013; Ribeiro, Lopes, and de Camargo 2007).

Table 5.3 Standardized Death Rates by Selected Amenable and Other Causes of Death, 1985 and 2010—Age Group 15–69 Years

		Argentina	Brazil	Chile	Colombia	Costa Rica	Guatemala	Mexico	Peru
Diabetes	1985	1.5	2.8	1.1	1.9	2.0	1.3	6.5	0.7
	2010	1.3	3.0	0.9	1.4	1.1	7.9	9.4	1.2
	Percent	14	5	18	26	45	526	46	78
Cerebrovascular disease	1985	45.0	75.0	44.4	44.1	21.6	12.2	24.8	18.5
	2010	19.6	32.0	17.9	16.6	10.9	8.1	15.4	8.5
	Percent	56	57	60	62	50	34	38	54
Ischemic heart disease	1985	46.9	66.0	43.4	65.4	54.8	22.1	32.4	15.3
	2010	22.4	41.6	21.7	34.8	29.8	19.1	36.2	8.0
	Percent	52	37	50	47	46	14	12	48
Hypertensive disease	1985	6.8	16.6	5.4	14.1	4.7	8.7	7.1	6.0
	2010	4.3	14.0	4.4	4.5	5.1	14.6	7.8	4.8
	Percent	37	16	18	68	9	68	9	20
Breast cancer	1985	36.9	26.9	27.3	21.9	28.9	5.2	18.1	24.2
	2010	28.5	27.2	21.6	23.2	20.3	12.9	21.8	12.4
	Percent	23	1	21	6	30	147	20	49
Uterine cancer	1985	12.7	14.2	20.1	23.4	15.6	15.6	22.5	21.4
	2010	9.6	8.7	7.3	10.4	7.3	17.0	9.4	11.1
	Percent	24	39	64	56	53	9	58	48
Colon cancer	1985	8.7	4.1	5.0	3.4	4.3	1.2	2.4	2.0
	2010	9.9	6.0	5.5	5.5	6.7	2.6	3.6	2.8
	Percent	14	45	11	59	56	113	52	36
Pneumonia and influenza	1985	5.8	14.2	20.9	8.5	2.7	67.7	12.5	24.4
	2010	20.0	13.5	6.6	7.1	6.1	30.5	6.6	11.9
	Percent	247	5	69	17	124	55	47	51
Amenable[a]	1985	110.6	159.3	117.4	120.8	78.6	109.7	84.8	74.3
	2010	81.8	101.7	57.7	63.9	52.9	83.0	71.3	41.7
	Percent	26	36	51	47	33	24	16	44
Other	1985	818.4	475.6	390.0	400.2	234.8	689.1	417.9	395.2
	2010	656.1	335.6	218.2	238.2	179.8	399.4	258.0	157.5
	Percent	20	29	44	40	23	42	38	60

Source: World Bank estimates with data from WHO Mortality Database, modified.
Note: The direct standardization method was applied using the 2000 WHO standard world population.
a. Amenable causes include hypertensive disease (ICD-9 401-5; ICD-10 I10-13, I15); cerebrovascular disease (ICD-9 430-38; ICD-60-69); ischemic heart disease (ICD-9 410-14; ICD-10 I20-25); malignant neoplasm of colon and rectum (ICD-9 53-54; ICD-10 C18-21); malignant neoplasm of breast and uterus (ICD-9 74, 179, 180, 182; ICD-10 C50, C53-55); and diabetes mellitus (ICD-9 250; ICD-10 E10-14).

In Conclusion

Indicators on coverage, utilization, and financial protection are likely to remain the mainstay of UHC monitoring. Yet traditional indicators have some important limitations. They shed little light on whether or not key health care needs are being effectively met, whether health care is being provided in a timely manner, and whether the quality of services is adequate—all factors that can drive a significant wedge between the use of health services and patient outcomes.

This chapter has demonstrated how survey and administrative data can provide important complementary insights on the performance of health systems and progress toward UHC. In recent years, many OECD countries have made significant investments in systems and capacity to systematically monitor unmet needs, waiting times, and health care quality. Such efforts in the LAC region are still in their infancy. However, many countries have mature administrative data systems—for example, cancer registries, health insurance claims, and hospital admissions data—that could be more extensively used to assess and monitor health system performance. Some countries are also investing in systems to monitor waiting times and health examination surveys with biomarkers. These are important steps. However, data quality and access, the lack of standardization, as well as capacity constraints in ministries of health often limit the extent to which data can be put to use to monitor the performance of the health system.

Notes

1. Although there are notable differences in terminology across assessment frameworks, health system performance is typically assessed in relation to intrinsic goals of improving the level and distribution of health outcomes, responsiveness, and financial protection. In addition to these intrinsic goals, most frameworks also highlight important intermediate outcomes, including access and coverage, efficiency, quality, and sometimes others, as well as key building blocks or factors for achieving intermediate outcomes and intrinsic goals (Hurst and Jee-Hughes 2001; OECD 2002; Roberts and others 2003; Smith, Mossialos, and Papanicolas 2008; WHO 2000, 2007).

2. Even with childhood immunizations, quality can be an important concern. For instance, the effectiveness of many vaccines depends on the production process, an intact cold chain from production to delivery of the vaccine, appropriate timing of doses, and other factors. These conditions are not met in many contexts, in which case immunized children may have limited or absent immunity despite having been vaccinated.

3. It is also related to the formula on community effectiveness from the health technology assessment literature: Effectiveness = Efficacy × Diagnostic Accuracy × Coverage × User Compliance × Provider Compliance.

4. In 2011, the number of deaths attributable to cardiovascular disease and diabetes has been estimated at around 100,000 and 350,000 respectively, with high fiscal and economic costs (WHO 2011). It is estimated that the cost attributable to CVDs to health systems in LAC was about US$10 billion and value of lost output was around US$19 billion (Bloom and others 2011).

5. Smaller studies from other countries confirm similar patterns of unmet need for both diagnosis and treatment. For instance, half the diabetic population in the Dominican Republic was found to be undiagnosed (Morales Peláez and others 1997).

6. A major problem with interpreting data on cancer in the region is that they are generally extrapolated from local hospital or regional databases, and only a small portion of the region's population is covered by national cancer registries, by contrast with 96 percent in the USA and 32 percent in Europe. See Centers for Disease Control and Prevention National Program of Cancer Registries (accessed August 22, 2013), http://www.cdc.gov/cancer/npcr/about.htm. Also see Goss and others (2013).

7. Late diagnosis tends to limit therapy options. For example, in the case of breast cancer, late-stage diagnosis, along with limited availability of other treatments, leads to higher rates of radical procedures such as mastectomy in low- and middle-income than in high-income countries. A report from the Mexican Cancer Institute (INCAN), for example, showed an 85 percent mastectomy rate at their institution, while in the United States breast-conserving surgery is more common and mastectomies performed in only 37 percent of cases (Chávarri-Guerra and others 2012).

8. The evidence is based on data from the payment system (*Autorização de Procedimento de Alta Complexidade*—APAC) and concerns all types of cancer for which radio- and/or chemotherapy were requested.

9. These differences are likely to reflect a host of factors, including disparities across groups in ease of access, quality of services, and demographic and socioeconomic conditions.

10. Survey estimates, which also take into account privately provided services administered over the last three years, suggest higher coverage of approximately 59 percent, although with significant disparities across socioeconomic groups (see chapter 4).

11. Evidence suggests that waiting times lead to poorer health outcomes, especially in the case of delayed attention in emergency situations (Guttmann and others 2011). In the case of breast cancer, time delays of longer than 12 weeks have been found to affect stage and consequently outcome and survival. (Richards and others 1999).

12. Opinion polls are often based on relatively small samples and answers tend to be very sensitive to how questions are asked. Results should hence be treated with some care.

13. The most important reason for not seeking care in both countries was that the individual thought they would get better without health care.

14. In the survey, 61 percent of respondents consider public health services bad or terrible, with 85 percent seeing no change or a worsening in the health system over the last three years. However, among those who actually used the national health system (SUS) in the last year, only 22 percent consider services bad or very bad.

15. In the Datafolha and IESS survey, household ranked private health insurance as the second most desired household assets, ahead of a car, life insurance, new household appliances, and a computer, with own house being the only item ranked as more important.

16. The index is based on Guidelines from the Program for Humanization of Prenatal Care and Childbirth established by the Brazilian Ministry of Health. The index evaluates the following criteria: (1) initiation of prenatal visits before the 16th gestational week; (2) minimum number of prenatal visits for gestational age; (3) results for the first round of routine exams (incl. glycaemia, Rh-factor, syphilis, HIV, etc.) from the 22nd gestational week; (4) tetanus vaccine from the 28th gestational week; (5) results for the second round of routine exams (glycaemia, urine sediment, and syphilis) after the 34th gestational week.

17. The study used the Adequacy of Prenatal Care Utilization Index (Kotelchuck 1994) to evaluate adequacy of prenatal care. Inadequate care was defined as prenatal care starting after the 15th week of gestation or a ratio of actual divided by expected number of visits below 50 percent.

18. Using 20 percent as the threshold rate to define the overuse of caesarean sections, or CS (WHO recommends not more than 15 percent), 4 million CS are in excess in 46 countries worldwide. According to WHO estimates, the global "excess" CS in 2008 was estimated to amount to approximately US$2.32 billion (all costs are denominated in 2005 constant $), while the cost of the global "needed" CS in 2008 was estimated

to amount to approximately US$432 million. CS are estimated to be about 2.8 times more expensive in countries with "excess" procedures than in those where procedures are "needed." Furthermore, the number of global "excess" CS in 2008 exceeded the number of "needed" ones by a factor of approximately 1.9 (Gibbons and others 2010).

19. The study involved a review of national statistics and hospital records, an inventory of facilities, and observations of peripartum client–provider interactions at 14 facilities.

20. Taking Brazil as an example—only 24 centers offer palliative care across the country and Brazil had the lowest ration of hospice or palliative care services per population in 21 countries in LAC (Wright and others 2008).

21. Morphine and other opioids are needed to manage severe pain, and WHO has included them on the list of essential medicines. WHO. *Health Topics. Essential Medicines* (accessed August 28, 2013). http://www.who.int/selection_medicines/list/en/.

22. While diagnostic criteria were largely consistent across national guidelines, there was considerable variation of treatment targets for blood glucose, as well as for rates of effective management of cardiovascular risk factors in individuals with diabetes.

23. The list of conditions for which mortality is considered amenable has varied significantly over time and across studies. In part, this reflects not only the introduction of new technology but also the extent to which the respective studies have focused on personal health care services or also broader primary-prevention interventions. For details, see Nolte and McKee (2003).

24. Of course, changes in amenable mortality reflect both changes in incidence and the effectiveness of health care (treatment as well as secondary and tertiary prevention). Hence, some care is needed in the interpretation of the data. Nolte and McKee (2003) note that "amenable mortality was never intended to be more than an indicator of potential weaknesses in health care that can then be investigated in more depth."

25. Selected amenable causes for the 0–14 age group include intestinal infectious disease (ICD-9 001-009;ICD-10 E40-56, D50-53); malnutrition and nutritional anemias (ICD-9 260-68; ICD-10 A00-9); pneumonia and influenza (ICD-9 480-86, 487; ICD-10 J10-18); for the 15–69 age group, amenable causes include hypertensive disease (ICD-9 401-5; ICD-10 I10-13, I15); cerebrovascular disease (ICD-9 430-38; ICD-60-69); ischemic heart disease (ICD-9 410-14; ICD-10 I20-25); malignant neoplasm of colon and rectum (ICD-9 53-54; ICD-10 C18-21); malignant neoplasm of breast and uterus (ICD-9 74, 179, 180, 182; ICD-10 C50, C53-55); and diabetes mellitus (ICD-9 250; ICD-10 E10-14). Unspecified causes were distributed proportionately according to the defined causes by country, year, and age group.

26. Cancer survival rates are defined as the proportion of patients with a particular cancer that are still alive after a defined time period (e.g., five years) compared with those still alive in the absence of a disease.

References

Abreu, Daisy Maria Xavier de, Cibele Comini César, and Elisabeth Barboza França. 2007. "Relação entre as causas de morte evitáveis por atenção à saúde e a implementação do Sistema Único de Saúde no Brasil." *Revista Panamericana de Salud Pública* 21 (5): 282–91.

———. 2009. "Diferencíais entre homens e mulheres na mortalidade evitável no Brasil (1983–2005)." *Cadernos de Saúde Pública* 25 (12): 2672–82.

Agurto, I., A. Bishop, G. Sanchez, Z. Betancourt, and S. Robles. 2004. "Perceived Barriers and Benefits to Cervical Cancer Screening in Latin America." *Preventive Medicine* 39 (1): 91–98.

AHRQ (Agency for Healthcare Research and Quality). 2013. *2012 National Healthcare Quality Report*. Rockville, MD. http://www.ahrq.gov/research/findings/nhqrdr/nhqr12/index.html.

Anderson, Benjamin O., Eduardo Cazap, Nagi S. El Saghir, Cheng-Har Yip, Hussein M. Khaled, Isabel V. Otero, Clement A. Adebamowo, Rajendra A. Badwe, and Joe B. Harford. 2010. "Optimisation of Breast Cancer Management in Low-Resource and Middle-Resource Countries: Executive Summary of Breast Health Global Initiative Consensus." *The Lancet Oncology* 12: 387–98.

Arah, Onyebuchi A., Gert P. Westert, Jeremy Hurst, and Niek S. Klazinga. 2006. "A Conceptual Framework for the OECD Health Care Quality Indicators Project." *International Journal for Quality in Health Care* 18 (Suppl. 1): 5–13.

Bargallo, Juan Enrique, Fernando Lara, Robin Shaw-Dulin, Victor Perez-Sánchez, Cynthia Villarreal-Garza, Hector Maldonado-Martinez, Alejandro Mohar-Betancourt, Carl Yoshizawa, Emily Burke, Timothy Decker, and Calvin Chao. 2015. "A Study of the Impact of the 21-Gene Breast Cancer Assay on the Use of Adjuvant Chemotherapy in Women with Breast Cancer in a Mexican Public Hospital." *Journal of Surgical Oncology* 111 (2): 203–07.

Barros, Fernando C., Cesar G. Victora, Aluisio J. D. Barros, Ina S. Santos, Elaine Albernaz, Alicia Matijasevich, Marlos R. Domingues, Iândora K. T. Sclowitz, Pedro C. Hallal, Mariângela F. Silveira, and J. Patrick Vaughan. 2005. "The Challenge of Reducing Neonatal Mortality in Middle-Income Countries: Findings from Three Brazilian Birth Cohorts in 1982, 1993, and 2004." *The Lancet* 365 (9462): 847–54.

Bitrán R., L. Escobar, and P. Gassibe. 2010. "After Chile's Health Reform: Increase in Coverage and Access, Decline in Hospitalization and Death Rates." *Health Affairs* 29: 2161.

Bloom, D. E., E. T. Cafiero, E. Jané-Llopis, S. Abrahams-Gessel, L. R. Bloom, S. Fathima, A. B. Feigl, T. Gaziano, M. Mowafi, A. Pandya, K. Prettner, L. Rosenberg, B. Seligman, A. Z. Stein, and C. Weinstein. 2011. *The Global Economic Burden of Noncommunicable Diseases*. Geneva: World Economic Forum.

Bright, Kristin, Maya Barghash, Martin Donach, Marcos Gutiérrez de la Barrera, Robert J. Schneider, and Silvia C. Formenti. 2011. "The Role of Health System Factors in Delaying Final Diagnosis and Treatment of Breast Cancer in Mexico City, Mexico." *The Breast* 20: S54–59.

Callaway, Mary, Kathleen M. Foley, Liliana De Lima, Stephen R. Connor, Olivia Dix, Thomas Lynch, Michael Wright, and David Clark. 2007. "Funding for Palliative Care Programs in Developing Countries." *Journal of Pain and Symptom Management* 33: 509–13.

Campbell, Stephen M., Martin O. Roland, and Stephen A. Buetow. 2000. "Defining Quality of Care." *Social Science & Medicine* 51 (11): 1611–25.

Cazap, E., A. Buzaid, C. Garbino, J. de la Garza, F. Orlandi, G. Schwartsmann, C. T. Vallejos, A. Gercovich, and G. Breitbart. 2010. "Breast Cancer in Latin America: Experts Perceptions Compared with Medical Care Standards." *The Breast* 19: 50–54.

Chávarri-Guerra, Y., C. Villarreal-Garza, P. Liedke, F. Knaul, A. Mohar, D. M. Finkelstein, and P. E. Goss. 2012. "Breast Cancer in Mexico: A Growing Challenge to Health and the Health System." *The Lancet Oncology* 13: e335–43.

CNI (Confederação Nacional da Indústria). 2012. "Retratos da sociedade brasileira: Saúde pública. Pesquisa CNI-IBOPE." CNI, Brasilia.

Concha, D. F., V. N. Pastén, F. V. Espinosa, and A. F. López. 2008. "Impacto de la Implementación del Plan AUGE en la detección antenatal de Cardiopatías Congénitas." *Revista Chilena de Obstetricia y Ginecología* 73: 163–72.

Das, Jishnu, and Jeffrey Hammer. 2014. "Practice Quality Variation in Low-Income Countries: Facts and Economics." *Annual Review of Economics* 6 (1).

DCCT/EDIC (Diabetes Control and Complications Trial/Epidemiology of Diabetes Interventions and Complications) Study Research Group. 2005. "Intensive Diabetes Treatment and Cardiovascular Disease in Patients with Type 1 Diabetes." *The New England Journal of Medicine* 353: 2643–53. doi:10.1056/NEJMoa052187.

Deloitte. 2011a. "2011 Survey of Health Care Consumers in Mexico: Key Findings, Strategic Implications." Deloitte Center for Health Solutions.

———. 2011b. "2011 Survey of Health Care Consumers in Brazil: Key Findings, Strategic Implications." Deloitte Center for Health Solutions.

Domingues, Rosa Maria Soares Madeira, Zulmira Maria de Araújo Hartz, Marcos Augusto Bastos Dias, and Maria do Carmo Leal. 2012. "Avaliação da adequação da assistência pré-natal na rede SUS do Município do Rio de Janeiro, Brasil." *Cadernos de Saúde Pública* 28: 425–37.

Donabedian, Avedis. 1980. *The Definition of Quality and Approaches to Its Assessment—Explorations in Quality Assessment and Monitoring, Vol. 1.* Ann Arbor: Health Administration Press.

Escarião, Paulo Henrique Gonçalves, Tiago Eugênio Faria de Arantes, Telma Lúcia Tabosa Florêncio, and Ana Lúcia de Andrade Lima Arcoverde. 2008. "Epidemiologia e diferenças regionais da retinopatia diabética em Pernambuco, Brasil." *Arquivos Brasileiros de Oftalmologia* 71 (2): 172–75.

Estado de São Paulo (newspaper). 2013. "SP tem 800 mil pedidos médicos na fila de espera." Estado de São Paulo.

Ferlay, J., H. R. Shin, F. Bray, D. Forman, C. Mathers, and D. M. Parkin. 2008. "Cancer Incidence and Mortality Worldwide: GLOBOCAN 2008" (accessed August 25, 2013), http://globocan.iarc.fr.

Gage, J. C., C. Ferreccio, M. Gonzales, R. Arroyo, H. Militza, and S. Robles. 2003. "Follow-up Care of Women with an Abnormal Cytology in a Low-Resource Setting.." *Cancer Detection and Prevention* 27: 466–71.

Gakidou, E., L. Mallinger, J. Abbott-Klafter, R. Guerrero, S. Villalpando, R. Lopez Ridaura, W. Aekplakorn, M. Naghavi, S. Lim, R. Lozanoa, and J. L. C. Murray. 2011. "Management of Diabetes and Associated Cardiovascular Risk Factors in Seven Countries: A Comparison of Data from National Health Examination Surveys." *Bulletin of the World Health Organization* 89: 172–83.

Gamba, M. A. 1998. "Amputações por diabetes mellitus, uma prática prevenível?" *Acta Paulista de Enfermagem* 11 (3): 92–100.

Gaziano, A. B., M. Mowafi, A. Pandya, K. Prettner, L. Rosenberg, B. Seligman, A. Z. Stein, and C. Weinstein. 2011. *The Global Economic Burden of Noncommunicable Diseases.* Geneva: World Economic Forum.

Gibbons, Luz, José M. Belizán, Jeremy A. Lauer, Ana P. Betrán, Mario Merialdi, and Fernando Althabe. 2010. "The Global Numbers and Costs of Additionally Needed and Unnecessary Caesarean Sections Performed Per Year: Overuse as a Barrier to Universal Coverage." World Health Report Background Paper, 1–31.

Gorgot, Luis Ramon Marques da Rocha, Iná Santos, Neiva Valle, Alicia Matisajevich, Aluisio J. D. Barros, and Elaine Albernaz. 2011. "Avoidable Deaths until 48 Months of Age among Children from the 2004 Pelotas Birth Cohort." *Revista de Saúde Pública* 45 (2): 334–42.

Goss, Paul E., Brittany L. Lee, Tanja Badovinac-Crnjevic, Kathrin Strasser-Weippl, Yanin Chavarri-Guerra, Jessica St. Louis, Cynthia Villarreal-Garza, Karla Unger-Saldaña, Mayra Ferreyra, Márcio Debiasi, Pedro E. R. Liedke, Diego Touya, Gustavo Werutsky, Michaela Higgins, Lei Fan, Claudia Vasconcelos, Eduardo Cazap, Carlos Vallejos, Alejandro Mohar, Felicia Knaul, Hector Arreola, Rekha Batura, Silvana Luciani, Richard Sullivan, Dianne Finkelstein, Sergio Simon, Carlos Barrios, Rebecca Kightlinger, Andres Gelrud, Vladimir Bychkovsky, Gilberto Lopes, Stephen Stefani, Marcelo Blaya, Fabiano Hahn Souza, Franklin Santana Santos, Alberto Kaemmerer, Evandro de Azambuja, Andres Felipe Cardona Zorilla, Raul Murillo, Jose Jeronimo, Vivien Tsu, Andre Carvalho, Carlos Ferreira Gil, Cinthya Sternberg, Alfonso Dueñas-Gonzalez, Dennis Sgroi, Mauricio Cuello, Rodrigo Fresco, Rui Manuel Reis, Guiseppe Masera, Raúl Gabús, Raul Ribeiro, Renata Knust, Gustavo Ismael, Eduardo Rosenblatt, Berta Roth, Luisa Villa, Argelia Lara Solares, Marta Ximena Leon, Isabel Torres-Vigil, Alfredo Covarrubias-Gomez, Andrés Hernández, Mariela Bertolino, Gilberto Schwartsmann, Sergio Santillana, Francisco Esteva, Luis Fein, Max Mano, Henry Gomez, Marc Hurlbert, Alessandra Durstine, and Gustavo Azenha. 2013. "Planning Cancer Control in Latin America and the Caribbean." *The Lancet Oncology* 14: 391–436.

Gragnolati, M., M. Lindelow, and B. Couttolenc. 2013. *20 Years of Health System Reform in Brazil: An Assessment of the Sistema Unico de Saude.* Washington, DC: World Bank.

Guanais, Frederico C., Ronald Gómez-Suárez, and Leonardo Pinzón. 2012. "Primary Care Effectiveness and the Extent of Avoidable Hospitalizations in Latin America and the Caribbean." IDB Discussion Paper Series IDB-DP-266, Inter-American Development Bank, Washington, DC.

Guttmann, Astrid, Michael J. Schull, Marian J. Vermeulen, and Therese A. Stukel. 2011. "Association between Waiting Times and Short-Term Mortality and Hospital Admission after Departure from Emergency Department: Population-Based Cohort Study from Ontario, Canada." *British Medical Journal* 342: d2983.

Hurst, J., and M. Jee-Hughes. 2001. "Performance Measurement and Performance Management in OECD Health Systems." Labour Market and Social Policy Occasional Paper 47, OECD Publishing, Paris.

IESS (Instituto de Estudos de Saúde Suplementar). 2011. "Pesquisa IESS/Datafolha aponta que o plan de saúde é uma necessidade e desejo do brasileiro." *Saúde Suplementar em Foco, Informativo Eletrônico* 2 (13).

INCA. 2010. "Análise da Atenção Oncológica no Brasil: Acesso, medicamentos e equipamentos." Presentation by Luiz Santini at Conselho Nacional de Saúde, Brasilia, July 7.

Institute of Medicine of the National Academies. 2001. *Crossing the Quality Chasm: A New Health System for the 21st Century.* Committee on Quality of Health Care in America. Washington, DC: National Academies Press.

IPEA (Instituto de Pesquisa Econômica Aplicada). 2011. *Sistema de indicadores de percepção social: Saúde.* Brasilia: IPEA.

Kelley, Edward, and Jeremy Hurst. 2006. "Health Care Quality Indicators Project: Conceptual Framework Paper." OECD Health Working Papers 23, OECD, Paris.

Kotelchuck, Milton. 1994. "An Evaluation of the Kessner Adequacy of Prenatal Care Index and a Proposed Adequacy of Prenatal Care Utilization Index." *American Journal of Public Health* 84 (9): 1414–20.

Lazcano-Ponce, Eduardo, Lina Sofía Palacio-Mejia, Betania Allen-Leigh, Elsa Yunes-Diaz, Patricia Alonso, Raffaela Schiavon, and Mauricio Hernandez-Avila. 2008. "Decreasing Cervical Cancer Mortality in Mexico: Effect of Papanicolaou Coverage, Birthrate, and the Importance of Diagnostic Validity of Cytology." *Cancer Epidemiology, Biomarkers and Prevention* 17: 2808–17.

Lee, B. L., P. Liedke, C. H. Barrios, S. D. Simon, D. M. Finkelstein, and P. E. Goss. 2012. "Breast Cancer in Brazil: Present Status and Future Goals." *The Lancet Oncology* 13: e95–102.

Lohr, Kathleen N., ed. 1990. *Medicare: A Strategy for Quality Assurance.* Vol. 1. Washington, DC: National Academies Press.

Lopez -Carrillo, L., L. Torres-Sanchez, M. Lopez-Cervantes, and C. Rueda-Neria. 2001. "Identification of Malignant Breast Lesions in Mexico." *Salud Pública de México* 43: 199–202.

Lora, Miranda, América Liliana, Marta Margarita Zapata Tarrés, Elisa María Dorantes Acosta, Alfonso Reyes López, Daniela Marín Hernández, Onofre Muñoz Hernández, and Juan Garduño Espinosa. 2011. "Estímulo iatrotrópico y tiempo al diagnóstico en pacientes pediátricos con leucemia linfoblástica aguda." *Boletín Médico del Hospital Infantil de México* 68 (6): 419–24.

Madrigal de la Campa, M. L., E. C. Lazcano Ponce, and C. Infante Castaneda. 2005. "Overuse of Colposcopy Service in Mexico." *Ginecología y Obstetricia de México* 73: 637–47.

Malta, Deborah Carvalho, Elisabeth Carmen Duarte, Juan José Corez Escalante, Márcia Furquim de Almeida, Luciana M. Vasconcelos Sardinha, Eduardo Marques Macário, Rosane Aparecida Monteiro, and Otaliba Libânio de Morais Neto. 2010. "Mortes evitáveis em menores de um ano, Brasil, 1997 a 2006: contribuições para a avaliação de desempenho do Sistema Único de Saúde." *Cadernos de Saúde Pública* 26 (3) 481–91.

Marinho, L. A., J. G. Cecatti, M. J. Osis, and M. S. Gurgel. 2008. "Knowledge, Attitude and Practice of Mammography among Women Users of Public Health Services." *Revista de Saúde Pública* 42: 200–07.

Marshall, Martin, Sheila Leatherman, and Soeren Mattke. 2004. "Selecting Indicators for the Quality of Health Promotion, Prevention and Primary Care at the Health Systems Level in OECD Countries." OECD Health Technical Papers 16, OECD, Paris.

McKee, Martin, and Anthony J. McMichael. 2008. "The Health of Nations." *BMJ* 337. http://www.bmj.com/content/337/bmj.a2811.

Miller, S., M. Cordero, A. L. Coleman, J. Figueroa, S. Brito-Anderson, R. Dabagh, V. Calderon, F. Caceres, A. J. Fernandez, and M. Nunez. 2003. "Averting Maternal Death and Disability. Quality of Care in Institutionalized Deliveries: The Paradox of the Dominican Republic." *International Journal of Gynecology and Obstetrics* 82: 89–103.

MinSalud. 2012. "Evaluación de la percepción social del sistema de salud y ordenamiento de las entidades promotoras de salud." Powerpoint presentation, October 2012, Oficina de Calidad.

Mohar, A., E. Bargallo, M. T. Ramirez, F. Lara, and A. Beltran-Ortega. 2009. "Available Resources for the Treatment of Breast Cancer in Mexico." *Salud Pública de México* 51: s263–69.

Morales Peláez, Eduardo, Méjico Angeles Suarez, Juan Batlle Pichardo, and Felix M. Escaño Polanco. 1997. "República Dominicana diabetes y ceguera: Resultados de una encuesta nacional realizada por Clubes de Leones Distrito Múltiple R." Clubes de Leones.

Murillo, R., C. Wiesner, R. Cendales, M. Pineros, and S. Tovar. 2011. "Comprehensive Evaluation of Cervical Cancer Screening Programs: The Case of Colombia." *Salud Pública de México* 53: 469–77.

National Cancer Institute. 2011. "SEER Cancer Statistics Review, 1975–2008." http://seer .cancer.gov/csr/1975_2008/.

Nazzal, N. C. T. P. Campos, H. R. Corbalán, Z. F. Lanas, J. J. Bartolucci, C. P. Sanhueza, C. G. Cavada, and D. J. C. Prieto. 2008. "The Impact of Chilean Health Reform in the Management and Mortality of ST Elevation Myocardial Infarction (STEMI) in Chilean Hospitals." *Revista Médica de Chile* 136 (10): 1231–39.

Nolte, E., and M. McKee. 2003. "Measuring the Health of Nations: How Much Is Attributable to Health Care ? An Analysis of Mortality Amenable to Medical Care." *BMJ* 327: 1129–32.

———. 2004. *Does Healthcare Save Lives? Avoidable Mortality Revisited.* London: Nuffield Trust.

———. 2012. "In Amenable Mortality—Deaths Avoidable through Health Care —Progress in the United States Lags that of Three European Countries." *Health Affairs* 31: 2114–22.

OECD (Organisation for Economic Co-operation and Development). 2002. *Measuring Up: Improving Health System Performance in OECD Countries.* Paris: OECD.

———. 2011. *Health at a Glance 2011.* Paris: OECD.

———. 2012. *Health at a Glance 2012.* Paris: OECD.

———. 2013. "Cancer Care: Assuring Quality to Improve Survival." OECD Health Policy Studies, Paris.

Palacio -Mejia, L. S., G. Rangel-Gomez, M. Hernandez-Avila, and E. Lazcano-Ponce. 2003. "Cervical Cancer, a Disease of Poverty: Mortality Differences between Urban and Rural Areas in Mexico." *Salud Pública de México* 45 (Suppl. 3): 315–25.

Paraje, Guillermo, and Felipe Vásquez. 2012. *Toward Universal Health Coverage: The Case of Chile.* Washington, DC: World Bank.

Perez-Cuevas, Ricardo, Svetlana V. Doubova, Marta Zapata-Tarres, Sergio Flores-Hernández, Lindsay Frazier, Carlos Rodríguez-Galindo, Gabriel Cortes-Gallo, Salomon Chertorivski-Woldenberg, and Onofre Muñoz-Hernández. 2013. "Scaling Up Cancer Care for Children without Medical Insurance in Developing Countries: The Case of Mexico." *Pediatric Blood and Cancer* 60: 196–203.

Pérez-Then, Eddy, Ana Gómez, Roberto Espinal, Jeannette Báez, Erwin Cruz Bournigal, Ceila Pérez-Ferrán, Rosa Abreu, Samuel Guerrero, Emilton López, Fátima Guerrero, and Equipo CENISMI. 2008. "Calidad de atención a la embarazada y al niño sano en centros de primer nivel de atención de las regiones de salud III, IV, V y VI de la República Dominicana." Informe final, Centro Nacional de Investigaciones en Salud Materno Infantil (CENISMI), Santo Domingo, República Dominicana.

Ribeiro, Eleonora R. O., Alzira Maria D. N. Guimarães, Heloísa Bettiol, Danilo D. F. Lima, Maria Luiza D. Almeida, Luiz de Souza, Antônio Augusto M. Silva, and Ricardo Q. Gurgel. 2009. "Risk Factors for Inadequate Prenatal Care Use in the Metropolitan Area of Aracaju, Northeast Brazil." *BMC Pregnancy and Childbirth* 9: 31.

Ribeiro, K. B., L. F. Lopes, and B. De Camargo. 2007. "Trends in Childhood Leukemia Mortality in Brazil and Correlation with Social Inequalities." *Cancer* 110: 1823–31.

Richards, M. A., P. Smith, A. J. Ramirez, I. S. Fentiman, and R. D. Rubens. 1999. "The Influence on Survival of Delay in the Presentation and Treatment of Symptomatic Breast Cancer." *British Journal of Cancer* 79: 858–64.

Roberts, M., W. Hsiao, P. Berman, and M. Reich. 2003. *Getting Health Reform Right: A Guide to Improving Performance and Equity*. New York: Oxford University Press.

Ross, Anna Gabriela, José Luis Zeballos, and Alberto Infante. 2000. "Quality and Health Sector Reform in Latin America and the Caribbean." *Revista Panamericana de Salud Pública* 8 (1–2): 93–98.

Salles, Marcio de Almeida, Agostinho Pinto Gouvêa, Daniela Savi, Marco Aurélio Figueiredo, Ramão Tavares Neto, Rodrigo Assis de Paula, and Helenice Gobbi. 2008. "Training and Standardized Criteria Improve the Diagnosis of Premalignant Breast Lesions." *Revista Brasileira de Ginecologia e Obstetrícia* 30: 550–5.

Santos, Iná S., Alicia Matijasevich, Aluísio J. D. Barros, Elaine P. Albernaz, Marlos Rodrigues Domingues, Neiva C. J. Valle, Deborah Carvalho Malta, Luís Ramón M. R. Gorgot, and Fernando C. Barros. 2011. "Avoidable Deaths in the First Four Years of Life among Children in the 2004 Pelotas (Brazil) Birth Cohort Study." *Cadernos de Saúde Pública* 27: s185–97.

Savedoff, William. 2009. "A Moving Target: Universal Access to Healthcare Services in Latin America and the Caribbean." IDB Research Department Working Paper 667, Washington, DC.

Schuster, Mark A., Elizabeth A. McGlynn, and Robert H. Brook. 2005. "How Good Is the Quality of Health Care in the United States?" *Milbank Quarterly* 83 (4): 843– 95.

Shengelia, Bakhuti, Chrisotpher J. L. Murray, and Orvill B. Adams. 2003. "Beyond Access and Utilization: Defining and Measuring Health System Coverage." In *Health Systems Performance Assessment: Debates, Methods and Empiricism*, edited by Christopher J. L. Murray and David B. Evans, 221–34. Geneva: WHO.

Siciliani, L., M. Borowitz, and V. Moran. 2013. "Waiting Time Policies in the Health Sector. What Works?" OECD Health Policy Studies, OECD, Paris.

Simon, S. D., J. Bines, C. H. Barrios, J. Nunes, E. Gomes, F. Pacheco, A. Santana Gomes, J. Segalla, S. Crocamo-Costa, D. Gimenes, B. van Eyll, G. Queiroz, G. Borges, L. Dal Lago, and C. Vasconcellos. 2009. "Clinical Characteristics and Outcomes of Treatment of Brazilian Women with Breast Cancer Treated at Public and Private Institutions—The AMAZONE Project of the Brazilian Breast Cancer Study Group (GBECAM)." Abstract 3082, San Antonio Breast Cancer Symposium December 11, San Antonio, TX.

Smith, P., E. Mossialos, and I. Papanicolas. 2008. "Performance Measurement for Health System Improvement: Experiences, Challenges, and Prospects." Background document, World Health Organization on behalf of the European Observatory on Health Systems and Policies, Copenhagen.

Sosa-Rubí, S. G., D. Walker, and E. Serván. 2009. "Performance of Mammography and Papanicolaou among Rural Women in Mexico." *Salud Pública de México* 51 (Suppl. 2): 236–45.

Staessen, Jan A., Ji-Guang Wang, and Lutgarde Thijs. 2001. "Cardiovascular Prevention and Blood Pressure Reduction: A Meta-Analysis." *The Lancet* 359: 1305–15.

TCU (Tribunal de Contas da União). 2011. *Política Nacional de Atenção Oncológica/ Tribunal de Contas da União; Relator: Ministro José Jorge.* Brasília: TCU, Secretaria de Fiscalização e Avaliação de Programas de Governo (Relatório de auditoria operacional).

Torres, V. I., L. A. Aday, L. De Lima, and C. S. Cleeland. 2007. "What Predicts the Quality of Advanced Cancer Care in Latin America? A Look at Five Countries: Argentina, Brazil, Cuba, Mexico, and Peru." *Journal of Pain and Symptom Management* 34: 315–27.

Vargas López, K. 2010. *El Desarrollo del Derecho a la Salud por Parte de la Sala Constitucional y Su Influencia en el Sistema Público de Salud en Costa Rica. Trabajo final de investigación aplicada sometido a la consideración de la Comisión del Programa de Estudios de Posgrado en Salud Pública para optar al grado y título de Maestría Profesional en Salud Pública con Énfasis en Gerencia de la Salud.* San Jose: Universidad de Costa Rica.

Victora, Cesar G., Estela M. L. Aquino, Maria do Carmo Leal, Carlos Augusto Monteiro, Fernando C. Barros, and Celia L. Szwarcwald. 2011. "Health in Brazil 2: Maternal and Child Health in Brazil: Progress and Challenges." *The Lancet* 377: 1863–76.

WHO (World Health Organization). 2000. *World Health Report 2000: Health Systems: Improving Performance.* Geneva: WHO.

———. 2006. *Quality of Care : A Process for Making Strategic Choices in Health Systems.* Geneva: WHO.

———. 2007. *Everybody's Business: Strengthening Health Systems to Improve Health Outcomes; WHO's Framework for Action.* Geneva: WHO.

———. 2011. "Global Health Observatory Data Repository. World Bank Regions: Latin America and Caribbean, Number of Deaths by Cause." http://apps.who.int/gho/data /node.main.CODWBDCPLAC?lang=en.

———. 2013. "Strengthening of Palliative Care as a Component of Integrated Treatment throughout the Life Course." EB134/28, WHO, Geneva.

WHO and World Bank. 2014. "Monitoring Progress toward Universal Health Coverage at Country and Global Levels: A Framework." Joint WHO/World Bank Group Discussion Paper, WHO and World Bank, Washington, DC.

Wright, Michael, Justin Wood, Thomas Lynch, and David Clark. 2008. "Mapping Levels of Palliative Care Development: A Global View." *Journal of Pain and Symptom Management* 35 (5): 469–85.

CHAPTER 6

Conclusions

Tania Dmytraczenko and Gisele Almeida

Introduction

During the past three decades, countries in Latin America and the Caribbean (LAC) have made progress toward the realization of the right to health. Countries have committed to protecting this right by ratifying international conventions and enacting constitutional provisions that guarantee access to health care for all. Consequently, there have been mounting demands for health systems to become more responsive in delivering affordable care that meets the needs of the population. The region's changing demographic and epidemiological profiles, notably the aging population and the shift of the burden of disease toward chronic illnesses, have put additional pressure on health systems to adapt.

In response, several countries in the region have implemented policies and programs to advance universal health coverage (UHC)—that is, "to ensure that everyone who needs health services is able to get them, without undue financial hardship" (WHO and World Bank 2014, 1). Social policies that encompass reforms in the health sector have been implemented in the context of recent redemocratization and stable economic growth, which in most countries has translated into rising household incomes, drastic drops in poverty, and declining inequality. A rising middle class and empowered electorate have demanded greater and more effective investments in health and other social sectors. When fulfilled, these have the potential to increase human capital and spur further economic growth and poverty reduction, creating a virtuous cycle.

Our examination reviewed LAC health care policies and applied an equity lens to assess changes in population coverage, service coverage, and financial protection. Advances toward the goal of achieving UHC have been shown on many fronts. First, the share of the population covered by programs that have explicit entitlements to health care has increased considerably; since the early 2000s, 46 million more people in the countries analyzed are covered by health care programs and policies aimed toward advancing UHC. In addition, equity has improved. Several countries have implemented heavily subsidized programs to target specific populations, such as those not covered by contributory social health insurance schemes; these are primarily insurance schemes that require the enrollment of beneficiaries. Other countries have prioritized extending coverage to vulnerable groups within the construct of programs that are universal in nature. Even in countries that maintain health systems in which subsidized schemes coexist with separate, largely contributory social health insurance plans, the result is overall coverage that is fairly equally distributed among income groups. Although employment-based social health insurance remains heavily skewed toward the rich, subsidized schemes are well targeted to the poor and provide some degree of counterbalance, at least initially.

From a financing perspective, reforms have been accompanied by a rise in public spending on health and in most cases a decline in the share of out-of-pocket payments in total health expenditures. Although not all reforms had an explicit objective of extending financial protection, most countries saw a reduction in catastrophic health expenditures and impoverishment caused by outlays for health. No clear picture emerges regarding catastrophic payments and equity; this may reflect limitations in the measure, which does not capture those who did not seek care because of financial barriers or provide enough granularity on the nature of the expenditures, in particular whether the care paid for was necessary or elective. Note that even though impoverishment caused by health spending and catastrophic health expenditures are low in relative terms and generally declining in the region, in the countries analyzed 2 million to 4 million people still fall below the poverty line because of health spending. Despite the positive trends, the share of out-of-pocket payments in total spending is still relatively high compared to most countries in the Organisation for Economic Co-operation and Development (OECD). Expenditures for medicines absorb by far the largest share of direct payments across income groups, but they are a particularly heavy burden for the poor.

Service coverage has also expanded. Subsidized schemes cover at the very least maternal and child health interventions, and most go beyond that to include comprehensive primary care. Half the countries studied offer extensive benefits that include the spectrum from primary to high-complexity care. The evidence corroborates that investments in extending cost-effective health care, with particular attention to reaching vulnerable populations, yield results. Scale-up of programs to advance UHC has coincided with improvements in health equity, narrowing the gap between the rich and the poor in health outcomes, and service utilization, particularly as related to the targets of the Millennium Development Goals; however, a pro-poor gradient in adverse outcomes remains. Countries that have programs with greater population coverage and more extensive benefits packages have achieved near universality in the utilization of maternal health care services; they have high levels of utilization and virtually no difference among income quintiles. In countries where a pro-rich gradient in services utilization remains, it is narrowest and overall levels are highest for services delivered through traditionally vertical programs, such as immunization and family planning programs. This is followed by services that are provided mostly at the lower levels of the delivery network (for example, antenatal care or medical treatment of acute respiratory infections). Gaps among the rich and the poor are wider for deliveries, which are done in hospitals.

The picture of adult health status is more nuanced and not nearly as positive, especially regarding the chronic conditions and illnesses that are the leading causes of mortality and morbidity in the middle to late stages of the life course. The share of the population reporting less-than-good health status has not declined markedly or consistently in most countries; and the indicators are highly skewed, with the poor uniformly reporting the worst outcomes.[1] Further, diagnosed chronic conditions such as diabetes, ischemic heart disease, and asthma are increasing among all income groups in several countries, as are associated risk factors such as obesity and hypertension. Despite expectations based on strong evidence in the literature that disadvantaged socioeconomic and marginalized populations have a higher risk of dying from noncommunicable diseases when compared to other groups (Di Cesare and others 2013), in our analysis no clear gradient emerged in diagnosed chronic conditions and associated risk factors. This is likely because better access to health care among the rich, particularly for diagnostic services, masks differences in de facto prevalence among income groups. Indeed, evidence from cancer screenings suggests that this may be the case. Utilization of these diagnostics is generally pro-rich, and the gradient is particularly pronounced in breast cancer screenings, which require access to specialist care. The trend in level and equity is positive, however; with the exception of Brazil, countries that have high levels of population coverage have greatly reduced the gap between the rich and the poor, especially for cervical cancer screenings but in Colombia and Mexico also for mammographies.

The ultimate goal of UHC is to improve health outcomes for all segments of the population. Ensuring access to health care for all without financial hardship is an important means to achieve this end. However, to translate the availability of health care into improved health outcomes, countries need to address patient needs, provide quality services, and deliver care in a timely manner. Data from selected countries and available research demonstrate that many health systems face serious challenges in these areas, which are likely to gain importance as health care needs become more complex and population expectations grow. Because of data limitations, efforts to monitor progress toward UHC to date do not adequately capture dimensions of unmet need for health care, quality of health services, and timeliness of delivery to assess whether access to *effective* coverage is improving.

Looking Back: Lessons Learned

LAC countries have taken different paths in moving toward UHC, with varying levels of success. Some have achieved outcomes comparable to those of OECD countries despite getting a much later start on programs to extend coverage. Although the countries studied represent a diverse set of experiences, a review of the evidence and policies implemented to advance UHC reveals common features in the approaches taken.

Political Commitment Backed by Resource Allocation

The establishment of constitutional or legal rights to health in the majority of LAC countries reflects the political commitment to achieving UHC. But constitutional rights do not automatically translate into higher health care coverage and may not be a sufficient condition to achieve the goal of UHC. Indeed, countries in and outside the region that are considered to be farther along the path to UHC do not have constitutions that enshrine the right to health (for example, Costa Rica and Canada). What is clear from previous research (Savedoff and others 2012) and is confirmed by our findings, is that increased pooled financing is necessary, as is a focus on equity. All countries studied saw an increase in public financing for health as a share of gross domestic product (GDP), and most scaled up coverage of pooling mechanisms that are financed largely if not entirely from general revenues that prioritize or explicitly target the population without capacity to pay. In the majority of the countries, political commitment translated into increased temporal budget allocations and the passage of legislation that earmarks funding for health, sets minimum expenditure requirements, or labels levies for health. Even countries that did not take such permanent measures moved partially away from input-based, line-item budgets toward per capita transfers that are sometimes derived from actuarial cost calculations and reduce uncertainty in financing.

Reducing Segmentation in Separate and Unequal Subsystems

Few countries have followed the path toward full integration whereby all mandatory contributions—whether financed from payroll levies and general revenues (as in Costa Rica) or only the latter (as in Brazil)—are pooled to finance access for the entire population through a common network of providers. To a greater or lesser extent, most countries have opted to maintain a segmented system in which a subsidized subsystem exists in parallel with one financed entirely or mostly through payroll contributions, and beneficiaries generally have access to different networks of providers. Traditionally, large discrepancies in the benefits packages as well as the quality of care have been present across schemes. Pooling arrangements that broaden the risk pool and facilitate cross-subsidization between contributing and subsidized beneficiaries, regulations that equalize benefits packages, and explicit guarantees to timely access to services that comply with specified standards of care (and thereby close avenues used to ration care in the resource-poor public sector) have effectively reduced disparities in financing and service provision among subsystems—for example, in Chile, Colombia, and Uruguay.

Prioritizing Cost-Effective Primary Care

Diversity in the array of benefits covered under the various health care programs ranges from comprehensive packages that encompass primary to high-complexity care, to narrower ones that focus on primary care, or even more specifically within that packages that focus on maternal and child health care.

Prioritizing cost-effective primary care in the benefits packages is a common denominator among all countries. Some countries started on a small scale and gradually expanded benefits, such as Argentina and Peru; others offered comprehensive coverage from the onset, such as Brazil, Costa Rica, and Uruguay. Prioritizing primary care favors the poor, who were previously more likely than wealthier individuals to not have access to basic care. Benefits are more comprehensive in countries that have integrated health systems and those that are farther along the path to integration. Most countries have a positive list that defines which services are covered, though that is not universally the case; Brazil, Colombia, and Costa Rica, for example, have open-ended benefits.

Creating a Partial Split between Financing and Provision and Introducing Strategic Purchasing

Although there is wide variability in the extent to which countries have moved away from highly integrated service delivery and finance toward models that separate these functions, a common trend is to adopt purchasing methods that incentivize efficiency and accountability and give stewards of the health sector greater leverage to steer providers to deliver on public health priorities. One way in which countries have created a separation of functions is by establishing contractual relationships between financiers and providers either through legally binding contracts or explicit agreements that specify the roles and responsibilities of each party and expected results. Payment mechanisms vary considerably, from capitation to fee-for-services to case-based payments, but generally methods incentivize providers to satisfy demand by tying the flow of funds to the enrollment of beneficiaries and/or services actually rendered. Increasingly, countries are instituting pay-for-performance mechanisms that reward the achievement of specific targets linked to population health needs. By eliminating the rigidities of line-item budgets, the new financing modalities offer providers greater autonomy to manage inputs and achieve efficiency gains. In decentralized systems, similar arrangements that promote achieving national policy priorities are being applied to fund transfers to subnational governments. With few exceptions—Chile, Colombia, and Uruguay—reforms have not introduced competition with the private sector. Despite the move toward demand-side financing, in most countries a sizeable portion of the public sector continues to receive supply-side financing through line-item budgets. Nonetheless, even in countries where the volume of resources that flows through these new payment mechanisms may be relatively small, the reforms introduce a platform on which to build systems that rely more heavily on strategic purchasing.

Looking Ahead: The Unfinished Agenda

Countries in LAC have made important progress toward the realization of the right to health and toward fulfilling the promise of UHC, but the job is by no means done. Maintaining the achievements to date and tackling the challenges that remain will require sustained investments in health. Indeed, throughout the region countries have increased public financing for health; however, in half of the countries studied, as a share of GDP these expenditures still represent less than 5 percent.[2] Nonetheless, in 8 of the 10 countries studied, the health sector already absorbs more than 15 percent of the public budget (the OECD average); and in 3 of the 8 countries the share exceeds 20 percent. This is concerning, because middle-income countries may not have the fiscal space for the rise of health expenditures to outpace economic growth; this was the case for many years in high-income countries that had aging populations.

Delivering on the commitment to UHC will invariably require concerted efforts to improve revenue generation in a fiscally sustainable manner as well as the efficiency of expenditures. This will be particularly important as countries move further along the demographic transition and face challenges of gradually rising dependency ratios and eventually a shrinking tax base. As countries look for ways to finance public expenditures on health, it will be important to assess the effectiveness and fairness of financing measures. Many countries in the region rely on levies on wages to finance health, but it would be worth exploring options that have been implemented elsewhere. Including rental or interest income in these calculations simultaneously generates revenue while improving progressivity in financing, as nonwage earnings represent a larger share of the total revenue in wealthier households. Although earmarking taxes for health care has been widely used in the region to finance the expansion of coverage, there is concern that this measure reduces flexibility to reallocate resources to meet changing population needs among sectors. Regardless, levying new taxes for health will be difficult for countries where the tax burden is already at OECD levels, such as Argentina and Brazil.[3]

Although prioritizing cost-effective primary care and reforms to pooling and purchasing arrangements undoubtedly contribute to improving the effectiveness of investments in health, much more needs to be done to contain cost escalations and increase efficiency in spending. First, the strategic purchasing reforms that were started must be deepened and their scope extended beyond primary care to yield greater gains in technical and allocative efficiency. Second, countries must move away from ad hoc processes to select service coverage and establish formal, transparent systems that set public-sector priorities based on well-defined criteria grounded in scientific evidence on effectiveness and cost as well as societal preferences. In the absence of such systems, several countries in the region have experienced the judicialization of the right to health, whereby disputes about what the state must legally provide are often resolved though litigation. This can lead to the public subsidization of ineffective or inefficient care and have the added adverse effect of increasing inequality, because the wealthy can better afford legal counsel. Third, in many countries the share of out-of-pocket payments in total health expenditures still exceeds 30 percent, and therefore efforts to contain rising input costs in the public sector cannot work in isolation. This is particularly, though not exclusively, relevant in the adoption of new medical technologies in the private sector, an area where supplier-induced demand was shown to be an important driver of cost escalation in developed countries. Effective regulation of private health care providers and insurance is still a major challenge in the region (Atun and others 2015).

Achieving value for money will require alleviating current bottlenecks in delivering appropriate and timely care that responds to the needs of patients. Evidence is limited, but data from available research on selected countries indicate that despite advances made in the last decade, health systems in the region face serious challenges in this regard. The disadvantages encountered by the poor and other vulnerable groups are compounded by disparities in the quality of services they can access. Converting investments in health into improved outcomes will require addressing current weaknesses in primary care, access to diagnostic procedures, and specialist care. In addition, although some countries in the region are developing approaches to measure and monitor quality and timeliness of care, efforts to improve data and analysis on these critical aspects are still in their infancy compared with the more mature health systems in the OECD. In addition to strengthening quality assurance mechanisms and remedying supply-side constraints at specific levels of the delivery network—such as human resources, medicines, and other health technologies, among others—better integration and coordination across boundaries of care is needed to ensure that patients receive as comprehensive array of health services as needed across the continuum of care. Concerns about quality and timeliness of care are important, not only from a value-for-money perspective, but also because they are key drivers of the population's satisfaction with health systems. As health care needs become more complex and population expectations of the health system grows, these issues are likely to become increasingly important.

The existing gap in per capita financing and the quality of services delivered among the subsystems is suboptimal from an equity perspective, but it provides a powerful incentive for individuals to buy into contributory regimes that offer more generous benefits packages and better care. As the differences between subsystems narrow, there is a risk that this incentive will be eroded. Indeed, in Chile, where workers have an option to apply their mandatory contribution toward a private health care plan or enroll in the public plan, our data show a migration of people away from the first and into the second. The evidence thus far suggests that extending insurance coverage to those outside the formal sector, such as in Mexico's Seguro Popular, has only a marginal impact on informality (Reyes, Hallward-Driemeier, and Pages 2011). Nonetheless, to sustain efforts to provide affordable health care to the entire population, countries will need to remain vigilant about capturing contributions from those who can afford to pay but are unwilling to voluntarily do so and targeting public subsidies for those who cannot afford to pay. Compulsion and subsidization are necessary and sufficient conditions for UHC (Fuchs 1996).

Toward Universal Health Coverage and Equity in Latin America and the Caribbean
http://dx.doi.org/10.1596/978-1-4648-0454-0

Finally, we manage what we measure. Delivering on the promise of UHC will require regular measurement and monitoring of results, including whether benefits are being shared by the entire population irrespective of socioeconomic status, gender or place of residence. To achieve this, it will be paramount to strengthen data—countries' health information systems, civil registration and vital statistics, and statistical systems generally—while improving international comparability. In the digital age, the opportunities to collect and process massive amounts of information through administrative records, surveys and other sources have mushroomed. The complexity of managing large data systems from multiple institutions containing highly sensitive medical information makes this a difficult area to tackle within the resource-constrained public sector. Partnerships with research institutions domestically and abroad could be a way for the ministries of health to mine the vast amount of data being generated on health financing, service provision, and outcomes to inform policy decision making and strengthen governance over the sector, as well as enhance transparency and accountability to the public.

Notes

1. There are severe limitations to analyzing the differences in adult health outcomes by socioeconomic strata. Data for the analysis of mortality trends generally come from civil vital registration statistics that typically do not contain information about socioeconomic status. Educational attainment can be used as a proxy, but among the countries studied only Chile and Mexico had reliable data for this type of analysis to be carried out. Instead, self-assessed health status, an indicator that has its shortcomings, was measured in the surveys reviewed (Lora 2012).

2. Countries that are below the threshold of 5 percent to 6 percent of public expenditures as a share of GDP struggle to ensure health coverage for the poor (WHO 2010).

3. Tax revenue as a share of GDP is 36 percent and 37 percent in Brazil and Argentina, respectively, compared to the OECD average of 34 percent.

References

Atun, Rifat, Luiz Odorico Monteiro de Andrade, Gisele Almeida, Daniel Cotlear, Tania Dmytraczenko, Patricia Frenz, Patrícia Garcia, Octavio Gómez-Dantés, Felicia M. Knaul, Carles Muntaner, Juliana Braga de Paula, Felix Rígoli, Pastor Castell-Florit Serrate, and Adam Wagstaff. 2015. "Health-System Reform and Universal Health Coverage in Latin America." Series on Universal Health Coverage in Latin America. *The Lancet* 385: 1230–47.

Di Cesare, Mariachiara, Young-Ho Khang, Perviz Asaria, Tony Blakely, Melanie J. Cowan, Farshad Farzadfar, Ramiro Guerrero, Nayu Ikeda, Catherine Kyobutungi, Kelias P. Msyamboza, Sophal Oum, John W. Lynch, Michael G. Marmot, and Majid Ezzati, on behalf of The Lancet NCD Action Group. 2013. "Inequalities in Non-Communicable Diseases and Effective Responses." *The Lancet* 381 (9866): 585–97.

Fuchs, Victor. 1996. "What Every Philosopher Should Know about Health Economics." *Proceedings of the American Philosophical Society* 140 (2): 186–96.

Lora, Eduardo. 2012. "Health Perceptions in Latin America." *Health Policy and Planning* 27 (7): 555–69.

Reyes, A., M. Hallward-Driemeier, and C. Pages. 2011. "Does Expanding Health Insurance beyond Formal-Sector Workers Encourage Informality? Measuring the Impact of

Mexico's Seguro Popular." Policy Research Working Paper, WPS 5785, World Bank, Washington, DC.

Savedoff, William, David de Ferranti, Amy L. Smith, and Victoria Fan. 2012. "Political and Economic Aspects of the Transition to Universal Health Coverage." Series on Universal Health Coverage, *The Lancet* 380: 924–32.

WHO (World Health Organization). 2010. *The World Health Report—Health Systems Financing: The Path to Universal Coverage*. Geneva: WHO.

WHO, and World Bank. 2014. "Monitoring Progress toward Universal Health Coverage at Country and Global Levels: Frameworks, Measures and Targets." WHO/HIS/HIA/14.1, WHO, Geneva, Switzerland.

APPENDIX A

Methodology

Introduction

The horizontal inequity methodology calls for comparing the actual and the need-expected distribution to assess inequities in health care use. Income-related distribution of actual health care utilization reveals inequality in use, while need-standardized health care utilization reveals inequity in use (van Doorslaer and others 2004). In the case of health care utilization, the utilization variable was standardized for health care need in addition to age and sex. Usually, health care need is proxied by self-assessed health status, chronic conditions, and physical limitations when available. The indirect standardization method is preferred over the direct standardization method, given its greater accuracy when dealing with individual-level data. Indirect standardization for health status and health care utilization is calculated as follows:

$$\hat{y}_i^{IS} = y_i - \hat{y}_i^X + y^m$$

where

$\hat{y}_i^{IS}$ = standardized health status or health care utilization,

y_i = actual health status or health care utilization,

$\hat{y}_i^X$ = expected health status or health care utilization, and

y_m = sample mean.

In the case of health care utilization, the need-expected utilization is computed in two steps. Actual health care utilization is calculated by running a linear ordinary least-squares regression, which regresses health care utilization (y_i) on the logarithm of income (ln inc$_i$), a vector of need variables (χ_k), and a vector of nonneed variables (Zp) as follows:

$$y_i = \alpha + \beta \ln \text{inc}_i + \sum_k \gamma_k \chi_{k,i} + \sum_p \delta_p Z_{p,1} + \varepsilon_i$$

where

α, β, γ_k, and δ_p = parameters, and
ε_i = error term.

By combining the coefficients from the estimation above with the actual values of the need variables (χ_k) selected for standardization, the sample mean values of the logarithm of income (ln inc$_i$), and the sample mean values of the nonneed variables (Zp) selected to be controlled for, the need-expected health care utilization is obtained as follows:

$$\hat{y}_i^x = \hat{\alpha} + \hat{\beta} \ln \text{inc}^m + \sum_k \hat{\gamma}_k \chi_{k,i} + \sum_p \hat{\delta}_p Z_p^m$$

where

$\hat{\alpha}, \hat{\beta}, \hat{\gamma}_k,$ and $\hat{\delta}_p$ = parameters, and

m = mean value.

Since health care utilization values, such as physician visits and number of inpatient days, are binary or nonnegative integer counts and nonnormally distributed dependent variables with data presenting a very skewed distribution in the latter case (due to a large number of zero observations), nonlinear models are more appropriate than linear models for the indirect standardization process. Nevertheless, while estimations generated by linear models may be less robust and precise than those generated by nonlinear models, evidence in the literature indicates that the results are similar (van Doorslaer and others 2004; O'Donnell and others 2008).

In addition, linear models offer advantages over nonlinear methods for calculating horizontal inequity measures; for example, control variables included in the regression can be entirely neutralized when generating the need predictions by setting them equal to their mean values, which improves the accuracy of the measurement, and contributions to any observed inequity can be assessed, which allows for separation of the contribution of each of the variables included in the model and assessment of their impact on utilization. The latter feature is very useful in decomposition, which allows for identifying factors that contribute to inequity (O'Donnell and others 2008).

The indices and distributions obtained with linear and nonlinear models were compared to confirm that the selection of a linear model would not affect the results. Given the advantages of using the linear model and the similarity of results with nonlinear models for all countries, preference was given to presentation of the results of the linear models.

Concentration indices were used to measure inequality and inequity. Inequality was measured with concentration indices of the unstandardized distribution (CI) of the dependent variable. Inequity was measured with concentration indices of the standardized distribution of the dependent variable, also known as the horizontal inequity index (HI). Therefore, the HI is a summary measure of the magnitude of inequity in the dependent variable, taking into consideration demographic factors such as age and sex or morbidity characteristics that are known to influence health status and utilization patterns across income groups.

HI is equivalent to the CI of the need-standardized dependent variable, which is the difference between the concentration index of actual distribution and the need-expected distribution (O'Donnell and others 2008). The average relationship between need and the dependent variable is used as the norm to assess horizontal inequity. Systematic deviations from the established norm were calculated for health status and health care utilization variables for at least two years in each country.

The CI can also be calculated by using a simple convenience covariance formula for weighted data, which is the covariance between the dependent variable and the rank in income distribution scaled by 2 and divided by the mean of the dependent variable (O'Donnell and others 2008), as follows:

$$CI = \frac{2^{IS}}{\mu_i} \text{cov}_w(y_i, R_i)$$

where
μ = weighted sample mean of y,
cov_w = weighted covariance, and
R_i = relative fractional rank of ith individual.

The relative fractional rank indicates the weighted cumulative proportion of the population up to the midpoint of each individual weight, and is calculated as follows:

$$R_i = \frac{1}{n}\sum_{j=1}^{i-1} w_j + \frac{1}{2}w_i$$

where
n = sample size, and
w = sampling weight.

HI values are calculated from samples, requiring the calculation of standard errors to test their statistical significance. Because these studies considered samples from different years, the t-statistics test was performed to calculate the statistical significance of the difference between the HI for each survey year.

References

O'Donnell, Owen A., Eddy van Doorslaer, Adam Wagstaff, and Magnus Lindelow. 2008. *Analyzing Health Equity Using Household Survey Data: A Guide to Techniques and Their Implementation*. Washington, DC: World Bank.

van Doorslaer, Eddy, Cristina Masseria, and the OECD Health Equity Research Group. 2004. *Income-Related Inequalities in the Use of Medical Care in 21 OECD Countries*. OECD Working Papers No. 14. Paris: OECD. DELSA/ELSA/WD/HEA(2004)5.

Indicator Definitions

Dimension	Life cycle stage	Indicator	Definition	Comments where applicable
Outcome	Early years	Infant mortality rate	Number of deaths among children under 12 months of age per 1,000 live births	Mortality rate calculated using the true cohort life table approach; DHS reports use the synthetic cohort life table approach
		Under-five mortality rate	Number of deaths among children under 5 years of age per 1,000 live births	Mortality rate calculated using the true cohort life table approach; DHS reports use the synthetic cohort life table approach
		Acute respiratory infection (younger than 5 years of age)	Percentage of children with an episode of coughing and rapid breathing (past 2 weeks)	
		Diarrhea (younger than 5 years of age)	Percentage of children with diarrhea (past 2 weeks)	
		Stunting (younger than 5 years of age)	Percentage of children with a height-for-age z-score <-2 standard deviations from the reference median	z-score calculated using WHO 2006[a] child growth standards
	Youth to middle years	Intimate partner violence (women)	Prevalence of intimate partner violence in the past 12 months	
		Traffic accidents and injuries	Probability of being involved in a transportation accident with bodily injury	Brazil—past year, 18+ population Jamaica—past 4 weeks, 18+ population Mexico—past year, 20+ population
		Self-assessed health status	Percentage of adults who rate own health as less than good	This indicator was created from an ordinal variable with five categories.

table continues next page

Appendix B *(continued)*

Dimension	Life cycle stage	Indicator	Definition	Comments where applicable
	Middle years and beyond	Diagnosed asthma	Percentage of adults ever diagnosed with asthma	
		Diagnosed depression	Percentage of adults ever diagnosed with depression	
		Diagnosed diabetes	Percentage of adults ever diagnosed with diabetes	
		Diagnosed heart disease	Percentage of adults (40+ years) ever diagnosed with infarction, angina pectoris, heart failure, or other heart disease	
Risk factor	Youth to middle years	Alcohol consumption	Percentage of adults who consume ≥5 (4 for women) standard drinks on at least one day (past week)	
		Tobacco use (women)	Percentage of women ages 15–49 years who smoke cigarettes, pipe, or other tobacco	Costa Rica—18–44 years Guatemala—18–49 years
	Middle years and beyond	Diagnosed hypertension	Percentage of adults (40+ years) ever diagnosed with hypertension	
		Obesity (nonpregnant women)	Percentage of women aged 15–49 with a body mass index above 30	Costa Rica and Guatemala—18–49 years Mexico—20–49 years
		Obesity (men)	Percentage of men (18+) with body mass index above 30	
Service utilization	Early years	Full immunization	Percentage of children aged 12–23 months who received BCG, measles, and three doses of polio and DPT, either verified by card or by recall of respondent	Jamaica—younger than 5 years old
		Medical treatment of acute respiratory infection (under 5)	Percentage of children with a cough and rapid breathing who sought medical treatment for acute respiratory infection (past 2 weeks)	
		Treatment of diarrhea (under 5)	Percentage of children with diarrhea given oral rehydration salts (ORS) or home-made solution	
		Contraceptive prevalence rate	Percentage of women aged 15–49 years, married or in union, who are currently using, or whose sexual partner is using, at least one method of contraception, regardless of the method used	Costa Rica—18–49 years Mexico—20–49 years

table continues next page

Appendix B *(continued)*

Dimension	Life cycle stage	Indicator	Definition	Comments where applicable
	Youth to middle years	Antenatal care	Percentage of mothers ages 15–49 who received at least four antenatal care visits from any skilled personnel (as defined in the country's survey)	
		Skilled birth attendance	Percentage of mothers ages 15–49 years who were attended by any skilled personnel at child's birth (as defined in the country's survey)	Costa Rica—18–44 years
		Cervical cancer screening	Proportion of women aged 18–69 who received a Pap smear during last pelvic examination (past 3 years)	Brazil—25–69 years Costa Rica—18–44 (1999) and 18–49 (2006) Guatemala—18–49 years Mexico—20–69; 1-year survey recall period adjusted to a 3-year basis
	Middle years and beyond	Breast cancer screening	Proportion of women ages 40–69 years who received a mammogram (past 3 years)	Colombia—40–49 years Mexico—1-year survey recall period adjusted to a 3-year basis
	All adults	Outpatient care	Percentage of adults who used any outpatient health care in the past 2 weeks	Chile reports any physician visit only
		Inpatient care	Respondent reported being admitted to hospital at least once during previous 12 months	Guatemala—1-month survey recall period adjusted to a 12-month basis
		Preventive care	Percentage of adults who used any health care service for prevention or without being sick in the last 3 months	Brazil—2-week recall period adjusted to a 3-month basis Colombia—12-month recall period adjusted to a 3-month basis
		Curative care	Percentage of adults who received any health care service due to need in the last month	Brazil and Mexico—2-week recall period adjusted to a 1-month basis Chile—3-month recall period adjusted to a 1-month basis
Financial protection	Household	Impoverishment at $1.25-a-day	A household is classified as impoverished by out-of-pocket payments if its consumption *including* out-of-pocket payments is above the poverty line while its consumption *excluding* out-of-pocket payments is below the $1.25-a-day poverty line	

table continues next page

Appendix B *(continued)*

Dimension	Life cycle stage	Indicator	Definition	Comments where applicable
	Household	Impoverishment at $2-a-day	A household is classified as impoverished by out-of-pocket payments if its consumption *including* out-of-pocket payments is above the poverty line while its consumption *excluding* out-of-pocket payments is below the $2-a-day poverty line	
	Household	Catastrophic payments using 25% of total consumption	Household's out-of-pocket payments exceeded 25% of its total consumption in previous year	

Note: DHS = Demographic Health Survey; DPT = vaccine against diphtheria, pertussis, and tetanus; BCG = Bacillus Calmette-Guérin (vaccine against tuberculosis).
a. http://www.who.int/childgrowth/standards/en.

Results of Equity Analysis: National Mean, Quintile Means, and Concentration/Horizontal Inequity Index

Early years

Mortality rate (under 5)

Country	Year	Mean	Q1	Q2	Q3	Q4	Q5	Relative CI/HI	Absolute HI
Bolivia	1998	108.0	165.3	118.1	117.2	45.3	37.2	−0.2530***	−0.0273
Bolivia	2003	107.6	133.5	139.3	103.7	74.5	43.8	−0.1660***	−0.0179
Bolivia	2008	82.0	120.6	93.0	74.8	52.6	32.1	−0.2190***	−0.0180
Brazil	1996	63.5	106.4	61.1	44.4	32.8	47.6	−0.2200***	−0.0140
Brazil	2006	26.8	47.4	32.4	24.8	16.7	08.1	−0.3122***	−0.0084
Colombia	1995	39.8	55.2	44.0	27.0	44.2	17.7	−0.1400***	−0.0056
Colombia	2000	31.0	46.3	40.4	25.6	11.5	21.2	−0.1950***	−0.0060
Colombia	2005	28.8	45.9	28.2	25.2	17.8	20.1	−0.1860***	−0.0054
Colombia	2010	25.0	32.5	25.5	23.8	23.5	13.0	−0.1400***	−0.0035
Dominican Republic	2002	45.1	74.2	50.3	42.9	32.5	15.2	−0.2290***	−0.0103
Dominican Republic	2007	37.3	56.9	41.5	33.2	24.8	22.4	−0.1710***	−0.0064
Guatemala	1995	85.5	99.3	111.3	87.9	70.5	25.3	−0.1470***	−0.0126
Guatemala	1998	68.9	88.8	71.5	89.7	61.6	18.9	−0.1464***	−0.0101
Guatemala	2002	58.7	84.2	70.2	65.4	39.6	14.4	−0.0901***	−0.0053
Guatemala	2008–09	46.0	68.2	44.9	48.2	25.9	12.5	−0.2007***	−0.0092
Haiti	2000	144.7	186.1	134.4	135.6	127.4	130.8	−0.0670**	−0.0097
Haiti	2005–06	113.3	134.5	129.1	117.2	99.8	52.6	−0.1060***	−0.0120
Haiti	2012	98.7	108.0	104.7	103.4	97.3	64.0	−0.0579***	−0.0057
Peru	1996	76.6	121.4	83.5	51.8	56.9	19.0	−0.2440***	−0.0187
Peru	2004–08	40.8	60.6	51.1	31.8	22.1	15.5	−0.2510***	−0.0102
Peru	2012	27.6	43.5	34.1	18.4	16.4	14.3	−0.2484***	−0.0069

Acute respiratory infection (under 5)

Country	Year	Mean	Q1	Q2	Q3	Q4	Q5	Relative CI/HI	Absolute HI
Bolivia	1998	0.2450	0.2690	0.2720	0.2020	0.2510	0.2130	−0.0380***	−0.0093
Bolivia	2003	0.2290	0.2190	0.2100	0.2320	0.2660	0.2190	0.0230*	0.0053
Bolivia	2008	0.2010	0.2410	0.2010	0.0202	0.1700	0.1710	−0.0640***	−0.0129
Brazil	1996	0.2440	0.2630	0.2710	0.2340	0.2140	0.2090	−0.0490***	−0.0120

table continues next page

Appendix C *(continued)*

Country	Year	Mean	Q1	Q2	Q3	Q4	Q5	Relative CI/HI	Absolute HI
Brazil	2006	0.1457	0.1787	0.1591	0.1473	0.1274	0.1082	-0.0983***	-0.0143
Colombia	1995	0.2480	0.2810	0.2270	0.2220	0.2410	0.2700	-0.0170	-0.0042
Colombia	2010	0.0630	0.0690	0.0730	0.0700	0.0500	0.0390	-0.0940***	-0.0059
Costa Rica	1999	0.0916	0.0816	0.1010	0.0707	0.0971	0.1068	0.0847	0.0078
Dominican Republic	1996	0.1120	0.1170	0.1020	0.1310	0.1110	0.0910	-0.0270	-0.0030
Dominican Republic	2007	0.1240	0.1480	0.1320	0.1260	0.1150	0.0770	-0.0910***	-0.0113
Guatemala	1995	0.2220	0.2330	0.2170	0.2220	0.2370	0.1860	-0.0120	-0.0027
Guatemala	2008–09	0.2041	0.245	0.221	0.201	0.175	0.133	-0.0966***	-0.0197
Haiti	2000	0.4140	0.4860	0.4580	0.3870	0.3960	0.2960	-0.0780***	-0.0323
Haiti	2005–06	0.2900	0.3220	0.3360	0.2910	0.2560	0.2190	-0.0710***	-0.0206
Haiti	2012	0.3615	0.3590	0.3591	0.3873	0.3759	0.3122	-0.0091	-0.0033
Mexico	2006	0.2222	0.1945	0.2151	0.2444	0.2402	0.2247	0.0399***	0.0089
Peru	1996	0.2070	0.2520	0.2190	0.1900	0.1840	0.1370	-0.0980***	-0.0203
Peru	2000	0.2040	0.2140	0.2150	0.2070	0.1810	0.1840	-0.0330***	-0.0067
Peru	2004–08	0.1910	0.2340	0.1860	0.1730	0.1720	0.1630	-0.0780***	-0.0149
Peru	2012	0.1394	0.1673	0.1535	0.1344	0.1021	0.1219	-0.0921***	-0.0128
Diarrhea (under 5)									
Bolivia	1998	0.1930	0.2200	0.2030	0.2070	0.1760	0.1170	-0.0800***	-0.0154
Bolivia	2003	0.2260	0.2500	0.2340	0.2240	0.2340	0.1520	-0.0630***	-0.0142
Bolivia	2008	0.2620	0.3050	0.2710	0.2810	0.2180	0.1950	-0.0760***	-0.0199
Brazil	1996	0.1000	0.1410	0.0920	0.0950	0.0810	0.0570	-0.1530***	-0.0153
Brazil	2006	0.2128	0.3003	0.2041	0.2142	0.1703	0.1536	-0.1274***	-0.0271
Colombia	1995	0.1690	0.1880	0.1990	0.1710	0.1520	0.1030	-0.0900***	-0.0152
Colombia	2000	0.1410	0.1780	0.1620	0.1310	0.1040	0.1030	-0.1070***	-0.0151
Colombia	2005	0.1440	0.1770	0.1700	0.1290	0.1120	0.0880	-0.1230***	-0.0177
Colombia	2010	0.1270	0.1640	0.1450	0.1140	0.1070	0.0730	-0.1380***	-0.0175
Costa Rica	1999	0.0678	0.1250	0.0392	0.0521	0.0745	0.0505	-0.1110	-0.0075
Dominican Republic	1996	0.1050	0.1080	0.0930	0.1310	0.0990	0.0860	-0.0250	-0.0026
Dominican Republic	2007	0.1490	0.1680	0.1560	0.1450	0.1320	0.1340	-0.0500**	-0.0075

table continues next page

Appendix C *(continued)*

Country	Year	Mean	Q1	Q2	Q3	Q4	Q5	Relative CI/HI	Absolute HI
Guatemala	1995	0.2100	0.2290	0.2160	0.2360	0.1760	0.1630	−0.0540***	−0.0113
Guatemala	2008–09	0.2293	0.2440	0.2322	0.2500	0.2140	0.1798	−0.0411***	−0.0094
Haiti	2000	0.2680	0.2730	0.2540	0.3010	0.2840	0.2150	−0.0120	−0.0032
Haiti	2005–06	0.2430	0.2610	0.2490	0.2480	0.2540	0.1800	−0.0430**	−0.0104
Haiti	2012	0.2128	0.1864	0.2362	0.2436	0.2185	0.1686	−0.0079	−0.0017
Jamaica	2004	0.0452	0.0500	0.0630	0.0500	0.0290	0.0340	−0.1410	−0.0064
Jamaica	2007	0.0770	0.0800	0.1090	0.0690	0.0360	0.0910	−0.0290	−0.0022
Mexico	2000	0.1172	0.1280	0.1326	0.1218	0.0990	0.0899	−0.0817***	−0.0096
Mexico	2006	0.1283	0.1357	0.1399	0.1102	0.1162	0.1416	−0.0163	−0.0021
Mexico	2012	0.1102	0.1045	0.1126	0.1249	0.1042	0.1013	−0.0084	−0.0009
Peru	1996	0.1810	0.2160	0.2070	0.1840	0.1420	0.0940	−0.1210***	−0.0219
Peru	2000	0.1550	0.1870	0.1810	0.1630	0.1120	0.0760	−0.1320***	−0.0205
Peru	2004–08	0.1400	0.1690	0.1550	0.1440	0.1100	0.0850	−0.1170***	−0.0164
Peru	2012	0.1231	0.1276	0.1464	0.1298	0.1000	0.0938	−0.0838***	−0.0103
Full immunization									
Bolivia	1998	0.2559	0.2206	0.2489	0.2087	0.3386	0.3054	0.0750**	0.0192
Bolivia	2003	0.5085	0.4779	0.4984	0.4444	0.5932	0.5805	0.0367**	0.0187
Bolivia	2008	0.6723	0.6790	0.6798	0.6704	0.6838	0.6347	−0.0083	−0.0056
Brazil	1996	0.7308	0.5731	0.7394	0.8586	0.8310	0.7558	0.0760***	0.0555
Colombia	1995	0.6576	0.5406	0.6679	0.6846	0.7119	0.7457	0.0649***	0.0427
Colombia	2000	0.5239	0.4052	0.4994	0.5959	0.6328	0.5457	0.1011	0.0530
Colombia	2005	0.5995	0.4918	0.5747	0.6631	0.6506	0.7420	0.0758***	0.0454
Colombia	2010	0.6848	0.6524	0.6793	0.7269	0.6974	0.6704	0.0149	0.0102
Costa Rica	1999	0.7573	0.7000	0.7619	0.7500	0.8095	0.7619	0.0366	0.0277
Dominican Republic	1996	0.3886	0.2796	0.3082	0.4742	0.4217	0.5156	0.1417***	0.0551
Dominican Republic	2002	0.3570	0.2690	0.3300	0.4120	0.4290	0.3660	0.0820***	0.0293
Dominican Republic	2007	0.5462	0.4513	0.5230	0.5631	0.5590	0.7148	0.0878***	0.0480
Guatemala	1995	0.4277	0.4148	0.4359	0.4640	0.3864	0.4318	0.0057	0.0024
Guatemala	2008–09	0.7125	0.7442	0.7011	0.7061	0.7144	0.6547	−0.0199	−0.0142

table continues next page

Appendix C *(continued)*

Country	Year	Mean	Q1	Q2	Q3	Q4	Q5	Relative CI/HI	Absolute HI
Haiti	2000	0.3375	0.2557	0.3059	0.4234	0.3107	0.4235	0.1005***	0.0339
Haiti	2005–06	0.4143	0.3338	0.4125	0.4614	0.3572	0.5605	0.0716***	0.0297
Haiti	2012	0.4522	0.4251	0.4550	0.5229	0.4226	0.4090	−0.0059	−0.0027
Jamaica	2004	0.8656	0.7880	0.8030	0.9490	0.8980	0.8900	0.0310	0.0268
Jamaica	2007	0.7778	0.6110	0.7670	0.7540	0.8880	0.8690	0.0550*	0.0428
Mexico	2000	0.7092	0.6747	0.6985	0.7282	0.7021	0.7483	0.0169	0.0120
Mexico	2006	0.7474	0.7446	0.7952	0.7279	0.7570	0.6883	−0.0137	−0.0102
Mexico	2012	0.7675	0.7361	0.8277	0.7777	0.7471	0.7328	−0.0053	−0.0041
Peru	1996	0.6338	0.5566	0.6399	0.6443	0.7197	0.6680	0.0479***	0.0304
Peru	2004–08	0.5373	0.4867	0.5289	0.5278	0.5876	0.6072	0.0436***	0.0234
Peru	2012	0.6387	0.6151	0.6476	0.6089	0.6597	0.6846	0.0200	0.0128
Medical treatment of ARI									
Bolivia	1998	0.4250	0.2740	0.3740	0.4130	0.5890	0.6940	0.1870***	0.0795
Bolivia	2003	0.4830	0.3950	0.5420	0.4940	0.4680	0.5740	0.0490***	0.0237
Bolivia	2008	0.5090	0.4060	0.4920	0.5380	0.5500	0.6990	0.0980***	0.0499
Brazil	1996	0.4620	0.3300	0.4830	0.4820	0.5280	0.6470	0.1240***	0.0573
Brazil	2006	0.6372	0.6294	0.5120	0.5707	0.6846	0.8552	0.0578***	0.0368
Colombia	1995	0.4870	0.3490	0.4930	0.5060	0.5340	0.6770	0.1290***	0.0628
Colombia	2010	0.6470	0.5280	0.6780	0.6830	0.7650	0.6410	0.0590***	0.0382
Costa Rica	2006	0.1752	0.1626	0.1944	0.1790	0.2157	0.1235	0.0111	0.0019
Dominican Republic	1996	0.5040	0.4388	0.4643	0.5670	0.4895	0.6017	0.0581**	0.0293
Dominican Republic	2002	0.6460	0.6770	0.6120	0.7000	0.6630	0.5120	−0.0200	−0.0129
Dominican Republic	2007	0.6226	0.6132	0.6482	0.6219	0.6185	0.5901	−0.0104	−0.0065
Guatemala	1995	0.4052	0.2755	0.2981	0.4759	0.4687	0.7399	0.1925***	0.0780
Guatemala	2008–09	0.7598	0.6252	0.7822	0.7974	0.9239	0.8615	0.0781***	0.0594
Haiti	2000	0.3795	0.3345	0.3312	0.4343	0.3885	0.5032	0.0794***	0.0301
Haiti	2005–06	0.2479	0.1466	0.1847	0.2718	0.3613	0.4137	0.2209***	0.0548
Haiti	2012	0.3496	0.2295	0.3001	0.3598	0.4296	0.5028	0.1457***	0.0509
Mexico	2000	0.5755	0.5265	0.5618	0.5966	0.5745	0.6361	0.0280***	0.0161

table continues next page

Appendix C *(continued)*

Country	Year	Mean	Q1	Q2	Q3	Q4	Q5	Relative CI/HI	Absolute HI
Mexico	2006	0.5843	0.5209	0.6018	0.5639	0.6099	0.6634	0.0393***	0.0230
Mexico	2012	0.6365	0.6191	0.6196	0.6115	0.6522	0.6996	0.0197**	0.0125
Peru	1996	0.4602	0.3613	0.4489	0.5174	0.5717	0.5796	0.1113***	0.0512
Peru	2004–08	0.6652	0.6456	0.6816	0.6345	0.7193	0.6720	0.0117	0.0078
Peru	2012	0.5931	0.5878	0.6030	0.6195	0.6026	0.5261	−0.0014	−0.0008
Treatment of diarrhea									
Bolivia	1998	0.4840	0.4510	0.4720	0.4920	0.5050	0.5800	0.0420**	0.0203
Bolivia	2003	0.3820	0.3790	0.3700	0.3890	0.3860	0.4010	0.0070	0.0027
Bolivia	2008	0.4380	0.3850	0.4570	0.4700	0.4840	0.4060	0.0330*	0.0145
Brazil	1996	0.4360	0.4260	0.4790	0.5160	0.3730	0.2930	−0.0100	−0.0044
Brazil	2006	0.4050	0.5121	0.3035	0.4460	0.2879	0.4962	−0.0623***	−0.0252
Colombia	1995	0.4450	0.3440	0.4880	0.4680	0.4960	0.4990	0.0780***	0.0347
Colombia	2000	0.3210	0.3280	0.3460	0.3130	0.2940	0.2810	−0.0240	−0.0077
Colombia	2005	0.5550	0.5000	0.5910	0.5640	0.6440	0.4860	0.0350**	0.0194
Colombia	2010	0.6100	0.5790	0.6380	0.6470	0.5750	0.6230	0.0090	0.0055
Dominican Republic	2002	0.3301	0.4265	0.3040	0.2969	0.3477	0.1748	−0.1020***	−0.0337
Dominican Republic	2007	0.4686	0.5011	0.4606	0.4709	0.4768	0.3989	−0.0221	−0.0104
Guatemala	1995	0.5156	0.5467	0.4319	0.5682	0.5536	0.4482	−0.0002	−0.0001
Guatemala	2008–09	0.4511	0.4683	0.3984	0.4237	0.4754	0.5778	0.0179	0.0081
Haiti	2000	0.4076	0.3246	0.3709	0.4278	0.4900	0.4494	0.0871***	0.0355
Haiti	2005–06	0.4395	0.3295	0.3857	0.4867	0.5295	0.5487	0.1242***	0.0546
Haiti	2012	0.5787	0.5657	0.5212	0.6085	0.5870	0.6449	0.0265*	0.0154
Mexico	2000	0.3831	0.3955	0.3961	0.3907	0.3832	0.3082	−0.0225	−0.0086
Mexico	2006	0.5313	0.5506	0.5508	0.5431	0.4638	0.5258	−0.0165	−0.0088
Peru	1996	0.2624	0.2695	0.2917	0.2204	0.2969	0.1655	−0.0242	−0.0064
Peru	2004–08	0.3830	0.3127	0.3235	0.4435	0.4430	0.5976	0.1202***	0.0460
Peru	2012	0.3799	0.2961	0.3814	0.4471	0.3972	0.4040	0.0705**	0.0268

table continues next page

Appendix C *(continued)*

Country	Year	Mean	Q1	Q2	Q3	Q4	Q5	Relative CI/HI	Absolute HI
Stunting (under 5)									
Bolivia	1998	0.3350	0.4960	0.4010	0.3050	0.2020	0.1040	−0.2290***	−0.0767
Bolivia	2003	0.3250	0.4870	0.4150	0.2810	0.1880	0.0990	−0.2400***	−0.0780
Bolivia	2008	0.2710	0.4510	0.3440	0.2190	0.1510	0.0660	−0.2920***	−0.0791
Brazil	1996	0.1300	0.2700	0.1160	0.0740	0.0410	0.0360	−0.4150***	−0.0540
Brazil	2006	0.0656	0.0641	0.0928	0.0600	0.0399	0.0427	−0.1254***	−0.0082
Colombia	1995	0.1980	0.3000	0.2240	0.1730	0.1050	0.1050	−0.2220***	−0.0440
Colombia	2000	0.1860	0.2800	0.2250	0.1600	0.1040	0.0970	−0.2100***	−0.0391
Colombia	2005	0.1560	0.2490	0.1650	0.1290	0.1120	0.0880	−0.1230***	−0.0192
Colombia	2010	0.1280	0.1930	0.1280	0.1110	0.0930	0.0680	−0.1870***	−0.0239
Costa Rica	2008	0.0528	0.0842	0.0634	0.0424	0.0436	0.0309	−0.1696	−0.0090
Dominican Republic	1996	0.1370	0.2680	0.1270	0.1040	0.0750	0.0370	−0.3440***	−0.0471
Dominican Republic	2007	0.1010	0.1690	0.1000	0.0720	0.0800	0.0530	−0.2270***	−0.0229
Guatemala	1995	0.5520	0.7020	0.6670	0.5920	0.3890	0.1500	−0.1740***	−0.0960
Guatemala	1998	0.5182	0.6949	0.6665	0.5618	0.3315	0.1467	−0.2096***	−0.1086
Guatemala	2002	0.4965	0.6546	0.5911	0.5396	0.2637	0.1433	−0.1236***	−0.0613
Guatemala	2008–09	0.4767	0.690	0.600	0.450	0.255	0.150	−0.2331***	−0.1111
Haiti	2000	0.2730	0.3710	0.3430	0.2710	0.2150	0.0910	−0.1940***	−0.0530
Haiti	2005–06	0.2810	0.3860	0.3620	0.3040	0.2010	0.0610	−0.2220***	−0.0624
Haiti	2012	0.2107	0.3110	0.2521	0.2043	0.1408	0.0692	−0.2175***	−0.0458
Jamaica	2004	0.0432	0.0690	0.0580	0.0340	0.0070	0.0480	−0.2180	−0.0094
Jamaica	2007	0.0428	0.0410	0.0570	0.0220	0.0310	0.0630	−0.0070	−0.0003
Peru	1996	0.3110	0.5150	0.3690	0.2420	0.1350	0.0830	−0.2940***	−0.0914
Peru	2000	0.3120	0.5420	0.3740	0.2120	0.1180	0.0710	−0.3270***	−0.1020
Peru	2004–08	0.2840	0.5170	0.3800	0.1690	0.1240	0.0610	−0.3520***	−0.1000
Peru	2012	0.1817	0.3862	0.2030	0.1122	0.0620	0.0401	−0.3982***	−0.0724

table continues next page

Appendix C *(continued)*

Youth to middle years

Drinking (alcohol consumption)

Country	Year	Mean	Q1	Q2	Q3	Q4	Q5	Relative CI/HI	Absolute HI
Mexico	2000	0.4781	0.5527	0.5073	0.4993	0.4765	0.4413	−0.0450***	−0.0215
Mexico	2006	0.3026	0.2459	0.2950	0.3108	0.3166	0.3293	0.0482***	0.0146
Mexico	2012	0.3264	0.3078	0.2973	0.3055	0.3390	0.3673	0.0435***	0.0142

Smoking (women)

Country	Year	Mean	Q1	Q2	Q3	Q4	Q5	Relative CI/HI	Absolute HI
Argentina	2005	0.3090	0.3082	0.3016	0.3202	0.3140	0.3027	0.0145	0.0045
Argentina	2009	0.2823	0.2955	0.2431	0.2880	0.3119	0.2751	0.0522***	0.0147
Bolivia	2008	0.0860	0.0620	0.0540	0.0670	0.0810	0.1480	0.2260***	0.0194
Brazil	2003	0.1948	0.2735	0.2155	0.1419	0.1678	0.1670	−0.1102***	−0.0215
Brazil	2006	0.1521	0.1829	0.1662	0.1469	0.1514	0.1221	−0.0810***	−0.0123
Brazil	2008	0.1383	0.1771	0.1527	0.1378	0.1240	0.1001	−0.1107***	−0.0153
Chile	2009	0.3650	0.3634	0.3308	0.2957	0.3926	0.4506	0.1263***	0.0461
Costa Rica	1999	0.0613	0.0293	0.0631	0.0534	0.0922	0.0683	0.2141***	0.0131
Costa Rica	2006	0.1229	0.1169	0.1339	0.1044	0.1163	0.1418	0.0174	0.0021
Dominican Republic	2002	0.0860	0.1330	0.1100	0.0820	0.0690	0.0560	−0.1760***	−0.0151
Dominican Republic	2007	0.0670	0.1080	0.0840	0.0600	0.0460	0.0480	−0.1830***	−0.0123
Guatemala	2002	0.0263	0.0169	0.0063	0.0088	0.0262	0.0599	0.4920***	0.0129
Guatemala	2008–09	0.0155	0.0062	0.0018	0.0071	0.0138	0.0504	0.5410***	0.0084
Haiti	2005–06	0.0320	0.0460	0.0350	0.0290	0.0230	0.0350	−0.0660	−0.0021
Haiti	2012	0.0497	0.0673	0.0621	0.0553	0.0444	0.0309	−0.1601***	−0.0080
Peru	2004–08	0.0610	0.0140	0.0170	0.0420	0.0740	0.1320	0.4140***	0.0253
Peru	2012	0.0481	0.0100	0.0088	0.0279	0.0525	0.1280	0.4960***	0.0238

Contraceptive prevalence

Country	Year	Mean	Q1	Q2	Q3	Q4	Q5	Relative CI/HI	Absolute HI
Argentina	2005	0.5550	0.5050	0.5930	0.5860	0.5890	0.5110	0.0442***	0.0245
Argentina	2009	0.6280	0.5840	0.6710	0.6570	0.6110	0.6210	0.0087	0.0054

table continues next page

Appendix C (continued)

Country	Year	Mean	Q1	Q2	Q3	Q4	Q5	Relative CI/HI	Absolute HI
Bolivia	1994	0.1777	0.0191	0.0684	0.1538	0.2399	0.4204	0.4463***	0.0793
Bolivia	1998	0.2511	0.0708	0.1719	0.2231	0.3246	0.4555	0.3030***	0.0761
Bolivia	2003	0.3501	0.2244	0.2786	0.3178	0.4219	0.4954	0.1635***	0.0572
Bolivia	2008	0.3449	0.2249	0.2689	0.3428	0.4096	0.4676	0.1489***	0.0514
Brazil	1996	0.7006	0.5605	0.6857	0.7396	0.7368	0.7674	0.0554***	0.0388
Brazil	2006	0.8494	0.8334	0.8777	0.8384	0.8572	0.8412	−0.0019	−0.0016
Chile	2006	0.5850	0.5880	0.5580	0.5500	0.6920	0.5480	−0.0079	−0.0046
Colombia	1995	0.5921	0.4200	0.6012	0.6229	0.6462	0.6535	0.0723***	0.0428
Colombia	2000	0.6414	0.5431	0.6169	0.6724	0.7001	0.6688	0.0566***	0.0363
Colombia	2005	0.6781	0.6059	0.6681	0.6889	0.7140	0.7170	0.0353***	0.0239
Colombia	2010	0.7284	0.6831	0.7306	0.7327	0.7500	0.7481	0.0186***	0.0136
Costa Rica	2006	0.6681	0.6101	0.7188	0.6855	0.5850	0.7444	0.0139	0.0093
Dominican Republic	1996	0.5923	0.5117	0.6230	0.5791	0.6173	0.6338	0.0365***	0.0216
Dominican Republic	1999	0.6419	0.5423	0.6885	0.6762	0.6027	0.6833	0.0232	0.0149
Dominican Republic	2002	0.6583	0.5877	0.6494	0.6794	0.6695	0.6955	0.0299***	0.0197
Dominican Republic	2007	0.7009	0.6666	0.7164	0.7122	0.7134	0.6923	0.0083*	0.0058
Guatemala	1995	0.2633	0.0542	0.1029	0.2127	0.3764	0.5714	0.4101***	0.1080
Guatemala	2008–09	0.2983	0.0546	0.1408	0.2328	0.4574	0.5995	0.3980***	0.1187
Haiti	1994–95	0.1313	0.0456	0.0848	0.1300	0.2048	0.2149	0.2885***	0.0379
Haiti	2000	0.2282	0.1736	0.2243	0.2576	0.2429	0.2381	0.0543**	0.0124
Haiti	2005–06	0.2483	0.1470	0.2229	0.2623	0.2982	0.2922	0.1216***	0.0302
Haiti	2012	0.2161	0.2091	0.2061	0.2399	0.2334	0.1927	−0.0121	−0.0026
Mexico	2000	0.5402	0.5054	0.6031	0.5723	0.5032	0.5252	−0.0141	−0.0076
Mexico	2006	0.5378	0.5270	0.5511	0.5269	0.5780	0.5067	−0.0014	−0.0008
Mexico	2012	0.4833	0.4450	0.4601	0.4745	0.5083	0.5270	0.0353***	0.0171

table continues next page

Appendix C *(continued)*

Country	Year	Mean	Q1	Q2	Q3	Q4	Q5	Relative CI/HI	Absolute HI
Peru	1996	0.4131	0.2394	0.3808	0.4508	0.4898	0.5036	0.1281***	0.0529
Peru	2000	0.5037	0.3673	0.4602	0.5466	0.5633	0.5791	0.0845***	0.0425
Peru	2004–08	0.4826	0.3596	0.4447	0.5272	0.5431	0.5353	0.0771***	0.0372
Peru	2012	0.5168	0.4109	0.5185	0.5280	0.5431	0.5865	0.0590***	0.0305
Antenatal care (4+ visits)									
Bolivia	1998	0.4718	0.1784	0.3584	0.5218	0.7245	0.8631	0.2948***	0.1391
Bolivia	2003	0.5748	0.3071	0.4818	0.5938	0.7212	0.8922	0.1975***	0.1135
Bolivia	2008	0.7033	0.4432	0.6332	0.7578	0.8400	0.9157	0.1360***	0.0956
Brazil	1996	0.7889	0.5341	0.7952	0.9004	0.9518	0.9717	0.1305***	0.1030
Brazil	2006	0.9611	0.9482	0.9357	0.9677	0.9761	0.9977	0.0130***	0.0125
Colombia	1995	0.7091	0.4365	0.6582	0.8092	0.8971	0.9223	0.1523***	0.1080
Colombia	2000	0.8062	0.6024	0.7748	0.8716	0.9218	0.9097	0.0852***	0.0687
Colombia	2005	0.8432	0.6870	0.8315	0.8897	0.9134	0.9598	0.0661***	0.0557
Colombia	2010	0.8983	0.7894	0.8941	0.9253	0.9513	0.9729	0.0415***	0.0373
Costa Rica	1999	0.9570	0.9342	0.9308	0.9379	0.9932	0.9930	0.0190***	0.0182
Dominican Republic	1996	0.8863	0.7866	0.8681	0.9121	0.9468	0.9730	0.0455***	0.0403
Dominican Republic	1999	0.9350	0.8640	0.9300	0.9470	0.9340	1.0000	0.0220**	0.0206
Dominican Republic	2002	0.9500	0.8950	0.9410	0.9680	0.9640	0.9860	0.0190***	0.0181
Dominican Republic	2007	0.9107	0.8283	0.8990	0.9272	0.9533	0.9760	0.0327***	0.0298
Guatemala	1995	0.4194	0.2272	0.2791	0.3908	0.6282	0.8562	0.2808***	0.1178
Guatemala	2008–09	0.6730	0.5030	0.5923	0.7050	0.8539	0.9436	0.1312***	0.0883
Haiti	2000	0.4487	0.2495	0.3276	0.4551	0.5290	0.7341	0.2150***	0.0965
Haiti	2005–06	0.5398	0.3214	0.4344	0.5396	0.6489	0.8253	0.1878***	0.1014
Haiti	2012	0.6772	0.5050	0.5598	0.6942	0.7824	0.8895	0.1187***	0.0804
Mexico	2000	0.8459	0.7015	0.8252	0.8843	0.9002	0.9256	0.0453***	0.0383
Mexico	2006	0.8739	0.7724	0.8666	0.8929	0.9067	0.9745	0.0395***	0.0345
Mexico	2012	0.9256	0.9098	0.9202	0.9151	0.9421	0.9495	0.0083***	0.0077
Peru	1996	0.4948	0.1603	0.4164	0.6057	0.7477	0.8965	0.3000***	0.1484

table continues next page

Appendix C *(continued)*

Country	Year	Mean	Q1	Q2	Q3	Q4	Q5	Relative CI/HI	Absolute HI
Peru	2000	0.6825	0.4075	0.5914	0.7679	0.8845	0.9365	0.1680***	0.1147
Peru	2004–08	0.8759	0.7292	0.8580	0.9287	0.9552	0.9712	0.0592***	0.0519
Peru	2012	0.9248	0.8083	0.9191	0.9630	0.9731	0.9939	0.0403***	0.0373
Skilled birth attendance									
Bolivia	1998	0.5746	0.1899	0.4447	0.6893	0.8849	0.9843	0.2953***	0.1697
Bolivia	2003	0.6112	0.2510	0.4960	0.7115	0.8803	0.9858	0.2489***	0.1521
Bolivia	2008	0.7082	0.3597	0.6460	0.8145	0.9215	0.9873	0.1884***	0.1334
Brazil	1996	0.8875	0.7282	0.8953	0.9678	0.9790	0.9932	0.0710***	0.0630
Brazil	2006	0.9692	0.9465	0.9595	0.9765	0.9902	0.9921	0.0126***	0.0122
Colombia	1995	0.8409	0.5972	0.8546	0.9155	0.9864	0.9828	0.1010***	0.0849
Colombia	2000	0.8633	0.6393	0.8502	0.9508	0.9873	0.9864	0.0879***	0.0759
Colombia	2005	0.9047	0.7281	0.9357	0.9723	0.9894	0.9922	0.0652***	0.0590
Colombia	2010	0.9462	0.8373	0.9656	0.9870	0.9931	0.9937	0.0373***	0.0353
Costa Rica	1999	0.9743	0.9290	0.9880	0.9796	0.9934	0.9860	0.0110***	0.0107
Dominican Republic	1996	0.9500	0.8817	0.9652	0.9693	0.9815	0.9771	0.0222***	0.0211
Dominican Republic	1999	0.9780	0.9560	0.9970	1.0000	0.9820	0.9370	–0.0020	–0.0020
Dominican Republic	2002	0.9830	0.9450	0.9920	0.9930	0.9960	0.9980	0.0120***	0.0118
Dominican Republic	2007	0.9465	0.8859	0.9499	0.9621	0.9786	0.9870	0.0222***	0.0210
Guatemala	1995	0.3536	0.0936	0.1636	0.3277	0.6361	0.9193	0.4384***	0.0410
Guatemala	2008–09	0.5262	0.2176	0.4053	0.6243	0.8637	0.9446	0.2926***	0.1539
Haiti	2000	0.2456	0.0509	0.0876	0.1324	0.3947	0.7019	0.4987***	0.1225
Haiti	2005–06	0.2630	0.0675	0.1078	0.2045	0.4267	0.6669	0.4475***	0.1177
Haiti	2012	0.3768	0.0965	0.2132	0.3821	0.5647	0.7882	0.3648***	0.1375
Mexico	2000	0.9053	0.6800	0.8718	0.9415	0.9520	0.9909	0.0553***	0.0501
Mexico	2006	0.9335	0.8339	0.9181	0.9600	0.9934	0.9958	0.0343***	0.0321
Mexico	2012	0.9616	0.9057	0.9681	0.9706	0.9885	0.9862	0.0149***	0.0144
Peru	1996	0.5737	0.1395	0.4916	0.7573	0.9087	0.9699	0.3146***	0.1805
Peru	2000	0.5853	0.1701	0.4549	0.7956	0.9358	0.9845	0.3157***	0.1848

table continues next page

Appendix C *(continued)*

Country	Year	Mean	Q1	Q2	Q3	Q4	Q5	Relative CI/HI	Absolute HI
Peru	2004–08	0.7744	0.4405	0.7509	0.9333	0.9782	0.9926	0.1602***	0.1241
Peru	2012	0.8689	0.6103	0.8746	0.9730	0.9925	0.9930	0.0957***	0.0832
Cervical cancer screening									
Argentina	2005	0.4790	0.1690	0.3580	0.4990	0.6630	0.6310	0.2470***	0.1183
Argentina	2009	0.6570	0.4110	0.5710	0.6970	0.7820	0.7860	0.1360***	0.0894
Brazil	2003	0.7192	0.6021	0.6574	0.7077	0.7748	0.8540	0.0724***	0.0520
Brazil	2008	0.7730	0.6904	0.7219	0.7649	0.8130	0.8747	0.0496***	0.0384
Chile	2009	0.5704	0.5264	0.5441	0.5556	0.5719	0.7059	0.0953***	0.0544
Chile	2011	0.6618	0.6580	0.6529	0.6295	0.6562	0.7133	0.0135***	0.0089
Colombia	2005	0.9144	0.8885	0.9056	0.9060	0.9150	0.9455	0.0116***	0.0106
Colombia	2010	0.9470	0.9467	0.9425	0.9370	0.9467	0.9623	0.0035***	0.0033
Costa Rica	1999	0.6202	0.5659	0.6390	0.6293	0.6269	0.6404	0.0372***	0.0231
Costa Rica	2006	0.7842	0.7480	0.7994	0.8008	0.7538	0.8167	0.0136	0.0107
Guatemala	1998	0.2564	0.0371	0.0872	0.1927	0.3854	0.5075	0.4096***	0.1050
Guatemala	2008–09	0.3374	0.1854	0.2253	0.3319	0.4275	0.5104	0.2120***	0.0715
Mexico	2000	0.6658	0.6789	0.6729	0.6685	0.6069	0.6985	0.0119	0.0037
Mexico	2006	0.7523	0.8001	0.7599	0.7346	0.7173	0.7513	−0.0261***	−0.0097
Mexico	2012	0.8394	0.8765	0.8332	0.8318	0.8060	0.8457	−0.0164**	−0.0075
Middle years and beyond									
Self-assessed health (less than good)									
Argentina	2003	0.1831	0.2879	0.2503	0.1393	0.1721	0.0671	−0.1852***	−0.0339
Argentina	2005	0.1992	0.2865	0.2437	0.1805	0.1424	0.1430	−0.2170***	−0.0432
Argentina	2009	0.1925	0.2794	0.2157	0.1953	0.1360	0.1360	−0.2180***	−0.0420
Brazil	1998	0.2844	0.3724	0.3543	0.2957	0.2449	0.1547	−0.1593***	−0.0453
Brazil	2003	0.2764	0.3719	0.3379	0.2974	0.2343	0.1406	−0.1712***	−0.0473
Brazil	2008	0.2879	0.3910	0.3415	0.3114	0.2413	0.1542	−0.1668***	−0.0480

table continues next page

Appendix C *(continued)*

Country	Year	Mean	Q1	Q2	Q3	Q4	Q5	Relative CI/HI	Absolute HI
Chile	2003	0.3587	0.4766	0.4351	0.3850	0.3111	0.2033	−0.1400***	−0.0502
Chile	2009	0.3403	0.4153	0.3895	0.3512	0.3192	0.2408	−0.0937***	−0.0319
Chile	2011	0.3744	0.4230	0.4168	0.3893	0.3592	0.2835	−0.0745***	−0.0279
Colombia	2003	0.2068	0.3418	0.2545	0.2058	0.1542	0.0776	−0.0714***	−0.0148
Colombia	2008	0.3441	0.4724	0.4098	0.3588	0.2908	0.1889	−0.1661***	−0.0572
Colombia	2010	0.2867	0.3906	0.3468	0.3030	0.2320	0.1613	−0.1666***	−0.0478
Costa Rica	2005	0.2241	0.3173	0.2495	0.2004	0.1961	0.1598	−0.1243***	−0.0279
Jamaica	2004	0.2244	0.2804	0.2622	0.2005	0.2028	0.1769	−0.1073***	−0.0241
Jamaica	2007	0.2277	0.2923	0.2301	0.2279	0.2038	0.1845	−0.0916***	−0.0209
Jamaica	2009	0.1930	0.2384	0.1839	0.1853	0.1797	0.1780	−0.0625***	−0.0121
Mexico	2000	0.4572	0.5237	0.5117	0.4712	0.4257	0.3537	−0.0786***	−0.0359
Mexico	2006	0.3629	0.4203	0.3959	0.3774	0.3507	0.2704	−0.0828***	−0.0301
Diagnosed asthma									
Argentina	2003	0.0329	0.0313	0.0437	0.0331	0.0306	0.0261	−0.0193***	−0.0006
Argentina	2005	0.0487	0.0221	0.0874	0.0365	0.0603	0.0372	0.0920***	0.0045
Brazil	2003	0.0402	0.0356	0.0415	0.0430	0.0415	0.0433	0.0335***	0.0013
Brazil	2008	0.0396	0.0376	0.0402	0.0415	0.0406	0.0423	0.0227***	0.0009
Chile	2009	0.0628	0.0610	0.0370	0.0600	0.0610	0.0950	0.2200***	0.0138
Costa Rica	2006	0.0300	0.0340	0.0283	0.0243	0.0352	0.0284	−0.0119	−0.0004
Jamaica	2004	0.0047	0.0051	0.0065	0.0016	0.0065	0.0040	−0.0108	−0.0001
Jamaica	2007	0.0090	0.0164	0.0098	0.0068	0.0040	0.0078	−0.1639*	−0.0015
Jamaica	2009	0.0278	0.0268	0.0266	0.0375	0.0255	0.0230	−0.0194	−0.0005
Mexico	2006	0.0033	0.0029	0.0024	0.0030	0.0044	0.0036	0.0888**	0.0003
Mexico	2012	0.0024	0.0019	0.0019	0.0026	0.0028	0.0030	0.0964**	0.0002
Diagnosed depression									
Brazil	2003	0.0590	0.0560	0.0609	0.0608	0.0629	0.0567	0.0049***	0.0003
Brazil	2008	0.0574	0.0551	0.0568	0.0610	0.0602	0.0550	0.0055***	0.0003
Chile	2009	0.2160	0.2210	0.2230	0.1820	0.2320	0.2220	0.1330***	0.0287

table continues next page

Appendix C *(continued)*

Country	Year	Mean	Q1	Q2	Q3	Q4	Q5	Relative CI/HI	Absolute HI
Costa Rica	2006	0.0392	0.0690	0.0499	0.0163	0.0417	0.0197	-0.2171***	-0.0085
Mexico	2006	0.1094	0.0884	0.1031	0.1191	0.1154	0.1208	0.0566***	0.0062
Mexico	2012	0.1129	0.0991	0.1059	0.1191	0.1187	0.1219	0.0456***	0.0051
Diagnosed diabetes									
Argentina	2005	0.0848	0.0871	0.0943	0.0768	0.0820	0.0837	-0.0018	-0.0002
Argentina	2009	0.0964	0.0940	0.0926	0.1109	0.0944	0.0899	0.0260*	0.0025
Brazil	2003	0.0378	0.0358	0.0377	0.0414	0.0402	0.0368	0.0093***	0.0004
Brazil	2008	0.0498	0.0473	0.0507	0.0515	0.0526	0.0490	0.0095***	0.0005
Chile	2009	0.0676	0.1030	0.0760	0.0590	0.0540	0.0460	0.0749	0.0051
Costa Rica	2006	0.0550	0.0694	0.0580	0.0473	0.0523	0.0484	-0.0624	-0.0034
Jamaica	2004	0.0190	0.0188	0.0266	0.0198	0.0164	0.0136	-0.0887	-0.0017
Jamaica	2007	0.0323	0.0255	0.0310	0.0339	0.0432	0.0280	0.0526	0.0017
Jamaica	2009	0.0721	0.0726	0.0647	0.0765	0.0649	0.0816	0.0281	0.0020
Mexico	2000	0.0618	0.0690	0.0467	0.0664	0.0654	0.0616	0.0140	0.0009
Mexico	2006	0.0713	0.0569	0.0708	0.0820	0.0752	0.0716	0.0430***	0.0031
Mexico	2012	0.0899	0.0908	0.0913	0.0865	0.0884	0.0923	-0.0004	0.0000
Diagnosed heart disease (over 40)									
Argentina	2003	0.0456	0.0513	0.0128	0.0514	0.0338	0.0784	0.1454***	0.0066
Argentina	2005	0.0658	0.0886	0.0851	0.0760	0.0415	0.0378	-0.1106***	-0.0073
Brazil	2003	0.0995	0.0982	0.1038	0.1046	0.1041	0.0868	-0.0146**	-0.0015
Brazil	2008	0.0953	0.0910	0.1021	0.1006	0.0967	0.0861	-0.0108*	-0.0010
Chile	2009	0.1809	0.2531	0.2164	0.1513	0.1566	0.1256	0.0301	0.0054
Mexico	2006	0.0582	0.0535	0.0525	0.0536	0.0696	0.0571	0.0351	0.0020
Mexico	2012	0.0736	0.0708	0.0774	0.0715	0.0725	0.0755	0.0276	0.0020
Diagnosed hypertension (over 40)									
Argentina	2005	0.4442	0.4625	0.4724	0.4457	0.4376	0.4114	0.0087	0.0039
Argentina	2009	0.4537	0.4718	0.4608	0.4834	0.4480	0.4091	0.0088	0.0040
Brazil	2003	0.3308	0.3379	0.3536	0.3488	0.3262	0.2872	-0.0311***	-0.0103

table continues next page

Appendix C *(continued)*

Country	Year	Mean	Q1	Q2	Q3	Q4	Q5	Relative CI/HI	Absolute HI
Brazil	2008	0.3494	0.3527	0.3676	0.3606	0.3483	0.3176	−0.0202***	−0.0071
Chile	2009	0.4415	0.5037	0.4800	0.4336	0.4085	0.3814	0.0618***	0.0273
Jamaica	2004	0.0721	0.0666	0.0901	0.0643	0.0734	0.0663	−0.0112	−0.0008
Jamaica	2007	0.1147	0.1334	0.1239	0.1156	0.1179	0.0829	−0.0764**	−0.0088
Jamaica	2009	0.1682	0.1685	0.1535	0.1533	0.1751	0.1909	0.0367	0.0062
Mexico	2000	0.2626	0.2287	0.2142	0.2231	0.2399	0.2848	0.0607*	0.0159
Mexico	2006	0.2350	0.2117	0.2489	0.2425	0.2445	0.2417	0.0185	0.0043
Mexico	2012	0.2604	0.2528	0.2601	0.2537	0.2625	0.2630	0.0093	0.0024
Obesity among men									
Argentina	2005	0.0690	0.0536	0.0691	0.0798	0.0739	0.0687	0.0570***	0.0042
Argentina	2009	0.0858	0.0674	0.0994	0.0841	0.0909	0.0871	0.0440***	0.0041
Chile	2009	0.1938	0.1684	0.1597	0.2640	0.2292	0.1449	0.1817***	0.0437
Colombia	2005	0.0871	0.0309	0.0694	0.0865	0.1162	0.1322	0.4647***	0.0443
Colombia	2010	0.1227	0.0575	0.1082	0.1244	0.1561	0.1671	0.3664***	0.0512
Obesity among nonpregnant women									
Argentina	2005	0.0478	0.0673	0.0591	0.0402	0.0369	0.0283	−0.0599*	−0.0029
Argentina	2009	0.0656	0.1007	0.0756	0.0570	0.0447	0.0375	−0.1247***	−0.0082
Bolivia	1998	0.1140	0.0470	0.0990	0.1380	0.1490	0.1510	0.1970***	0.0225
Bolivia	2008	0.1740	0.0820	0.1580	0.2010	0.2320	0.1680	0.0840***	0.0146
Brazil	1996	0.0980	0.0630	0.0990	0.1200	0.1210	0.0950	0.0970***	0.0095
Brazil	2006	0.2099	0.1941	0.2067	0.2315	0.2310	0.1933	−0.0016	−0.0003
Chile	2009	0.3071	0.3506	0.3512	0.3407	0.2608	0.2130	0.0230	0.0071
Colombia	1995	0.0930	0.0700	0.1210	0.0850	0.0820	0.1160	0.0450	0.0042
Colombia	2000	0.1070	0.0770	0.0880	0.1240	0.1180	0.1330	0.1420***	0.0152
Colombia	2005	0.1160	0.0970	0.1150	0.1230	0.1280	0.1120	0.0270**	0.0031
Colombia	2010	0.1420	0.1400	0.1600	0.1470	0.1390	0.1190	−0.0380***	−0.0054
Costa Rica	2006	0.1480	0.1714	0.1308	0.1530	0.1720	0.1188	−0.0362	−0.0054
Guatemala	1998	0.1267	0.0243	0.0659	0.1309	0.1488	0.3008	0.3992***	0.0506

table continues next page

Appendix C *(continued)*

Country	Year	Mean	Q1	Q2	Q3	Q4	Q5	Relative CI/HI	Absolute HI
Guatemala	2002	0.1389	0.0730	0.0938	0.1377	0.1799	0.1760	0.2499***	0.0347
Guatemala	2008–09	0.1702	0.0833	0.1119	0.1731	0.2229	0.2323	0.1941***	0.0330
Haiti	1994–95	0.0270	0.0080	0.0100	0.0000	0.0250	0.1170	0.5820***	0.0157
Haiti	2005–06	0.0620	0.0060	0.0180	0.0310	0.0710	0.1300	0.4370***	0.0271
Haiti	2012	0.0776	0.0118	0.0397	0.0506	0.0869	0.1508	0.3670***	0.0285
Mexico	2006	0.1029	0.0623	0.0813	0.1204	0.1084	0.1419	0.1588***	0.0163
Peru	1996	0.0960	0.0300	0.0730	0.1160	0.1350	0.1610	0.2750***	0.0264
Peru	2000	0.1300	0.0360	0.0970	0.1590	0.1790	0.1410	0.1540***	0.0200
Peru	2004–08	0.1420	0.0500	0.1220	0.1700	0.1780	0.1500	0.1110***	0.0158
Peru	2012	0.1787	0.0853	0.1610	0.2170	0.2153	0.1849	0.0975***	0.0174
Breast cancer screening									
Argentina	2005	0.5520	0.4000	0.5020	0.5900	0.6900	0.6210	0.1390***	0.0767
Argentina	2009	0.7060	0.5870	0.6640	0.7290	0.8080	0.7670	0.0830***	0.0586
Brazil	2003	0.4780	0.2360	0.3304	0.4545	0.5899	0.7790	0.2355***	0.1126
Brazil	2008	0.5918	0.3639	0.4651	0.5472	0.6649	0.8401	0.1470***	0.0870
Chile	2009	0.3740	0.2830	0.2540	0.3980	0.4280	0.5070	0.2205***	0.0825
Chile	2011	0.5714	0.5009	0.5156	0.5328	0.5981	0.7039	0.0662***	0.0378
Colombia	2005	0.7695	0.6986	0.6829	0.6934	0.7516	0.8269	0.0463***	0.0356
Colombia	2010	0.8001	0.7324	0.8194	0.7845	0.7683	0.8284	0.0169***	0.0136
Costa Rica	2006	0.3276	0.2362	0.2870	0.3469	0.3691	0.3990	0.0912***	0.0299
Mexico	2000	0.3871	0.3492	0.3382	0.3457	0.3219	0.4804	0.0884	0.0133
Mexico	2006	0.5177	0.4443	0.4593	0.4898	0.4945	0.6390	0.0978***	0.0211
Mexico	2012	0.8141	0.8383	0.8336	0.8128	0.7691	0.8239	−0.0082	−0.0035
Outpatient visits									
Argentina	2003	0.4598	0.3354	0.4484	0.4298	0.4926	0.5928	0.1140***	0.0524
Argentina	2005	0.5147	0.3875	0.5202	0.5222	0.6142	0.5289	0.0918***	0.0473
Brazil	1998	0.2468	0.1818	0.2121	0.2388	0.2639	0.3331	0.1321***	0.0175
Brazil	2003	0.2699	0.2248	0.2356	0.2594	0.2841	0.3423	0.0981***	0.0143

table continues next page

Appendix C *(continued)*

Country	Year	Mean	Q1	Q2	Q3	Q4	Q5	Relative CI/HI	Absolute HI
Brazil	2008	0.2685	0.2242	0.2379	0.2615	0.2820	0.3345	0.0928***	0.0134
Chile	2003	0.1125	0.1099	0.1097	0.1085	0.1117	0.1228	0.0682***	0.0205
Chile	2009	0.1160	0.1139	0.1161	0.1103	0.1112	0.1288	0.0602***	0.0186
Chile	2011	0.1354	0.1433	0.1408	0.1258	0.1252	0.1421	0.0433***	0.0153
Guatemala	2006	0.1871	0.1341	0.1715	0.1875	0.2123	0.2397	0.1137***	0.0213
Guatemala	2011	0.1474	0.1073	0.1355	0.1375	0.1602	0.2026	0.1208***	0.0178
Mexico	2006	0.1708	0.1515	0.1665	0.1643	0.1757	0.1957	0.0538***	0.0048
Mexico	2012	0.1645	0.1456	0.1556	0.1635	0.1716	0.1861	0.0526***	0.0045
Inpatient (admission)									
Argentina	2003	0.0775	0.0976	0.0358	0.0921	0.0785	0.0829	0.0467***	0.0036
Argentina	2005	0.0769	0.0743	0.0883	0.0475	0.0855	0.0886	0.0436***	0.0034
Brazil	1998	0.0842	0.0938	0.0843	0.0790	0.0777	0.0861	−0.0193***	−0.0016
Brazil	2003	0.0804	0.0876	0.0757	0.0754	0.0764	0.0868	0.0007	0.0001
Brazil	2008	0.0804	0.0841	0.0780	0.0753	0.0778	0.0870	0.0073	0.0006
Chile	2000	0.0680	0.0770	0.0670	0.0650	0.0620	0.0680	0.0200***	0.0014
Chile	2003	0.0729	0.0776	0.0706	0.0709	0.0704	0.0751	0.0681***	0.0050
Chile	2009	0.0574	0.0605	0.0577	0.0558	0.0545	0.0586	0.0322***	0.0018
Chile	2011	0.0681	0.0750	0.0714	0.0651	0.0614	0.0675	0.0307***	0.0021
Colombia	2003	0.0784	0.0628	0.0728	0.0810	0.0808	0.0948	0.0773***	0.0061
Colombia	2008	0.0747	0.0684	0.0752	0.0657	0.0845	0.0798	0.0361**	0.0027
Colombia	2010	0.0773	0.0660	0.0773	0.0775	0.0825	0.0832	0.0473***	0.0037
Costa Rica	2006	0.0522	0.0491	0.0469	0.0459	0.0706	0.0482	0.0403	0.0021
Guatemala	2006	0.1067	0.0610	0.0489	0.1210	0.1378	0.1711	0.2400***	0.0022
Guatemala	2011	0.0636	0.0436	0.0346	0.0602	0.0896	0.0929	0.2175***	0.0012
Jamaica	2004	0.0650	0.0325	0.0627	0.0589	0.0781	0.0933	0.1645	0.0107
Jamaica	2007	0.0449	0.0057	0.0321	0.0480	0.0577	0.0805	0.3314***	0.0149
Jamaica	2009	0.0433	0.0301	0.0587	0.0476	0.0702	0.0102	−0.0419	−0.0018
Mexico	2000	0.0618	0.0521	0.0598	0.0689	0.0658	0.0623	0.0324***	0.0020
Mexico	2006	0.0457	0.0438	0.0466	0.0440	0.0456	0.0487	0.0201*	0.0009

table continues next page

Appendix C *(continued)*

Country	Year	Mean	Q1	Q2	Q3	Q4	Q5	Relative CI/HI	Absolute HI
Mexico	2000	0.0472	0.0483	0.0474	0.0511	0.0423	0.0472	−0.0101	−0.0005
Peru	2004	0.0476	0.0354	0.0461	0.0468	0.0586	0.0513	0.0666***	0.0032
Peru	2008	0.0533	0.0358	0.0506	0.0579	0.0574	0.0650	0.0927***	0.0049
Peru	2011	0.0606	0.0459	0.0591	0.0662	0.0620	0.0697	0.0664***	0.0040
Preventive visits									
Argentina	2003	0.6018	0.6311	0.6269	0.4643	0.5409	0.7041	0.0293	0.0077
Argentina	2005	0.7753	0.7278	0.7705	0.8096	0.8111	0.7312	0.0298	0.0117
Brazil	1998	0.1012	0.0574	0.0787	0.1001	0.1146	0.1530	0.1961***	0.0035
Brazil	2003	0.2630	0.2051	0.2146	0.2418	0.2723	0.3707	0.1464***	0.0073
Brazil	2008	0.2030	0.1589	0.1618	0.1843	0.2143	0.2892	0.1487***	0.0055
Chile	2003	0.1669	0.1870	0.1823	0.1666	0.1558	0.1426	0.0024	0.0004
Chile	2009	0.1832	0.2014	0.2015	0.1794	0.1680	0.1658	0.0020	0.0004
Chile	2011	0.2139	0.2584	0.2427	0.2054	0.1841	0.1788	−0.0239***	−0.0051
Colombia	2003	0.1472	0.0924	0.1175	0.1374	0.1745	0.2357	0.1450***	0.0683
Colombia	2008	0.1756	0.1253	0.1560	0.1807	0.1951	0.2326	0.0913***	0.0491
Colombia	2010	0.1736	0.1230	0.1490	0.1723	0.1976	0.2408	0.1000***	0.0534
Peru	2004	0.1044	0.0977	0.1145	0.1182	0.1025	0.0889	−0.0334**	−0.0035
Peru	2008	0.1637	0.1594	0.1765	0.1657	0.1643	0.1529	−0.0129*	−0.0021
Peru	2011	0.1525	0.1609	0.1615	0.1529	0.1469	0.1404	−0.0288***	−0.0044
Curative visits									
Argentina	2003	0.7077	0.6749	0.7014	0.7829	0.7444	0.6424	0.0000	0.0000
Argentina	2005	0.5336	0.5462	0.5255	0.5570	0.5096	0.5316	0.0072	0.0038
Brazil	1998	0.2232	0.1704	0.1987	0.2151	0.2358	0.2931	0.1163***	0.0138
Brazil	2003	0.1991	0.1746	0.1807	0.1959	0.2110	0.2324	0.0674***	0.0071
Brazil	2008	0.2144	0.1841	0.1962	0.2146	0.2242	0.2518	0.0701***	0.0080
Chile	2003	0.0652	0.0552	0.0567	0.0616	0.0692	0.0839	0.1285***	0.0235
Chile	2009	0.0737	0.0638	0.0679	0.0691	0.0730	0.0955	0.1115***	0.0229
Chile	2011	0.0927	0.0890	0.0879	0.0857	0.0888	0.1125	0.0980***	0.0248

table continues next page

Appendix C *(continued)*

Country	Year	Mean	Q1	Q2	Q3	Q4	Q5	Relative CI/HI	Absolute HI
Colombia	2003	0.6859	0.6046	0.6395	0.6464	0.7193	0.8033	0.0576***	0.0395
Colombia	2008	0.7847	0.6949	0.7751	0.7801	0.8299	0.8404	0.0373***	0.0293
Colombia	2010	0.7801	0.7129	0.7595	0.7344	0.8301	0.8635	0.0404***	0.0315
Guatemala	2006	0.1947	0.1391	0.1751	0.1963	0.2232	0.2501	0.1164***	0.0227
Guatemala	2011	0.1517	0.1108	0.1372	0.1397	0.1672	0.2100	0.1251***	0.0190
Jamaica	2004	0.6724	0.6182	0.6958	0.7043	0.6701	0.6752	0.0146	0.0098
Jamaica	2007	0.6777	0.4817	0.6726	0.7020	0.7687	0.7611	0.0808***	0.0548
Jamaica	2009	0.7808	0.7017	0.7683	0.7760	0.7931	0.8632	0.0375**	0.0293
Mexico	2006	0.8253	0.7692	0.8353	0.7964	0.8369	0.8700	0.0369**	0.0215
Mexico	2012	0.8584	0.8505	0.8402	0.8327	0.8665	0.8904	0.0245*	0.0153
Peru	2004	0.1429	0.0896	0.1233	0.1392	0.1649	0.1976	0.1440***	0.1440
Peru	2008	0.1645	0.1382	0.1501	0.1576	0.1821	0.1945	0.0721***	0.0721
Peru	2011	0.1880	0.1623	0.1795	0.1826	0.1973	0.2185	0.0610***	0.0610

Source: DHS—Equity Datasheet. Otherwise, study estimates based on Argentina—ENFR 2005 and 2009; Brazil—PNDS 2006, PNAD 2003 and 2008; Chile—ENS 2009, CASEN 2003, 2009, and 2011, ENCAVI 2006; Colombia—ENDS 2005 and 2010, ECV—2003, 2008, and 2010, ENSIN 2005 and 2010; Costa Rica—ENSSR 1999, ENSA 2006, ENANU 2008; Guatemala—ENSMI 2008–09, ENCOVI 2006 and 2011; Haiti—DHS 2012; Jamaica—JSLC 2004, 2007, and 2009; Mexico—ENSA 2000, ENSANUT 2006 and 2012; Peru—DHS 2012, ENAHO 2004, 2008, and 2012.

Note: Mean and Q1 through Q5 show deaths per 1,000 live births.

Significance level: * = 10 percent, ** = 5 percent, *** = 1 percent.

Environmental Benefits Statement

The World Bank Group is committed to reducing its environmental footprint. In support of this commitment, the Publishing and Knowledge Division leverages electronic publishing options and print-on-demand technology, which is located in regional hubs worldwide. Together, these initiatives enable print runs to be lowered and shipping distances decreased, resulting in reduced paper consumption, chemical use, greenhouse gas emissions, and waste.

The Publishing and Knowledge Division follows the recommended standards for paper use set by the Green Press Initiative. Whenever possible, books are printed on 50 percent to 100 percent postconsumer recycled paper, and at least 50 percent of the fiber in our book paper is either unbleached or bleached using Totally Chlorine Free (TCF), Processed Chlorine Free (PCF), or Enhanced Elemental Chlorine Free (EECF) processes.

More information about the Bank's environmental philosophy can be found at http://crinfo.worldbank.org/wbcrinfo/node/4.

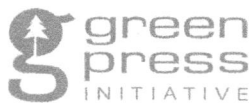

green
press
INITIATIVE

www.ingramcontent.com/pod-product-compliance
Lightning Source LLC
Chambersburg PA
CBHW080417270326
41929CB00018B/3064